Predicting Dependence Liability of Stimulant and Depressant Drugs

Predicting Dependence Liability of Stimulant and Depressant Drugs

edited by

Travis Thompson, Ph.D.

Professor, Departments of Psychology and Psychiatry, University of Minnesota

and

Klaus R. Unna, M.D.

Professor, Department of Pharmacology, University of Illinois at the Medical Center, Chicago

UNIVERSITY PARK PRESS

Baltimore • London • Tokyo

UNIVERSITY PARK PRESS
International Publishers in Science and Medicine
Chamber of Commerce Building
Baltimore, Maryland 21202

Typeset by American Graphic Arts Corporation and Alpha Graphics, Inc.
Manufactured in the United States of America by Universal Lithographers, Inc., and The Optic Bindery Incorporated

Library of Congress Cataloging in Publication Data:

Conference on Prediction of Abuse Liability of Stimulant and Depressant Drugs, National Academy of Sciences, 1976.
Predicting dependence liability of stimulant and depressant drugs.

"Conference sponsors: Committee on Problems of Drug Dependence, NAS-NRC," and others.
Includes index.
1. Drug abuse—Congresses. 2. Stimulants—Congresses. 3. Tranquilizing drugs—Congresses. 4. Sedatives—Congresses. 5. Drugs—Side-effects—Congresses. I. Thompson, Travis I. II. Unna, Klaus R. III. National Research Council. Committee on Problems of Drug Dependence. IV. Title. [DNLM: 1. Drug dependence—Congresses. 2. Analeptics—Pharmacodynamics—Congresses. 3. Psychotropic drugs—Pharmacodynamics—Congresses. 4. Hypnotics and sedatives—Pharmacodynamics—Congresses. QV100 C748p 1976]

RC566.AlC66 1976 615′.782 77-7581
ISBN 0-8391-1147-9

31186

Proceedings of the "Conference on Prediction of Abuse Liability of Stimulant and Depressant Drugs," held April 19–21, 1976, at the National Academy of Sciences, Washington, D.C.

CONFERENCE SPONSORS

Committee on Problems of Drug Dependence, NAS-NRC, Drug Enforcement Administration, Food and Drug Administration, and National Institute on Drug Abuse

CONFERENCE SUPPORT

The Conference was supported by the Drug Enforcement Administration, the Food and Drug Administration, and the National Institute on Drug Abuse under Contract No. 271-76-3322.

CO-CHAIRMEN OF THE CONFERENCE

Dr. Travis Thompson
Professor, Departments of
Psychology and Psychiatry
Minneapolis, Minnesota

Dr. Klaus R. Unna
Professor,
Department of Pharmacology
University of Illinois
at the Medical Center
Chicago, Illinois

COMMITTEE ON PHYSICAL DEPENDENCE

Dr. Klaus R. Unna, *Chairman*
Professor,
Department of Pharmacology
University of Illinois
at the Medical Center
Chicago, Illinois

Dr. Everette L. May, *Rapporteur*
Chief, Section on Medicinal
Chemistry
National Institutes of Health
Bethesda, Maryland

Dr. Gerald A. Deneau
Associate Research Scientist
Testing and Research Laboratory
New York State Office of Drug Abuse
Services
Brooklyn, New York

Dr. Dora B. Goldstein
Adjunct Professor
Department of Pharmacology
Stanford University School of
Medicine
Stanford, California

Dr. Louis S. Harris
Professor and Chairman, Department
of Pharmacology
Medical College of Virginia
Richmond, Virginia

Dr. Billie E. Jones
Chief of Psychophysiology Section
NIDA Addiction Research Center
Lexington, Kentucky

Dr. William R. Martin
Director, NIDA Addiction Research
Center
Lexington, Kentucky

Dr. Tomoji Yanagita
Director, Division of Medical Science
Central Institute for Experimental
Animals
Kawasaki, Japan

177

COMMITTEE ON BEHAVIORAL TOXICOLOGY AND BEHAVIORAL PREDICTIVE METHODS

Dr. Bernard Weiss, *Chairman*
Professor, Department of Radiation Biology and Biophysics
University of Rochester School of Medicine
Rochester, New York

Dr. Stephen G. Holtzman, *Rapporteur*
Associate Professor
Department of Pharmacology
Emory University
Atlanta, Georgia

Dr. Everett Ellinwood
Professor of Psychiatry
Duke University Medical Center
Durham, North Carolina

Dr. Douglas Ferraro
Associate Professor of Psychology
The University of New Mexico
Albuquerque, New Mexico

Dr. Leon S. Otis
Director, Departments of Psychobiology and Physiology
Stanford Research Institute
Menlo Park, California

Dr. Donald A. Overton
Associate Professor of Psychiatry
Temple University Health Sciences Center
Philadelphia, Pennsylvania

Dr. Walter A. Pieper
Professor of Psychology
Georgia State University
Atlanta, Georgia

COMMITTEE ON SELF-ADMINISTRATION OF DRUGS

Dr. Travis Thompson, *Chairman*
Professor, Departments of Psychology and Psychiatry
Minneapolis, Minnesota

Dr. Charles R. Schuster, *Rapporteur*
Professor of Psychiatry
The University of Chicago
Chicago, Illinois

Dr. Robert L. Balster
Assistant Professor of Pharmacology
Medical College of Virginia
Richmond, Virginia

Dr. Joseph V. Brady
Professor and Director of Behavioral Biology
The Johns Hopkins University School of Medicine
Baltimore, Maryland

Dr. Steven R. Goldberg
Assistant Professor of Psychobiology
Department of Psychiatry
Harvard Medical School
Boston, Massachusetts

Dr. Friedrich Hoffmeister
Director of Medicine
Institut für Pharmakologie
Bayer A. G.
Wuppertal, Republic of West Germany

Dr. Chris E. Johanson
Research Associate
Department of Psychiatry
The University of Chicago
Chicago, Illinois

Dr. James H. Woods
Assistant Professor
Department of Pharmacology
The University of Michigan Medical School
Ann Arbor, Michigan

Dr. Tomoji Yanagita
Director, Division of Medical Science
Central Institute for Experimental Animals
Kawasaki, Japan

COMMITTEE ON CLINICAL EVALUATION

Dr. Leo E. Hollister, *Chairman*
(Chairman, Committee on Problems of Drug Dependence)
Medical Investigator
Veterans Administration Hospital
Palo Alto, California

Dr. Roy W. Pickens, *Rapporteur*
Professor, Department of Psychiatry
University of Minnesota
Minneapolis, Minnesota

Dr. George Bigelow
Baltimore City Hospitals
Baltimore, Maryland

Dr. Dale C. Cameron
12546 Plaza Centrada
Rancho Bernardo
San Diego, California

Dr. John D. Griffith
Chief, Stimulant and Hallucinogen Drug Unit
NIDA Addiction Research Center
Lexington, Kentucky

Dr. Donald R. Jasinski
Chief, Clinical Pharmacology Section
NIDA Addiction Research Center
Lexington, Kentucky

Dr. Jack H. Mendelson
Professor of Psychiatry
Harvard Medical School
McLean Hospital
Belmont, Massachusetts

Dr. Marian W. Fischman
Research Associate
Department of Psychiatry
The University of Chicago
Chicago, Illinois

BANQUET SPEAKER

Dr. Abraham Wikler
Professor of Psychiatry and Pharmacology
Department of Psychiatry
University of Kentucky Medical Center
Lexington, Kentucky

NATIONAL ACADEMY OF SCIENCES-NATIONAL RESEARCH COUNCIL

Mr. Duke C. Trexler
Executive Secretary
Committee on Problems of Drug Dependence

Contents

Contributors

Satish K. Batta
Research Associate
Temple University Health Sciences Center
Philadelphia, Pennsylvania 19122

Joseph V. Brady
Professor and Director of Behavioral Biology
The Johns Hopkins School of Medicine
Baltimore, Maryland 21205

Gerald A. Deneau
Associate Research Scientist
Testing and Research Laboratory
New York State Office of Drug Abuse Services
Brooklyn, New York 11202

Peter Dews
Professor of Psychiatry and Psychobiology
Harvard University Medical School
Boston, Massachusetts 02115

Everett Ellinwood
Professor of Psychiatry
Department of Psychiatry
Duke University Medical Center
Durham, North Carolina 27710

Marian W. Fischman
Research Associate
Department of Psychiatry
The University of Chicago
Chicago, Illinois 60637

Dora B. Goldstein
Adjunct Professor of Pharmacology
Stanford University School of Medicine
Stanford, California 94305

Roland R. Griffiths
Assistant Professor of Behavioral Biology
The Johns Hopkins School of Medicine
Baltimore, Maryland 21205

Friedrich Hoffmeister
Director of Medicine
Institut für Pharmakologie
Bayer A. G.
Wuppertal, Republic of West Germany

Donald R. Jasinski
Chief, Clinical Pharmacology Section
NIDA Addiction Research Center
Lexington, Kentucky 40507

Chris E. Johanson
Research Associate
Department of Psychiatry
The University of Chicago
Chicago, Illinois 60637

Billie E. Jones, Jr.
Chief of Psychophysiology Section
NIDA Addiction Research Center
Lexington, Kentucky 40507

Thomas J. Kennedy, Jr.
American Association of Medical Colleges
1 Dupont Circle
Washington, D.C.

M. Marlyne Kilbey
Assistant Professor of Medical Psychology
Department of Psychiatry
Duke University Medical Center
Durham, North Carolina 27710

William R. Martin
Director, NIDA Addiction Research Center
Lexington, Kentucky 40507

Nancy K. Mello
Associate Director, Alcohol and Drug Abuse Research Center
Harvard Medical School
McLean Hospital
Belmont, Massachusetts 02178

Jack H. Mendelson
Professor of Psychiatry
Alcohol and Drug Abuse Research Center
Harvard Medical School
McLean Hospital
Belmont, Massachusetts 02178

Michiko Okamoto
Associate Professor of Pharmacology
Cornell University Medical College
New York, New York 10021

Donald A. Overton
Associate Professor of Psychiatry
Temple University Health Sciences Center
Philadelphia, Pennsylvania 19122

Walter A. Pieper
Professor of Psychology
Georgia State University
Atlanta, Georgia 30303

Charles R. Schuster
Professor, Department of Psychiatry
The University of Chicago
Chicago, Illinois 60637

Travis Thompson
Professor, Departments of Psychology and Psychiatry
University of Minnesota
Minneapolis, Minnesota 55455

Abraham Wikler
Professor of Psychiatry and Pharmacology
University of Kentucky
Lexington, Kentucky 40507

Tomoji Yanagita
Director
Division of Medical Science
Central Institute for Experimental Animals
Kawasaki, Japan

Welcome

Thomas J. Kennedy, Jr.

I am pleased to welcome you here for what all of us connected with the Assembly of Life Sciences feel is a most significant and timely program—the Conference on Prediction of Abuse Liability of Stimulant and Depressant Drugs. Dr. Travis Thompson and Dr. Klaus Unna have given their leadership as co-chairmen, and I would like to express my own congratulations to them for their development of an outstanding program. Represented here today are the sponsor agencies that have made the conference possible by their support and by their participation in the various planning groups: the Drug Enforcement Administration, the Food and Drug Administration, and the National Institute on Drug Abuse. Some thirty pharmaceutical firms have also sent their representatives. These are the firms that have supported the Committee on Problems of Drug Dependence over the years. Their participation in this conference is still another instance of their ongoing aid in the Committee's programs and activities. The members of the panels, the panel reporters, and the committees that will draw up the final report are also with us from many parts of the world. To all of you, may I extend our cordial welcome.

In 1972, the Committee on Problems of Drug Dependence published in the UN Bulletin of Narcotics its report "Testing for Dependence Liability in Animals and Man." That report dealt principally with narcotics rather than with stimulant and depressant drugs. As the Committee on Problems of Drug Dependence has expanded its programs, and as it currently explores alternative auspices, it has broadened its objectives to include in its area of interest the stimulant and depressant drugs. This conference is the first step in that direction. The conference objective is to outline the methods to be used in animal screening programs aimed at finding the dependence liability of amphetamines and barbiturates, and also to recommend whether or not a screening program is needed, similar to that which the Committee has conducted so effectively with narcotics for the past thirty years. They are important objectives in the national interest, and your group has the thanks of the Assembly of Life Sciences of the Academy Research Council for your efforts leading to this conference.

Your plans to publish the proceedings here are of great value in preserving and extending the conference findings. All of you will receive a copy after publication, and I hope you will find the recommendations developed of equal interest and application in the councils of the pharmaceutical industry, government, and the medical sciences. Certainly, if the findings of the conference indicate that effective evaluative procedures do currently exist in this category of drugs, it will have decided implications for all these groups.

I welcome you, and I hope you will have a pleasant and profitable three days with us.

Predicting Dependence Liability of Stimulant and Depressant Drugs

Predicting Abuse Liability of Sedatives and Stimulants

Travis Thompson

BACKGROUND

Nathan B. Eddy[1] wrote a definitive history of the attempt by the National Research Council—National Academy of Sciences to protect the public from drugs proposed for therapeutic usage which possessed dangerous properties. That document records the development of the Committee on Problems of Drug Dependence in 1956, from what had originally been the Advisory Committee on Drug Addiction in 1929. One of the major contributions of the Advisory Committee and its successor committees was to provide an unbiased clearing house for the evaluation of new analgesic compounds for dependence liability.

The Committee dealt mostly with opiate and opioid drugs. The physical dependence screening programs at The University of Michigan and later at the University of Virginia evaluated countless new compounds in monkeys, under the Committee's auspices. The human testing program, using former heroin addicts at Lexington, provided validation of these physical dependence programs. During the thirty years of this program no new compound possessing the virulent dependence potential of heroin found its way into the market.

Over the years increasing attention has been shifted to other aspects of drug dependence, and to dependence on nonopiate drugs. Over the past decade consideration has been given repeatedly to developing screening programs for drugs of both the sedative-hypnotic type and the stimulant type. The absence of physical dependence with drugs of the latter category posed screening problems for investigators working with opiates and barbiturates. Moreover, the newer sedative drugs, such as chlordiazepoxide and diazepam, appeared to have somewhat different properties from those of the short acting barbiturates. These facts, combined with the progressive concern over psychological and behavioral aspects of drug dependence, led many pharmacologists to doubt the value of delving into these areas. Some investigators felt the time was premature, others maintained that we must wait until more refined biochemical or physiological tests of dependence potential were developed.

Individual scientists went about their tasks without regard to such admonitions, and between 1960 and the present a vast body of scientific literature has emerged concerning new quantitative methods of assessing dependence liability of depressant and stimulant drugs in animals and man. It was in the light of these developments that the Committee on Problems of Drug Dependence, at its Spring meeting in 1975, began the task of reviewing the current state of knowledge concerning preclinical methods of predicting dependence liability of drugs, with special reference to sedative-hypnotics and stimulants. The papers in this volume and the summary chapter provide an indication of the current state of knowledge in this important area.

Before embarking on a review of the findings two issues must be clarified: 1) What do we mean by the term "drug dependence"? and 2) What is the best estimate of the extent of drug dependence in the United States? There have been many definitions of drug dependence, beginning with that of Tatum, Seevers, and Collins[2] and including the recent World Health Organization Definition.[3] Different authors have given varying emphasis to physical dependence, psychological and behavioral dependence, social consequences, and other forms of toxicity.

Recent findings (such as those reviewed in the present volume) suggest our concept of drug dependence is gradually changing, placing greater emphasis on the control the dependence-producing drug gains over the user's behavior. As a working definition, by *drug dependence* we mean a state of a person or animal produced by repeated administration of a drug, such that the drug user will engage in substantial amounts of behavior over an extended period with such behavior leading specifically to further administration of the drug. Physical dependence and other toxic side effects are important to the degree that they exacerbate or reduce the user's tendency to continue to administer the drug. Tolerance is significant as far as it leads to the user's tendency to self-administer the drug with greater frequency and at higher dosages, thus producing greater risks of toxicity or untoward effects on the user.

Early discussions of screening for opiate or barbiturate dependence focused on testing for physical dependence. Typically animals were chronically administered the test compound; observations for illness after discontinuing drug administration confirmed whether or not the animals had become physically dependent. When standardized screening programs emerged, colonies of monkeys chronically maintained on daily doses of morphine were used to test for substitutability of new drugs. Daily morphine administration was interrupted and the test drug was administered after the monkey had begun to show signs of withdrawal. If the test drug ameliorated the withdrawal signs and symptoms, it was presumed to have dependence potential of the morphine type.

In the early 1960s several reports indicated that another set of procedures could be used to assess dependence potential. Animals were surgically fitted with a chronic venous catheter through which drug solutions could be administered. The animals were then provided with a switch that they could operate to infuse a small quantity of drug solution through the catheter. This method permitted a direct quantitative method of assessing drug-seeking, which had previously been a largely subjective and unmeasurable disposition.

RELIABILITY AND VALIDITY

In any scientific enterprise, replicability of results is prerequisite to any statements about the meaningfulness of the outcome. Reliability measures in the physical dependency screening procedures have been high, with findings in one laboratory being readily reproduced in others. Until recently the predictive validity of physical dependence in monkeys for abuse potential in humans was considered virtually perfect—that is, if a drug substituted for morphine in a physically dependent monkey, it had abuse potential in man. This isomorphism has been recently called into question. The synthetic compound, 1-α-5,9-Diethyl-2^1-hydroxy-2-methyl-6,7-benzomorphan has an analgesic potency approximately equivalent to that of morphine, but it failed to support physical dependence in the monkey. In fact, the drug produced a mild withdrawal syndrome in physically dependent monkeys.[4] Yet when tested in an intravenous self-administration procedure with monkeys, the drug was highly effective in maintaining and controlling behavior (Balster and Harris, personal communication). These findings are of special significance, because this drug has been demonstrated to have substantial abuse potential in man. In other words, the absence of physical dependence in the monkey was not valid in predicting the absence of human abuse potential. However, maintenance of intravenous self-administration by monkeys

Self-admin. better predictor than dependence

was an effective predictor of abuse potential in man. It remains to be seen whether this relation will continue to hold as more synthetic analgesics and less common sedatives are developed.

THE EXTENT OF DRUG DEPENDENCE

The extent of drug dependence in the United States is difficult to document accurately. It has been estimated that the peak incidence of heroin dependence occurred in 1972 with approximately 2 million users.[5] It has also been noted that there was a decline in heroin use in major metropolitan areas between 1972 and 1974, followed by a resurgence.[6] Whatever the case, dependence of the opiate type seems to have increased to more than 2 million users, and has fluctuated in that vicinity over the past 4 to 5 years.

The use of sedative-hypnotics is more widespread. Benvenuto, Lau, and Cohen[7] studied polydrug abuse in five states selected to be as geographically diverse as possible. Extrapolating from their data, Benvenuto and co-workers concluded that nearly 7.5 million Americans use nonopiate drugs nonmedically. These investigators found there are about 14 million users of minor tranquilizers, of whom 3.5 million persons use these drugs nonmedically. Another 8.6 million people use other sedative drugs, with about 1 million persons using them nonmedically. In sum, nearly 4.5 million Americans use *some* sedative or minor tranquilizing drug nonmedically.

Numbers of this magnitude are mind boggling, so perhaps it would be useful to attempt to put them in perspective. According to these figures, there are as many nonmedical users of nonopiate drugs in the United States as the entire population of Chicago. Clearly, the nonmedical use of depressants and stimulants is no small problem.

Considering the extent of the use of depressant and stimulant drugs, it is somewhat surprising that our problems with these agents are not more severe than they appear to be. This is not to say, however, that depressant and stimulant drugs do not present problems. Barbiturates and minor tranquilizers in particular are often implicated in suicide and automobile accidents, especially in combination with alcohol. Perhaps some of the reasons these compounds have not had more serious, deleterious effects has to do with their *relative* abuse potential. That is, although some of the minor tranquilizers are used widely, and may lead to relatively low degrees of dependence in many users, they seldom gain extensive control over the patient's behavior or have widespread toxic effects. This suggests that part of the solution to identifying safer drugs may be to find agents with demonstrated efficacy but that have very limited disposition to produce toxic effects (including physical dependence) and that possess little or no reinforcing effects.

The foregoing suggestion implies that as far as drug dependence risk is concerned, three factors must be considered: 1) therapeutic efficacy, 2) reinforcing efficacy, and 3) toxicity (including propensity to produce physical dependence). One might reasonably ask what properties the "ideal" stimulant or depressant compound would possess with regard to these factors. One way of thinking about the question is to speculate about the dose-response curves of therapeutic efficacy, reinforcing efficacy, and toxicity. The "ideal" drug would presumably be therapeutically effective at doses that would (a) not be reinforcing and (b) would not produce toxic effects. Moreover, if reinforcing doses of the drug *were* reached in nontherapeutic (i.e.,

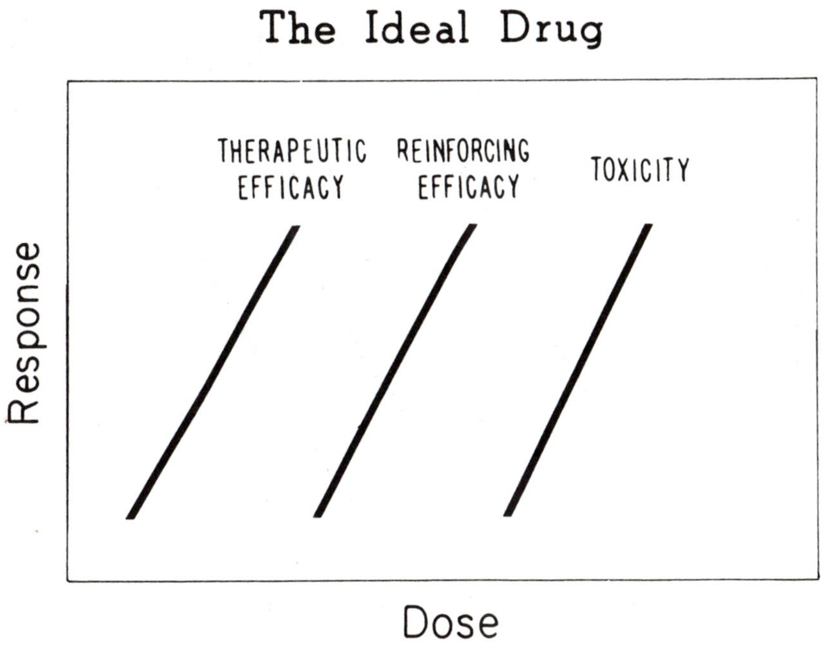

Figure 1. The hypothetical dose-reponse curves of therapeutic efficacy, reinforcing efficacy, and toxicity of the "ideal" stimulant or depressant drug—i.e., a drug with no reinforcing or toxic effects at any therapeutic dose.

nonmedical) use, such effects would be well below those producing toxic side effects (Figure 1). In practice such drugs are very hard to come by.

If these are the features of the "ideal" drug, what would the high risk drug profile look like? The cardinal feature would be that the lowest doses producing reinforcing effects would be below those of therapeutic effects (Figure 2). Thus, *any and all* therapeutic use of the drug would involve dose levels that would be reinforcing; thus it would gain control over the patient's behavior. In addition, at modest to high therapeutic dose levels, toxic manifestations would appear (e.g., tolerance and physical dependence). In all likelihood a drug with such a profile would not be marketed unless it possessed such unique therapeutic effects that most practicing physicians would be unable to conduct reasonable and responsible patient care without it.

Finally, what profile would the "*typical*" sedative or stimulant drug present (Figure 3)—i.e., the drugs we currently see on the

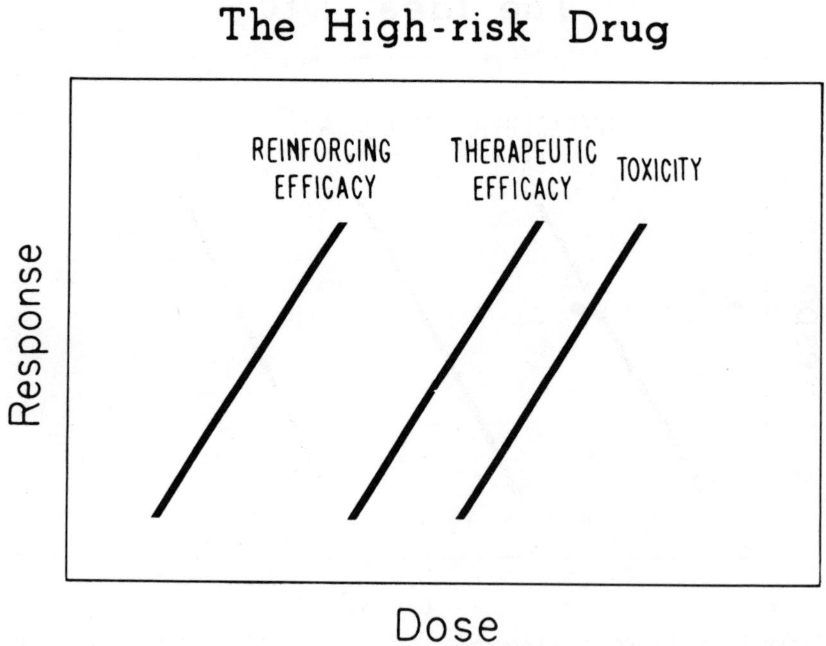

Figure 2. The hypothetical dose-response curves of therapeutic efficacy, reinforcing efficacy, and toxicity of the "high risk" stimulant or depressant. Notice that at *all* therapeutic dosages significant reinforcing effects would obtain.

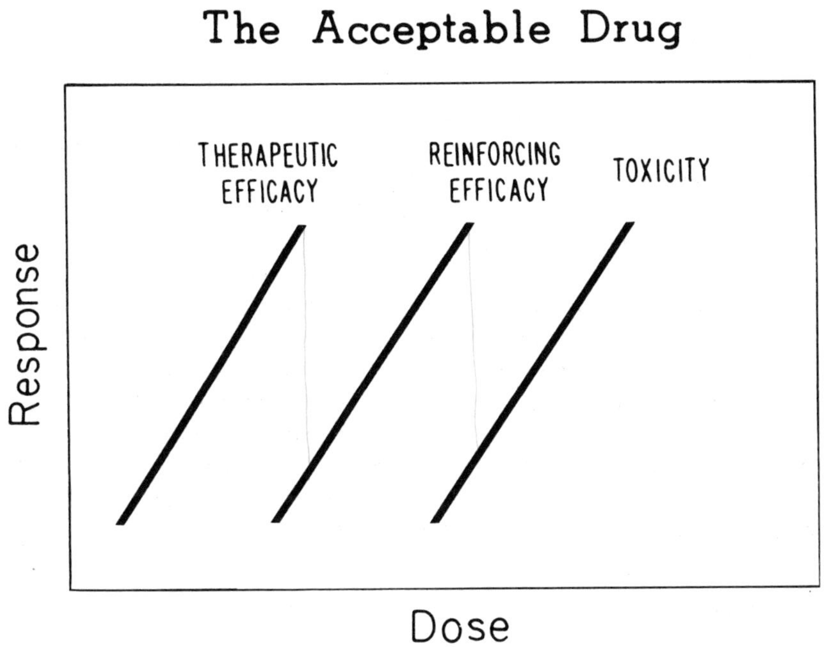

Figure 3. The hypothetical dose-response curves of therapeutic efficacy, reinforcing efficacy, and toxicity of the "typical" stimulant or depressant.

market? First, low and moderate therapeutic dosages would be free of reinforcing effects. At high therapeutic doses there are more reinforcing effects. Moreover, high reinforcing doses of the drug would have to be reached before toxic effects would ensue. The more commonly marketed drugs generally conform to this picture.

SHORT TERM AND LONG TERM SOLUTIONS

Drug screening programs, especially those in larger industrial and governmental laboratories, have tended to use large numbers of animals administered single or several drug doses, with testing lasting from several minutes to several days. Expediency and cost considerations have led to the conclusion that any effective screening program must be rapid and inexpensive. As the study of drug dependence has become increasingly sophisticated this conventional wisdom has come under scrutiny. The issue really becomes balancing the advantages of rapid and inexpensive screening methods against the risk of toxicity or dependence liability that only becomes evident on more careful investigation of drugs in more complex situations over an extended period. One need only think of the relatively late discovery of tardive dyskinesia produced by haloperidol to become a little more sympathetic to the view that speed and economy may not always be of the essence. On the other hand, many early screening procedures can certainly be accomplished relatively inexpensively. However, it is almost certainly unrealistic to expect any single test, conducted on a few subjects (e.g., mice) over a few experimental days, to possess sufficient predictive validity to satisfy any discerning scientist. More carefully thought out procedures that are sensitive to the variables operating in human drug dependence must be devised. In the succeeding pages four approaches to this problem are discussed: 1) Physical dependence methods in animals and man; 2) Human psychological and behavioral methods; 3) Animal behavioral predictors and toxicological tests; and 4) Infrahuman self-administration procedures. Our conclusions based on a review of the evidence are contained in Chapter 22.

LITERATURE CITED

1. Eddy, N. B. 1973. The National Research Council Involvement in the Opiate Problem. National Academy of Sciences, Washington, D.C.
2. Tatum, A. L., Seevers, M. H., and Collins, K. H. 1929. Morphine addiction and its physiological interpretation based on experimental evidence. J. Pharm. Exp. Therap. 36:447.
3. World Health Organization Report. 1975. Evaluation of Dependence Liability and Dependence Potential of Drugs: Report, WHO Scientific Committee, Technical Report, Series 577, WHO, Geneva.
4. Villareal, J. 1970. Recent advances in the pharmacology of morphine-like drugs. In: Drug Dependence, R. T. Harris, W. M. McIsaac, and C. R. Schuster (eds.), University of Texas Press, Austin.
5. National Commission on Marijuana and Drug Abuse. 1973. Reported in *The New York Times,* March 3, 1973.
6. Kaufman, E. 1975. Multi-drug abuse: Definition and determinants. Presented at the Meeting of the Committee on Problems of Drug Dependence, Washington, D.C., May, 1975.
7. Benvenuto, J. A., Lau J., and Cohen, R. 1975. Patterns of nonopiate/polydrug abuse: Findings of a National Collaborative Research Project. Presented at the Meeting of the Committee on Problems of Drug Dependence, Washington, D.C., May, 1975.

Assessment of Depressant Abuse Potentiality

William R. Martin

I have never measured the physical dependence-producing capability of a depressant. Some years ago, however, I initiated experiments in man with the end of measuring and validating methods for the primary reinforcing properties of barbiturates and other types of drugs of abuse in man. Dr. Jasinski has continued these experiments and his results are reported in another chapter. Thus, when preparing this paper, I realized that I had little advice to give concerning the practicalities of measuring the abuse potentiality of depressants. I have, however, given much thought to the general problem of assessing the abuse potentiality of psychoactive drugs and would like to share some of my views with you as they relate to depressants.

IMPORTANCE OF VALIDITY

It is of importance that methods for assessing the abuse potentiality of depressants and stimulants be well validated. (The issue of validity and methods that may help in this task are discussed subsequently.) The primary role of the Federal government in the assessment of the abuse potentiality of drugs is: 1) to protect public health by preventing the introduction of psychoactive drugs into the practice of medicine without foreknowledge of their addiction liability; and 2) to assist in the development of safe, nonaddicting efficacious drugs for treating disordered brain function. This endeavor should not inhibit the development of new useful therapeutic modalities in either the area of psychiatry or other medical disciplines. For this reason, data bearing on the abuse potentially of new drugs should not be overinterpreted until they are well validated.

PHARMACOLOGICAL EQUIVALENCE

The abuse potentiality of a drug can be most easily and reliably assessed when it can be shown to be pharmacologically equivalent to a standard drug that is known to be abused. A variety of techniques have been used to establish pharmacological equivalence both in animals and in man. For the depressants, these include production of motor incoordination, sleep, EEG changes, depression of the reticular activating system, and spinal cord reflex activity. Further, depressants induce tolerance and dependence, and through the use of cross-tolerance, suppression, and direct addiction studies, more data can be acquired that bear on the issue of pharmacological equivalence.

HOW SELECTIVE ARE OUR METHODOLOGIES?

The mode of action of depressant drugs is not understood. It is not known whether or not they are agonists acting on selective receptors. There is, however, clear cut evidence that there are differences between depressants in their pharmacological effects. For example, there are differences between the effects of diazepam and pentobarbital on both the EEG and spinal cord reflex activity. Do these differences have relevance with regard to their abuse potential? As Dr. Jones discusses in his chapter, there is reason to believe that the perniciousness of abuse of secobarbital but not pentobarbital is greater than that of diazepam, despite the fact that diazepam is used clinically 10 to 20 times more frequently than pentobarbital and secobarbital. Are these differences a consequence of their pharmacology and selectivity of action? It is well within the realm of probability that we will develop increasingly selective depressants that will have greater safety and efficacy and lesser abuse potentiality. The development of drugs with these characteristics should be encouraged.

We have yet, however, to determine how selective our methods are for identifying abuse potentiality. The systematic studies of the abuse potentiality of narcotics and narcotic antagonists, which now have extended over 40 years, have disclosed several important variables that relate to specificity.

Species

There is now a large body of evidence that suggests that prototypic receptors may differ from species to species. Thus, man, monkeys, dogs, rats, and mice differ in their reactivity to benzomorphans, meperidine, and normorphine but not to morphine and certain of its close congeners. It is also well known that there are marked differences in drug metabolism between species and that metabolites may be active.

Agonists

Agonists can be strong, partial, or competitive antagonists. The identification of partial agonists or drugs with a ceiling effect has provided a circumstance whereby both toxicity and abuse potential may be reduced. Methods should thus have the capability of identifying partial agonists.

Receptor Dualism

It has now been demonstrated that for several types of agonists, there are distinguishable types of receptors that have diverse pharmacological effects. These include noradrenergic, cholinergic, and histaminergic drugs as well as narcotic analgesics. With regard to abuse potentiality, receptor dualism has proven to have some interesting implications. Thus, three narcotic type receptors have been identified, two whose occupancy leads to reinforcing effects (μ and κ), and a third that gives rise to aversive effects (σ). It is evident that drugs can have varying degrees of reinforcing and aversive effects and that through a proper balance of these agonistic effects, drugs of varying abuse potentiality can be developed.

THE RELATIONSHIP BETWEEN THE MARKET PLACE AND ABUSE POTENTIAL

The market place and patient acceptance play a large role in the decisions of drug manufacturers and developers about which drugs are brought to the NDA (New Drug Application) state of development. It is and has been obvious that drugs with reinforcing properties have greater patient acceptance than drugs with aversive properties. A pharmaceutical firm's judgment on whether to seek a very expensive IND (Investigational New Drug) must take predicted customer acceptance into consideration. This type of consideration may not be consonant, however, with minimizing drug abuse. Thus, the effort to minimize drug abuse through the development of therapeutic agents of low abuse potentiality must be accompanied by efforts not only to bring effective drugs with minimal abuse potentiality into the hands of the practitioner but also to educate the practitioner about their use.

RELEVANT POPULATIONS FOR HUMAN STUDIES

It is also important to consider the relevance of the population to the properties of drugs that one is investigating. Although this area has not been systematically explored, it would appear from the work of Lasagna et al.[1] that normal volunteers liked the effects of amphetamine and pentobarbital but did not like the effects of morphine or heroin. Postaddicts also like the subjective effects produced by amphetamine[2] and pentobarbital,[3] but, in contrast to control subjects, they also like the effects of morphine and heroin.[4] Many studies conducted at the Addiction Research Center as well as in other laboratories have indicated that a large portion of addicts have an antisocial personality, one aspect of which is the prevalance of feelings of hypophoria. The cardinal dimensions of hypophoria are feelings of unpopularity, ineptness, and inefficiency. All drugs of abuse decrease these hypophoric feelings in addicts but not necessarily in individuals who have a normal range of feelings (euphoria). It is important to determine if normal subjects can identify the euphoric properties of drugs. To state the question differently—can the ability of a drug to relieve feelings of hypophoria in individuals with an antisocial personality be identified in normal subjects? It is suggested as a possibility that the reinforcing properties of drugs of abuse can be reliably identified only in individuals with an antisocial personality. A similar question is relevant to studies measuring reinforcing properties of drugs in animals.

WHAT IS PHYSICAL DEPENDENCE?

It is not amiss to reexamine the importance of physical dependence in assessing the abuse potentiality of the depressants in order to avoid developing an inappropriate strategy based on an anachronistic vocabulary. The term "physical dependence" was initially used to designate an abstinence syndrome that could be characterized by physical signs and in which the dependence was identified by drug-seeking behavior. Except for those who are committed to a philosophy of dualism, the organicity and physicalness of behavior and feeling states are neither less nor more than those of autonomic and somatomotor signs.

As tolerance and physical dependence as they relate to drug abuse are usually described to sophomore medical students, the drug abuser experiences a feeling of well-being following his initial injections, but with repeated administration tolerance to this effect develops. To recapture these effects, more and more of the drug is taken, which produces physical dependence. The symptoms and related signs of the abstinence syndrome are discomforting to the addict and he continues to take drugs to avoid abstinence signs.

Whether this scenario corresponds to reality is not known. No one has systematically studied the effects of depressants on feeling states and drug need through a cycle of addiction. To our knowledge this has only been done for the narcotics.[5] When narcotics are administered chronically, they fail not only to produce euphoria but also to enhance the negative feeling state, hypophoria. Secondly, it is not clear that convulsions and delirium tremens are discomforting to the addict and are of importance in the genesis of an increased need to use depressants. There are several reasons for questioning the importance of convulsions and delirium in drug-seeking behavior: 1) The fact that abusers of meperidine and propoxyphene use convulsant dose levels argues that the convulsions are not highly aversive to addicts. 2) Further, amphetamines and cocaine are self-administered by both man and animals to the extent that they produce both a psychosis and delirium. 3) LSD-like hallucinogens and hallucinogenic anesthetics such as phencyclidine and ketamine are also abused, and their abuse would also argue against the point that distortions of perception and intellectual function are aversive to drug abusers. 4) Finally, drug-seeking behavior on the part of both barbiturate-dependent and alcohol-dependent subjects most commonly precedes by many hours the emergence of these life-threatening signs of abstinence.

It is therefore suggested that convulsions and delirium may be unrelated to an induced need that gives rise to continuing depressant-seeking behavior and that the suppression of these signs should not be interpreted as need reduction. Rather, the only significance of suppression of delirium and convulsions may be to provide supporting evidence establishing pharmacological equivalence. Because there are demonstrated differences in the pharmacology of the various depressants, it would be unwarranted at this time to suggest that they produce physical dependence through a common mechanism of action and that suppression indicates a common mode of action.

WHY IS PHYSICAL DEPENDENCE BAD?

The perniciousness of physical dependence is threefold. First, in the case of the depressants, abstinence signs may be life-threatening. Secondly, with the emergence of tolerance and physical dependence, the subjective effects produced by the depressants may change, as they do with narcotics, and chronic administration of these agents may result in the exacerbation of the negative feeling states of the addict. Thirdly, depressants may also produce a protracted abstinence syndrome that may predispose addicts to relapse. These latter variables may be of importance in defining the abuse potentiality of depressants. In this regard, the fact that a drug has reinforcing properties is not in itself an undesirable property. It is well within the realm of probability that drugs that may allow the definitive treatment of hypophoric aspects of the addict's pathology will have reinforcing properties. Thus, if a reinforcing drug has therapeutic efficacy and causes little or no harm, it should not be considered addicting.

VALIDATION REVISITED

Our efforts to assess the abuse potentiality of depressants are in their infancy. The perniciousness of the abuse of depressants must be more clearly identified and defined and be placed on some sort of continuum. The analysis of Dr. Jones suggests that depressants are probably less likely to place the abuser in an emergency room or in the cool anteroom of the coroner than are narcotics and stimulants. It is important that their harmfulness also be compared with alcohol.

There are many ways that experimental methods for measuring abuse potentiality can be validated:

1) There must be some sort of concordance between both the incidence and perniciousness of street abuse, on the one hand, and the results of both animal and clinical studies, on the other. Because faddism plays, at times, a prominent role in drug abuse patterns, a good concordance can be expected only for those drugs whose street abuse is well established.

2) There must be concordance between animal and clinical results. In the past little effort has been devoted to explaining discordant results. In order to define the limitations of our methods, more effort should be placed on determining the reasons for discrepancies.

3) The establishment of covariation between measures also helps establish the validity of methods. This principle has been in use for many years at the Addiction Research Center. Fraser and Isbell[6] first showed that the miotic effects and the subjective effects of narcotic analgesics were associated. Subsequently, it was shown that elevation of blood pressure for amphetamines[2] and enhancement of postrota-

tional nystagmus for pentobarbital[3,7,8] were associated with changes in subjective effects.

SUMMARY AND CONCLUSIONS

It may be that in our effort to assess the abuse potentiality of depressant drugs we are embarking on an adventure that may well have as many if not more complexities than have been encountered in our assessment of the abuse potentiality of narcotic analgesics and related drugs. It is apparent from the chapters in this text that the state of the art with regard to the assessment of the abuse potentiality of depressants will be well described. I would like to urge upon my colleagues the philosophy that it is at least equally and perhaps more important to pay attention to inconsistencies of data as it is to attend to similarities. It is through examining dissimilarities that we will gain insight into the development of better drugs for the treatment of anxious and sleepless patients as well as those who suffer from an antisocial personality. These diseases of feeling states certainly stand among the most common of all psychiatric disorders and deserve the attention of the most imaginative of neuroscientists.

LITERATURE CITED

1. Lasagna, L., von Felsinger, J. M., and Beecher, H. K. 1955. J. Amer. Med. Assoc. 157:1007.
2. Martin, W. R., Sloan, J. W., Sapira, J. D., and Jasinski, D. R. 1971. Clin. Pharmacol. Ther. 12:245.
3. Martin, W. R., Thompson, W. O., and Fraser, H. F. 1974. Clin. Pharmacol. Ther. 15:623.
4. Fraser, H. F., Van Horn, G. D., Martin, W. R., Wolbach, A. B., and Isbell, H. 1961. J. Pharmacol. Exp. Ther. 133:371.
5. Martin, W. R., Jasinski, D. R., Haertzen, C. A., Kay, D. C., Jones, B. E., Mansky, P. A., and Carpenter, R. W. 1973. Arch. Gen. Psychiat. 28:286.
6. Fraser, H. F., and Isbell, H. 1960. Bull. Narcot. 12:15.
7. Martin, W. R., Fraser, H. F., and Isbell, H. 1962. Fed. Proc. 21:326.
8. McClane, T. K., and Martin, W. R. 1976. Clin. Pharmacol. Ther. 20:198.

Characteristics of Ethanol Physical Dependence

A Basis for Quantitative Comparison of Sedative Drugs

Dora B. Goldstein

There exists a group of sedative-hypnotic drugs, loosely identified as the alcohol-barbiturate group. These drugs share a spectrum of dose-related actions, from sedation through ataxia, hypnosis, anesthesia, and respiratory depression. They are not good analgesics. This chemically diverse group includes alcohol, paraldehyde, and chloral hydrate, as well as the barbiturates, the "non-barbiturate hypnotics" (methaqualone, glutethimide, etc.) and the minor tranquilizers such as meprobamate and the benzodiazepines.

Within the sedative-hypnotic group there is a variable incidence of reported abuse. Addiction to alcohol is obviously a major problem, and abuse of barbiturates is also important, but there are relatively few reports of abuse of the other compounds. There is indeed evidence that physical dependence on all these compounds can arise. Ethanol and the barbiturates are well known to produce a withdrawal reaction characterized by hallucinations, convulsions, and delirium. A similar withdrawal reaction, most easily recognized by convulsions, has been reported after chronic use of nonbarbiturate hypnotics, meprobamate, and the benzodiazepines.[1-4] Experimental physical dependence on these drugs has been produced in animals.[1,5-7] Is their different incidence of abuse merely a matter of fashion within the street culture or are there really differences in abuse liability among these drugs? How would we assess this type of hazard in a new sedative-hypnotic drug? I will discuss here one aspect of these questions, namely the attributes

---

This study supported in part by United States Public Health Service Grant AA 01066.

of physical dependence that might influence addiction liability. The methods and concepts developed in our recent attempts to characterize alcohol physical dependence in mice should be applicable to comparative studies. Some interesting questions arise when we attempt to apply our alcohol results to other drugs.

EVALUATION OF WITHDRAWAL REACTIONS

We start with the testable hypothesis that all the drugs produce the same type of withdrawal reaction. Skipping for the moment the important problem of how and in what quantity to administer the drugs, let us consider how to compare the withdrawal reactions quantitatively, using the well-defined alcohol withdrawal reaction in mice as a prototype. Freund[8] was the first to describe this syndrome and to grade it by stages of increasing severity. Freund's Stage I includes intermittent tremor and overactivity, especially in response to sensory stimuli. Stage II is characterized by a variety of abnormal movements such as retropulsion, tail arching, and repetitive, stereotyped motions. Stage III includes generalized tonic-clonic convulsions and Stage IV is death, often during a convulsion. We have seen a similar syndrome in our mice and established a grading system[9] based on the intensity or frequency of seven signs, namely lethargy, tremor, startle to noise, tail lift, convulsions elicited by handling (see below), spontaneous convulsions, and death. As soon as a strong withdrawal reaction can be observed with a new drug, one can determine whether or not the syndrome resembles this typical alcohol withdrawal reaction. If so, we are ready to begin quantitative comparisons. We can choose a single quantifiable sign as an index of the overall syndrome. Loss of body weight or some type of seizure threshold would be appropriate objective measures. Preferably, however, the index should be a test that is repeatable at intervals in the same animals so that the time course of the withdrawal reaction can be estimated. For this purpose, we have used a specific type of convulsion elicited by picking up the mice by the tail. Such convulsions occur only very rarely in normal mice (less than 1% in our hands). These convulsions on handling are a prominent feature of the alcohol withdrawal reaction in randomly bred Swiss-Webster mice and in the DBA/2J and BALB/cJ inbred strains, but not in C57BL/6J mice.[10] We score these convulsions on a scale of 1 to 4 points according to intensity.[11] Although these numbers are arbitrary, they turn out to have such good linearity with alcohol dose that we treat the scores like real numbers, using t-tests, etc., for com-

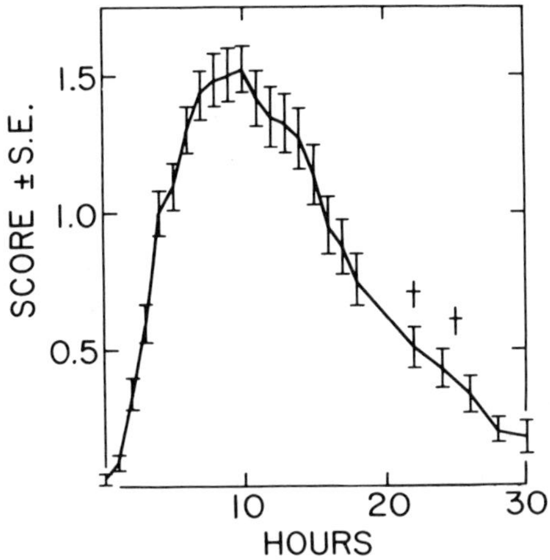

Figure 1. Scores for convulsions on handling in Swiss-Webster mice exposed to alcohol (by inhalation) at a mean blood level of 2 mg/ml for three days. The curve represents eleven experiments combined, with a total of 95 mice. *Abscissa:* Hours after removing the mice from the vapor chamber. *Ordinate:* Mean scores for convulsions on handling, based on a standard rating system with a range of 0 to 4 points. *Vertical bars* represent standard errors, and *dagger symbols* represent deaths. Reproduced from Reference 12, by permission. Copyright 1973, The Williams & Wilkins Co., Baltimore.

parisons between groups. Nonparametric statistical tests would also be appropriate.

Figure 1 shows a typical curve for seizure scores (convulsions on handling) against hours after withdrawal, indicating the time course. This curve represents several different experiments combined, with the same exposure to alcohol, and the small standard errors show that the curve is easily reproducible.[12] We estimate the severity of alcohol withdrawal reactions in different groups of mice either by the peak height of such curves or by the area under them. Figure 2 shows curves for groups of mice given alcohol for 1 to 9 days. It is clear that we can distinguish between withdrawal reactions of different intensity, such as those that might be produced by different drugs.

EQUIVALENT EXPOSURE TO DIFFERENT DRUGS

The next problem is to establish how much drug is necessary to produce a given intensity of withdrawal reaction. For alcohol, this is a matter of blood concentrations and the time for which they are maintained. With short durations of alcohol administration, the simple

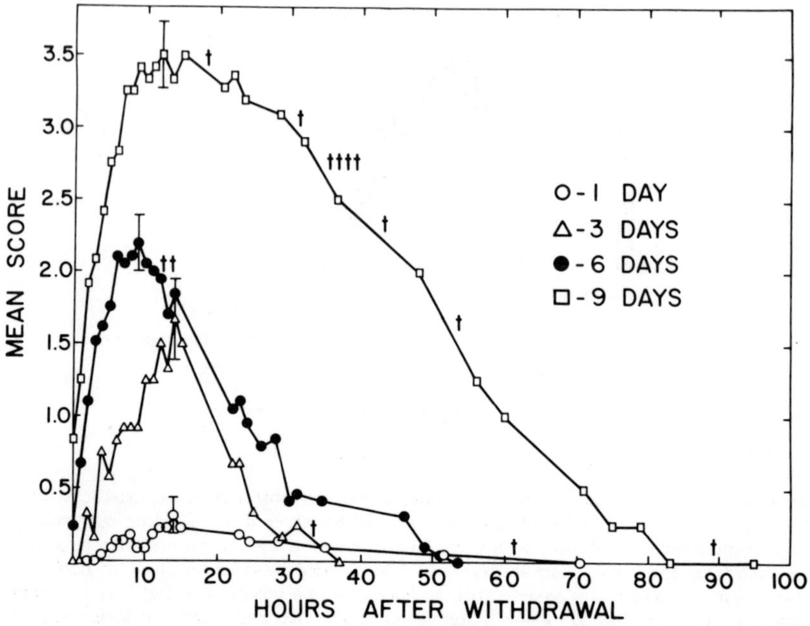

Figure 2. Withdrawal scores of Swiss-Webster mice given alcohol by inhalation for one to nine days. After withdrawal, the 12 to 23 surviving mice in each group were scored for convulsions on handling. The *points* are means, *vertical bars* represent standard errors, and *dagger symbols* represent deaths. Reproduced from Ref. 11, by permission. Copyright 1972, The Williams & Wilkins Co., Baltimore.

product of blood levels and duration correlates very well with withdrawal scores. We call this product the "exposure" to alcohol. If ethanol is administered by inhalation (in a vapor chamber where mice are housed for a few days) and pyrazole is injected daily, very stable blood alcohol concentrations are maintained and we can estimate the alcohol exposure by measuring the blood alcohol each day. Figure 3 shows the peak height of withdrawal reactions that result from various combinations of blood level and time. Here only the product is shown. An alcohol exposure of 6 could be obtained by maintaining a blood level of 1 mg/ml for 6 days, 2 mg/ml for 3 days, or any other such combination. The figure shows that the seizure scores increased linearly with alcohol exposure.

This is one way that drugs could be compared for relative potency in eliciting physical dependence. However, here we encounter the first difficulty. Obviously we cannot maintain the same absolute blood levels with the different drugs, most of which are lethal at the concentrations used for ethanol. We must use units of blood concentration that are in some way equivalent, and it is not a simple matter to define such equivalence. What we are interested in, in the context of abuse liability, is some relation between the exposure that produces physical dependence and the exposure that people might reasonably attain. Lacking a way to assess euphoria in mice, we might choose the mildest objective sign of intoxication, ataxia, representing an appreciable behavioral effect very roughly in the range that people might consider pleasurable. Mice could feasibly be maintained at an ataxic blood level for several days. We know that alcohol physical dependence develops under these conditions. So a good first step

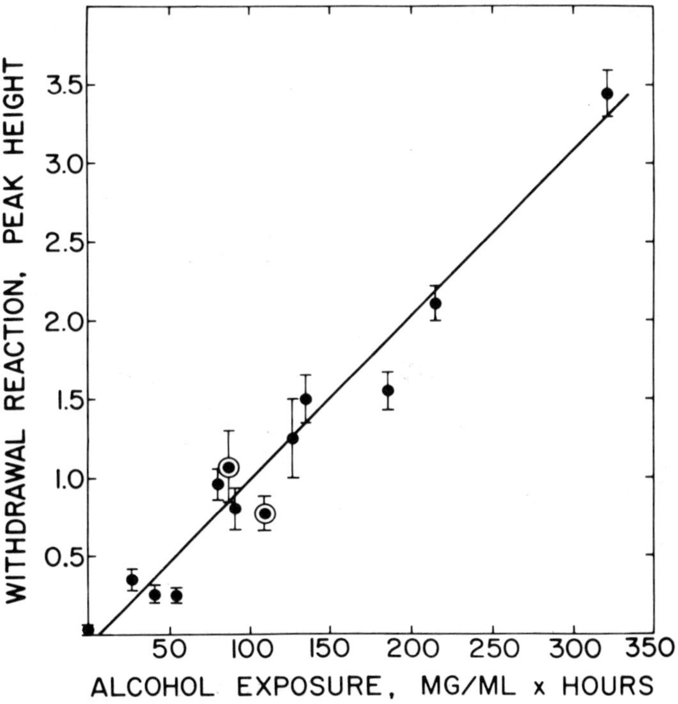

Figure 3. Relation of the severity of withdrawal reactions to the total exposure to alcohol. The *abscissa* represents the product of mean blood alcohol levels and the number of days of intoxication. The *ordinate* is the peak height of withdrawal-score curves, such as those in Figures 1 and 2. Each *point* is a separate experiment. *Vertical bars* represent standard error of the mean. Reproduced from Ref. 11, by permission. Copyright 1972, The Williams & Wilkins Co., Baltimore.

would be to determine the ataxic blood level of another drug, establish units of drug exposure comparable to those used for ethanol, and see whether equivalent exposures give the same severity of withdrawal reaction.

TIME COURSE OF PHYSICAL DEPENDENCE

The linear relationship between alcohol exposure and withdrawal scores holds only for short durations of intoxication. We examined the time of onset of physical dependence by exposing animals to constant blood alcohol concentrations for different lengths of time.[13] Figure 4 shows that the severity of withdrawal reactions begins to level off after a week or two of alcohol administration. There seems to be a maximum that would not be exceeded even with prolonged exposure. Furthermore, the plateau is dose-related, being higher in mice kept at

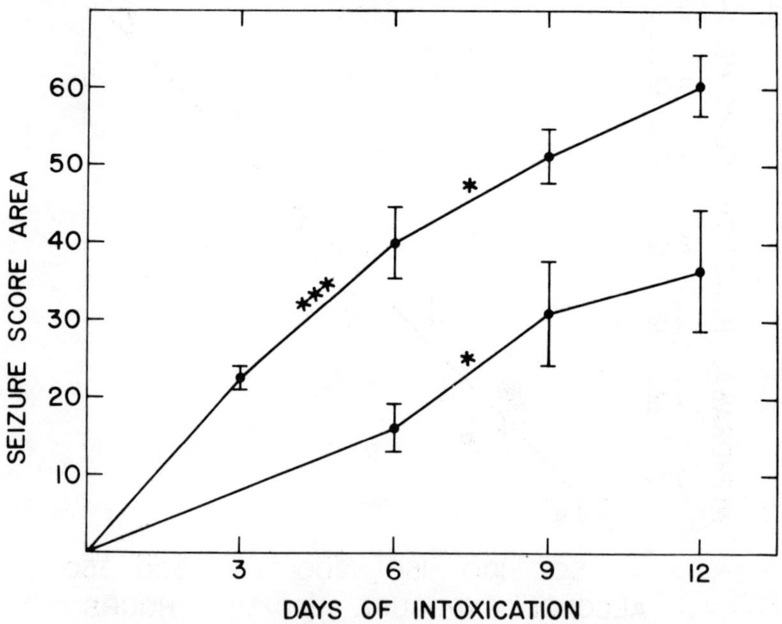

Figure 4. Rate of onset of physical dependence. Mice were exposed to alcohol by inhalation so as to maintain mean blood levels of 2.0 (*upper curve*) or 1.0 (*lower curve*) mg/ml for three to twelve days and the withdrawal reaction was scored as in Figure 1. The *ordinate* is the area under the withdrawal-score curve up to 24 hours after withdrawal. Adjacent points differ significantly where indicated by *, $p < 0.05$ (one-tailed t-test) or **, $p < 0.001$. Reproduced from Ref. 13, by permission. Copyright 1974, The Williams & Wilkins Co., Baltimore.

Table 1. Failure of physical dependence to cumulate when intoxication is interrupted[a]

	Withdrawal Area	
Duration (days)	Continuous Intoxication	Interrupted Intoxication
3	22	24
6	40	32
9	51	30
12	60[b]	32[c]

[a] Swiss-Webster mice were maintained at a mean blood level of 2 mg/ml by inhalation for a total of twelve days. The column labeled "continuous intoxication" represents the same mice as in the upper curve of Figure 4. The column labeled "interrupted intoxication" represents mice that were removed from the vapor chamber for one day after each three days of intoxication. The data are areas under the curve for seizure scores versus hours, as in Figure 4.

[b] $p < 0.001$ versus 3 days.

[c] Not significantly different from 3 days.

2 mg/ml than at 1 mg/ml. Such curves offer more options for comparing drugs. One might ask whether the plateau and the time course would be the same with any sedative drug maintained at the ataxic concentration. One might expect on theoretical grounds[14] that the half-time for approach to the plateau would be a property of the drug receptor or target system and therefore that all drugs that elicit physical dependence by the same mechanism should have the same time course, even though they might differ in potency. Different time courses would suggest that the drugs elicit physical dependence by different mechanisms.

Another factor that must be considered is the reversibility of the dependent stage. If instead of maintaining a constant level of intoxication for three to twelve days, as just described, we interrupted the alcohol administration for one day after every three days of intoxication, we found that the withdrawal scores did not increase with time but instead stayed the same, as if the mice had undergone only a single three-day intoxication period (Table 1). This means that the physical dependence developed during each three-day cycle must have decayed, essentially completely, during the one-day sober intervals. Such a rapid disappearance of physical dependence was unexpected (although a similar time course had been reported for opiate dependence in mice[15]). We have recently confirmed this finding with quite a different model. Administering alcohol to mice in a liquid diet, we found that the animals often drank heavily (over 25 g/kg per day) for a few days and then reduced their intake sharply for one day. Withdrawal scores of individual mice correlated well with the final period of uninterrupted alcohol intake, rather than with the cumulative dose, indicating that a one-day break in intake had abolished the effect of the previous drinking period. Thus the inhalation model and the liquid diet model agree that 24 hours is enough for mice to recover from physical dependence.*

This lability of the dependent state means that experiments comparing different drugs should be done in such a way that fluctuations in drug concentration are prevented. We can do this with alcohol by inhalation if we use pyrazole as a blood alcohol stabilizer, but we cannot do it without pyrazole in either the inhalation or liquid diet models. A method for continuous intraperitoneal infusion, developed by Teiger[17] for rats, is being set up in our laboratory with mice and may prove to be a good way to maintain intoxication with some drugs.

My concern about temporal patterns of voluntary alcohol consumption led me to examine the circadian rhythm of diet intake in mice. It is known that many circadian variations can be well described by a cosine curve,[18] where some physiological function varies as the cosine of time, with a certain amplitude. Light is a very strong synchronizer for such rhythms[19] so we can be quite sure that the period of the rhythm will be 24 hours if we use a 24-hour light-dark cycle in the mouse room. Assuming for the moment that the rate of drinking is indeed a cosine function of time, we can fit a few daily observations (at convenient times) to the best cosine curve, which will show the daily peak time and the amplitude. Three observations a day sufficed to show that the mice drank both day and night (although more at night) and never sobered up, even between observation times. Using data of Kakihana (personal communication) and from the literature,[20] with six or eight observations per day, we could show that the intake data do indeed fit well to cosine curves. We have not yet checked the fit of the blood alcohol data, but we would expect, as a first approximation, that it would follow the intake curve. However, circadian rhythms in alcohol metabolism rates superimposed on the intake pattern could well distort this curve. The reason we want to

---

* It should be noted that an experiment by Branchey et al.[16] does not agree. They found more severe withdrawal reactions after a second cycle of intoxication than after one cycle, even with an interval of a few weeks between cycles.

know about the circadian pattern of drug intake is that we believe that fluctuations in drug concentrations may affect the development of physical dependence. Analysis of dips in the blood levels should be a part of the comparison of dependence potency.

RATE OF DRUG ELIMINATION

Theoretically, the severity of the withdrawal reaction should be affected by the rate of elimination of the drug. If two groups of animals have achieved the same magnitude of physical dependence with two different drugs, we expect that the shorter-acting drug would produce the stronger withdrawal reaction. The extreme case would be a drug that left the body instantly at the end of its administration period, suddenly revealing the whole amount of dependence existing at that moment. Alternatively, a slowly eliminated drug would suppress the withdrawal reaction during the time necessary for recovery from the dependent state. Thus we can predict a priori (now that we know how rapidly physical dependence decays) that long-acting drugs will be less of a problem than short-acting drugs with respect to the severity of withdrawal reactions. However, there is a trade-off between the advantages of long- and short-acting drugs. Long-acting drugs are more likely to produce physical dependence because continuous maintenance of effective blood levels is easier with these agents, but long-acting drugs are unlikely to produce dangerous withdrawal reactions because they cannot be abruptly withdrawn. From a practical point of view, we really don't care whether physical dependence exists as long as there is no withdrawal reaction. This is all that really matters when we are considering physical dependence as a factor in abuse liability for people. But as pharmacologists we would like to know whether a dependent state exists, regardless of whether or not this state is overtly displayed as a withdrawal reaction. To do these experiments properly, we would have to find some way to modify the elimination rate so that it is the same for the drugs we are comparing.

GENETIC CORRELATIONS

Finally, in comparative studies we can use genetic variability to examine whether or not different drugs have a common mechanism. This approach has recently given very interesting results with respect to acute hypnotic actions of alcohol and bariturates. Among inbred strains of mice, the C57BL mice are relatively insensitive to central effects of alcohol compared to other strains, such as BALB,[21] but they are more sensitive to barbiturates.[22] Similarly, the strains of mice developed by selective breeding by McClearn and Kakihana[23] for different sensitivity to alcohol, the "short-sleeping" and "long-sleeping" lines, do not show a differential effect of barbiturates.[24] This indicates that there are some genetically controlled sites of acute action that are different for the two drugs. An analogous experiment could be done with withdrawl reactions. We already know that there is an easily measurable difference in alcohol withdrawal scores among inbred mouse strains[10] and between the short-sleeping and long-sleeping lines.[25] As soon as we have a good model for barbiturate dependence it will be useful to test these same strains. If the strains that show strong alcohol withdrawal reactions do not show strong barbiturate withdrawal reactions, we would have evidence that there is some step in the path between the primary drug action and the withdrawal reaction that is not shared by alcohol and barbiturates.

CONCLUSIONS

Both concentration and time are important variables in the study of physical dependence. Comparison of drugs for potency in eliciting physical dependence should take them both into account. Blood concentrations of the drugs should be equieffective with respect to some suitable acute action that both drugs share. If feasible, the drug concentrations should be maintained constant, day and night, for several days. After withdrawal, the abstinence syndrome should be measured as quantitatively as possible. The methods available to date are still rather crude; better techniques would be welcome.

LITERATURE CITED

1. Essig, C. F. 1964. Addiction to nonbarbiturate sedative and tranquilizing drugs. Clin. Pharmacol. Ther. 5:334–343.
2. Ewart, R. B. L., and Priest, R. G. 1967. Methaqualone addiction and delirium tremens. Br. Med. J. 3:92–93.
3. Hollister, L. E., Motzenbecker, F. P., and Degan, R. O. 1961. Withdrawal reactions from chlordiazepoxide ("Librium"). Psychopharmacologia 2:63–68.
4. Wikler, A., and Essig, C. F. 1970. Withdrawal seizures following chronic intoxication with barbiturates and other sedative drugs. Epilepsie Prob. Actuels Pharmacopsychiat. 4:170–184.
5. Kohli, R. P., Singh, N., and Kulshrestha, V. K. 1974. An experimental investigation of dependence liability of methaqualone in rats. Psychopharmacologia 35:327–334.

6. Yanagita, T., and Takahashi, S. 1971. Dependence liability of several hypnotic-antianxiety agents evaluated in monkeys. Reported to the Committee on Drug Dependence, February, 1971.
7. Yanaura, S., Tagashira, E., and Suzuki, T. 1975. Physical dependence on morphine, phenobarbital and diazepam in rats by drug-admixed food ingestion. Japan J. Pharmacol. 25:453–463.
8. Freund, G. 1969. Alcohol withdrawal syndrome in mice. Arch. Neurol. 21:315–320.
9. Goldstein, D. B., and Pal, N. 1971. Alcohol dependence produced in mice by inhalation of ethanol: Grading the withdrawal reaction. Science 172:288–290.
10. Goldstein, D. B., and Kakihana, R. 1974. Alcohol withdrawal reactions and reserpine effects in inbred strains of mice. Life Sci. 15:415–425.
11. Goldstein, D. B. 1972. Relationship of alcohol dose to intensity of withdrawal signs in mice. J. Pharmacol. Exp. Ther. 180:203–215.
12. Goldstein, D. B. 1973. Alcohol withdrawal reactions in mice: Effects of drugs that modify neurotransmission. J. Pharmacol. Exp. Ther. 186: 1–9.
13. Goldstein, D. B. 1974. Rates of onset and decay of alcohol physical dependence in mice. J. Pharmacol. Exp. Ther. 190:377–383.
14. Goldstein, D. B. 1975. Testing the homeostat hypothesis of drug addiction. In: H. D. Cappell and A. E. LeBlanc (eds.), Biological and Behavioral Approaches to Drug Dependence, pp. 1–11. Addiction Research Foundation, Toronto.
15. Cheney, D. L., and Goldstein, A. 1971. Tolerance to opioid narcotics: Time course and reversibility of physical dependence in mice. Nature 232:477–478.
16. Branchey, M., Rauscher, G., and Kissin, B. 1971. Modifications in the response to alcohol following the establishment of physical dependence. Psychopharmacologia 22:314–322.
17. Teiger, D. G. 1974. Induction of physical dependence on morphine, codeine and meperidine in the rat by continuous infusion. J. Pharmacol. Exp. Ther. 190:408–415.
18. Halberg, F., Tong, Y. L., and Johnson, E. A. 1967. Circadian system phase—an aspect of temporal morphology: Procedures and illustrative examples. In: H. von Mayersbach (ed.), The Cellular Aspects of Biorhythms. Springer-Verlag, New York.
19. Pittendrigh, C. S. 1975. Circadian oscillations in cells and the circadian organization of multicellular systems. In: C. S. Pittendrigh (ed.), Circadian Oscillations and Organization in Nervous Systems, pp. 437–458. MIT Press, Cambridge.
20. Freund, G. 1970. Alcohol consumption and its circadian distribution in mice. J. Nutr. 100:30–36.
21. Kakihana, R., Brown, D. R., McClearn, G. E., and Tabershaw, I. R. 1966. Brain sensitivity to alcohol in inbred mouse strains. Science 154:1574–1575.
22. Randall, C. L., and Lester, D. 1974. Differential effects of ethanol and pentobarbital on sleep time in C57BL and BALB mice. J. Pharmacol. Exp. Ther. 188:27–33.

23. McClearn, G. E., and Kakihana, R. 1973. Selective breeding for ethanol sensitivity in mice. Behavior Genetics 3:409–410.
24. McClearn, G. E. 1975. Genetics and the pharmacology of alcohol. Proc. VI Internat. Congr. Pharmacol. 3:59–66.
25. Goldstein, D. B., and Kakihana, R. 1975. Alcohol withdrawal reactions in mouse strains selectively bred for long or short sleep times. Life Sci. 17:981–986.

Preclinical Assessment of the Physiological Dependence Capacity of Depressant Drugs

Gerald A. Deneau

We are addressing ourselves in this chapter to the subject of the assessment of the physiological dependence capacity of drugs that depress the central nervous system. There was a time when physiological dependence was considered to be synonymous with "Addiction Liability." We all know today that this is not so. The only factor common to all forms of drug abuse or addiction is the reinforcing property of a drug's ability to alter the subject's appreciation of the environment. With the depressant drugs (alcohol, sedatives, hypnotics, etc.) physiological dependence is an unfortunate consequence of chronic toxicity which serves as a secondary reinforcement to the continued abuse of this class of drugs.

The first laboratory demonstration of physiological dependence to the depressants (barbiturates) was performed by Hoff and Kauders in the late 20s. Independently, Seevers and Tatum reported a more detailed study of the same phenomenon. This was, in fact, the subject of Seevers' doctoral thesis. During the 30s, many investigators studied this fascinating phenomenon and the following characteristics were illustrated.

1) Physiological dependence develops more readily when a constant drug effect is maintained than it does when the dosage is intermittent.
2) The degree of physiological dependence that develops is a function of daily dosage and of the duration of chronic intoxication. That is, at a constant daily dosage the severity of the dependence will increase over a period of several months and then it will plateau, but higher dosages will induce a more severe state of dependence.
3) The classical studies of Isbell, Fraser et al. at Lexington demonstrated that alcohol dependence was essentially the same as barbiturate dependence. In more recent times, Essig has shown that many of the newer sedatives (minor tranquilizers, etc.) are inter-

changeable with the barbiturates with respect to their physiological dependence-producing capacities.

From the work of Himmelsbach with opiates, there are three ways of assessing physiological dependence capacity:

1) The direct development of physiological dependence upon chronic administration of a drug.
2) Substitution: If a subject is dependent upon a drug and the substitution of another drug maintains the dependence (i.e., prevents abstinence) then the substitute drug may be assumed to possess the same dependence-producing properties as the primary drug.
3) Single-Dose Suppression: If a subject who is physiologically dependent upon a drug is experiencing abstinence signs and the administration of another drug relieves those signs specifically, the second drug may be assumed to be acting on the same pathway as the drug of primary dependence.

In more recent years, self-administration procedures have been developed such that laboratory animals may demonstrate, by their behavior, whether or not a drug has reinforcing properties—i.e., whether or not it induces psychogenic dependence.

Several years ago, in collaboration with Weiss, we developed a substitution method for assaying barbiturate-like physiological dependence in the dog. The dog was selected as the test subject because of its gentle nature, highly developed behavioral repertoire, and ease of dosing. The drug can be wrapped in a small amount of moist, commercial dog food and the subjects will swallow it in one gulp. This eliminates the need of stomach tubing or parenteral injection.

Sodium barbital was chosen as the primary drug of dependence because of its long duration of action—one dose per day was sufficient to develop and maintain dependence. A dose of 100 mg/kg/day was chosen because former studies indicated that this dose would induce dependence of moderate severity, but fatalities during untreated withdrawals would not be expected.

Under this regimen, it was found that maximal dependence did not develop until more than one year of treatment, as is illustrated by the following data:

Months of Treatment	% Convulsions	% Delirium
1–3	20	0
4–6	40	20
7–12	90	40
13–24	100	100

When test drugs were studied, they were substituted for a period of five days. The dosage was adjusted so that no abstinence signs appeared, but the subjects were not so intoxicated that they could not eat or drink water in amounts consistent with the maintenance of health. The frequency of administration was adjusted to be consonant with each drug's duration of action.

After five days of substitution, all treatment was withdrawn for five days and the ensuing abstinence syndrome was graded for intensity and duration. If the test drug maintained dependence through the five days of treatment and a typical abstinence syndrome developed during the withdrawal period, the substitute drug was assumed to have barbiturate-like properties.

A point-score system, as developed by Himmelsbach for the opiates, was used to grade the intensity of the abstinence syndrome. Each sign was graded from one to four, depending upon its severity, as follows:

Delirum:

1. Dog fails to respond or responds abnormally to the observer.
2. Dog displays poor judgment, or aggressiveness, or maintains a strange posture for minutes, or barks at no apparent object.
3. Dog displays purposeless jumping, unprovoked attacks on other dogs or observers, moving the head and eyes as if seeing an imaginary object.
4. Dog displays continuous bizarre behavior, searching for an imaginary object.

Tremor:

1. Palpable tremor of the extremities.
2. Periodic visible tremor of the extremities.
3. Continuous tremor of the extremities.
4. Gross tremors involving the entire body.

Mydriasis:

1. 1 mm
2. 2 mm
3. 3 mm
4. 4 mm

Fever (Fahrenheit):

1. 0.2–0.4°
2. 0.5–0.9°
3. 1.0–1.9°
4. 2.0–3.6°

Sleeplessness:

1. Less than 6 hours sleep in 24 hours.
2. Less than 4 hours sleep in 24 hours.
3. Less than 2 hours sleep in 24 hours.
4. No sleep in 24 hours.

Tachycardia:

1. 5–9
2. 10–19
3. 20–29
4. 30–150

Weight Loss:

1. 3%
2. 6%
3. 10%
4. 15%

Using this procedure, we found that the following drugs would substitute for sodium barbital:

Phenobarbital sodium	30 mg/kg q 12 hr.
Pentobarbital sodium	15 mg/kg q 6 hr.
Chloral hydrate	500 mg/kg q 12 hr.
Paraldehyde	1 cc/kg q 12 hr.
Ethyl alcohol	8 mg/kg q 12 hr.
Bromural	450 mg/kg q 6 hr.
Carisoprodal	200 mg/kg q 6 hr.
Meprobamate	150 mg/kg q 6 hr.
Chlordiazepoxide	100 mg/kg q 12 hr.
Glutethimide	125 mg/kg q 6 hr.
Methyprylon	80 mg/kg q 6 hr.
Methaqualone	300 mg/kg q 12 hr.

By the substitution technique, a test drug can be assayed in a 2-week period as opposed to the several months required for direct dependence studies. The substitution technique also permits better quantification than could be obtained by single dose suppression studies.

One must be cautious in the interpretation of these data, however; they *are not* synonymous with abuse liability. In subsequent direct dependence studies, we have determined that carisoprodal, in doses up to 900 mg/kg/day for 6 months, does not induce primary physiological dependence. Other studies using the self-administration technique with monkeys have shown that monkeys will not intoxicate themselves with dosages of phenobarbital or chlordiazepoxide sufficient to induce physiological dependence. This indicates that the latter drugs are not sufficiently reinforcing to possess major abuse potential.

Of all the available laboratory techniques, the self-administration procedure with the monkey would seem to be the most informative. With this technique, one can observe the psychogenic dependence capacity (reinforcing properties) of the drug. Tolerance-inducing potential is also readily seen, and, finally, by withdrawal of the drug, its physiological dependence capacity can be determined. The most serious drawback with this technique is that for intravenous administration the drug must be water soluble. For insoluble drugs, Yanagita has developed a technique employing naso-gastric infusion. More recently, Altshuler and myself have used a direct gastric cannula.

To date, all techniques with modest predictive reliability are expensive in terms of subjects, maintenance, and technical time. It is only if an adequate number of test drugs are to be studied that any degree of efficiency can be realized.

Predicting Abuse Liability of Depressant Drugs

Billie E. Jones, Jr.

Whether or not a drug can produce physical dependence of the barbiturate or alcohol type can be determined with confidence. While such information is necessary, it alone will not predict the extent to which a drug will be abused, or the relative abuse liability.

In regard to determining the dependence-producing ability of a depressant drug, there are ample data. Since the early work of Seevers and Tatum[1] with dog, and of Isbell et al.[2] and Fraser et al.[3] with man, there have been a substantial number of experimental studies demonstrating the effects of abstinence from depressant drugs or substituting one drug for another.[4-26] These experiments have employed a variety of subjects, drugs, and methods of observation. Table 1 gives a summary of many of the signs of abstinence that have been reported and the drugs studied. While the listing in Table 1 is not exhaustive it demonstrates that many minor and major signs of abstinence are commonly observed across species and depressant drugs. The most common signs appear to be: 1) anorexia, 2) tremor, 3) startle, 4) weight loss, and 5) convulsion. Depending on the particular depressant on which the subjects are dependent, the signs in Table 1 have a time of onset from the start of abstinence of a few hours to a few days. Typically, the earliest signs are anorexia and tremor and the latest are convulsions and delirium. The absence of a particular sign in Table 1 does not necessarily mean that it does not occur, only that it was not commonly reported. The quantification of the signs varies widely, often only reported as observed, occasionally objectively measured.

Extending the substitution method Himmelsbach developed for opiates, a large number of drugs have been tested for their ability to substitute for barbital or pentobarbital. Table 2 shows drugs that have been studied; those that substituted satisfactorily and those that did not. Of the drugs in Table 2 that did substitute satisfactorily, only one, carisoprodol, has failed to produce dependence when administered chronically.

Table 1. Observed signs of abstinence from depressant drugs[a]

Sign	Man	Dog, Cat, Rat, Mouse, Monkey
Anorexia	2, 3, 6	5, 17, 19, 24, 26, 25 (pheno)
Vomiting	2, 3, 6	9, 24, 26
Tremor	2, 3, 6, 8	1, 5, 9, 15, 19, 20, 22, 23, 24, 26
Twitching	2, 3	23, 26
Startle Reflex	2	9, 15, 22, 23, 25, 26
Hyperflexia	2, 6	
Convulsion	2, 3, 6, 8	1, 5, 9, 14, 15, 17, 19, 20, 22, 23, 24, 25
Convulsion Threshold		15
Weight Loss	2, 3, 8	5, 17, 19, 20, 24, 25 (pheno), 26
Anxiety	2, 3	
Weakness	2, 3, 6, 8	5
Insomnia	2, 3, 6, 8	20, 26
Tracking		19, 20, 24
Delirium	2, 3, 6, 8	19, 20
Tachycardia	2	20
Hyperthermia	2, 3, 6	5, 20, 24, 25 (pheno)
Tachypnea	2	
Orthostatic Hypotension	2, 3, 6	
Mydriasis	2	20
EEG Paroxysmal Spikes and Slow Waves	2, 3, 10	12

Barbital	1, 17, 20, 24	Alcohol	6, 8, 19, 22, 23
Secobarbital	2, 3, 5, 10	Meprobamate	9
Pentobarbital	2, 5, 10, 15, 26	Methaqualone	25
Amobarbital	2, 5	Glutethimide	14
Phenobarbital	25		

[a] Numbers give references in which signs and drugs were reported.

Table 2. Drugs tested for substitution for barbital or pentobarbital in dogs or monkeys (Refs. 18, 20, 24, 26)

Suppressed Abstinence Signs	Did Not Suppress Abstinence Signs
Secobarbital	Promethazine
Phenobarbital	Chlorpromazine
Pentobarbital	Potassium Bromide
Chloral Hydrate	Benzoctamine
Paraldehyde	Perlapine
Ethyl Alcohol	Diphenylhydantoin Sodium
Bromural	Barbituric Acid
Carisoprodol[a]	Scopolamine
Meprobamate	Hydrazine
Chlordiazepoxide	Iproniazid
Diazepam	Reserpine
Glutethimide[b]	Pyrabenzamine
Methyprylon	α-Methyldopa
Methaqualone	L-Glutamine
Chloroform	L-Arginine
Oxazolam	L-Glutamate
	L-Tryptophane

[a] Does not produce dependence on direct addiction test (11, 20).
[b] High toxicity during direct addiction (14, 20).

We have recently reported an efficient method for the bioassay of physical dependence on sedative drugs in the dog.[26] This method differs from previous methods in two respects. First, the dogs are maintained on the relatively short-acting pentobarbital administered automatically through an indwelling venous catheter, and second, *t*-score scales were developed that lend themselves to parallel line assays of relative potency and to determining differences in the profile of effects of different drugs.

Figure 1 shows the degrees of abstinence on several subscales during graded reductions of the pentobarbital maintenance dose. Figure 2 illustrates for approximately equipotent doses of pentobarbital and secobarbital that the profile across scales is similar, while methaqualone has a different profile of effects. Parallel line assays of the complete data in that experiment indicated that compared to pentobarbital, the relative potency for secobarbital was 0.85 (0.60–1.20) and for methaqualone 0.14 (0.05–0.24).

If the automatic infusions of the pentobarbital maintenance dose are interrupted daily for a period of six hours and the dog allowed to self-administer drugs during that time, dose-related response rates use-

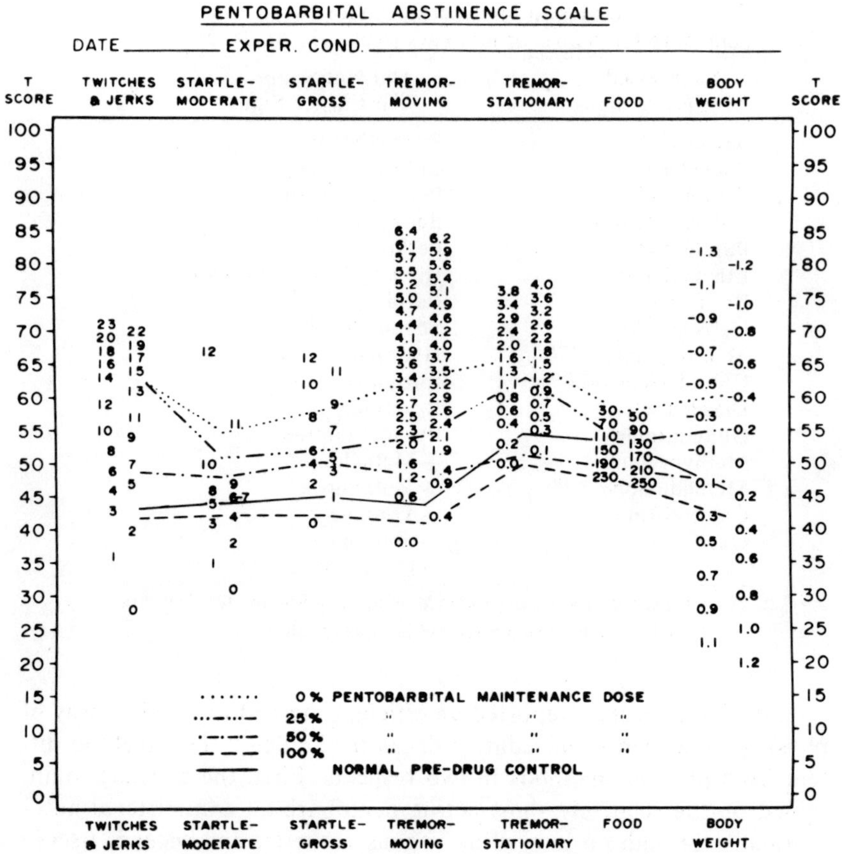

Figure 1. Raw scores and *t*-scores on seven abstinence subscales for eight dogs, before being dependent on pentobarbital sodium and at 20 to 26 hours after graded reductions of the maintenance dose (200 mg/kg/day).

ful for comparing drugs are obtained. Figure 3 shows an example of such responding.

When we turn to the question of the extent to which the various depressant drugs are abused, the exact information we need is not available. There are, however, several kinds of data that may be useful. Table 3 shows the depressant drugs on the November 1975 list of the Drug Abuse Warning Network (DAWN).[27] In column 1 the percentage of the total drug incidents associated with a particular drug is given. In column 2 the total kilograms prescribed are given based on the IMS America[28] data for Jan.–Sept. 1975. In column 3 estimated relative potency for each drug compared to pentobarbital is shown. Column 4 gives an estimate of the equivalent amounts for each drug by multiplying column 2 (kg prescribed) by column 3 (estimated relative potency). By using the estimated equivalent amounts (column 4) and the percent mentioned in the DAWN data (column 1), a ratio is determined and shown in column 5. This ratio can be used as a relative abuse index for comparing the drugs. It relates the frequency of

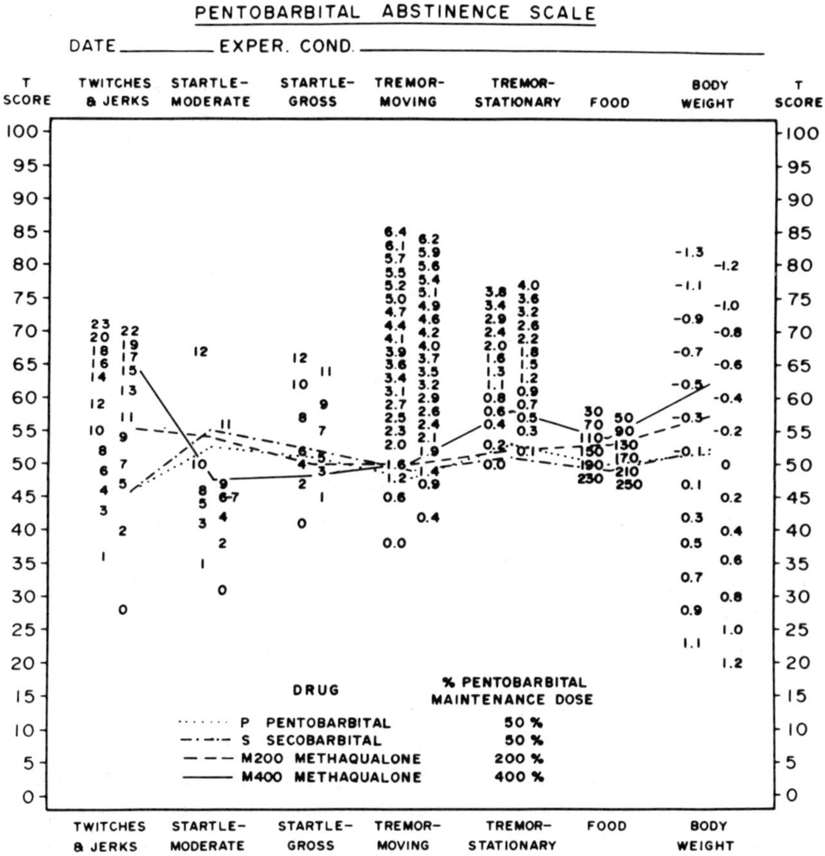

Figure 2. Comparison of the profiles of abstinence scores for pentobarbital, secobarbital and methaqualone substituted in graded amounts for the pentobarbital maintenance dose (200 mg/kg/day). $N = 5$.

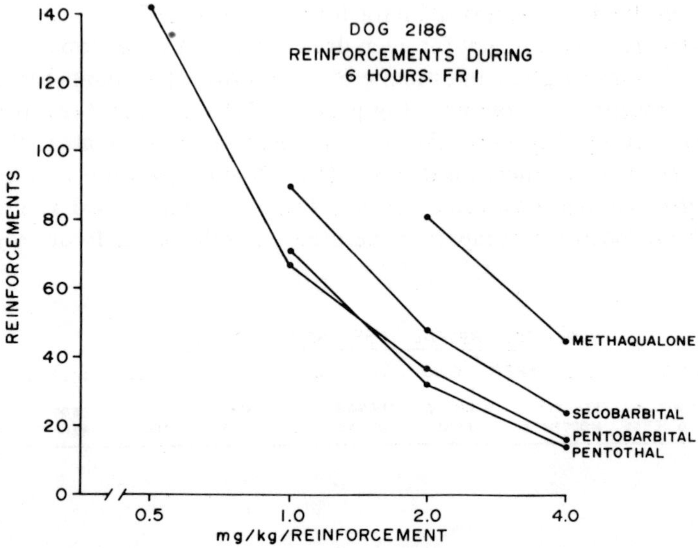

Figure 3. Number of intravenously self-administered reinforcements for different unit doses of methaqualone, secobarbital, pentobarbital and pentothal during a 6-hour period that the passively administered pentobarbital maintenance dose (200 mg/kg/day) was stopped.

occurrence of a drug in the DAWN list to the equivalent amount of the drug prescribed, compared to pentobarbital.

Looking at Table 3, we see that diazepam has the highest percent mentions in the DAWN list (10.3%), and has a relative abuse index in column 5 of 0.79, while secobarbital has a DAWN percent of 2.6 but a relative abuse index of 4.24. Thus, while diazepam has the highest observed abuse rate, its abuse rate relative to the amount prescribed is lower than secobarbital.

Tables 4 and 5 show the same kinds of data for the stimulant and narcotic drugs from the DAWN list.

Table 6 shows a selected list of drugs from Tables 3, 4 and 5 for comparison of the depressant, stimulant, and narcotic drugs. In Table 6 we see that, as a category, the stimulant drugs have the highest relative abuse index. The depressant drugs have the lowest relative abuse index but the highest percent mentions in the DAWN data.

The lack of correlation between the DAWN percent mentions and the estimated abuse index raises the question of what kind of drug abuse is represented by the DAWN data. We compared the percent

Table 3. Abuse estimates of depressants

Drug	1 DAWN Nov. 1975 Percent Mentions	2 Kilograms Prescribed Jan.–Sept. 1975 (IMS America)	3 Estimated Relative Potency[a]	4 Estimated Equivalent (kg)	5 $\frac{\text{Col 1}}{\text{Col 4}} \times 10^4$
Diazepam	10.3	13,118	10[b]	131,180	0.79
Secobarbital	2.6	6,127	1	6,127	4.24
Chlordiazepoxide	1.9	8,247	5[b]	41,235	0.46
Methaqualone	1.7	14,826	0.5	7,413	2.29
Flurazepam	1.6	6,612	3[b]	19,836	0.81
Seco-Amobarbital	1.6	7,112	1[b]	7,112	2.25
Phenobarbital	1.2	14,490	0.25	3,622	3.31
Ethchlorvynol	0.9	26,104	0.2[b]	5,220	1.72
Pentobarbital	0.9	9,188	1	9,188	0.98
Meprobamate	0.8	189,000	0.07	13,293	0.60
Chorazepate	0.5	1,395	7[b]	9,765	0.51

[a] Relative potency compared to pentobarbital.

[b] Relative potency estimate not based on assay.

Table 4. Abuse estimates of stimulants

Drug	1 DAWN Nov. 1975 Percent Mentions	2 Kilograms Prescribed Jan.–Sept. 1975 (IMS America)	3 Estimated Relative Potency[a]	4 Estimated Equivalent (kg)	5 $\frac{\text{Col 1}}{\text{Col 4}} \times 10^4$
Amphetamine and *d*-Amphetamine	1.9	1,988	1	1,988	9.56
Methamphetamine	0.4	194	1	194	20.62
Methylphenidate	0.4	1,410	0.5	705	5.67

[a] Relative potency compared *d*-amphetamine.

Table 5. Abuse estimates of narcotics

Drug	1 DAWN Nov. 1975 Percent Mentions	2 Kilograms Prescribed Jan.–Sept. 1975 (IMS America)	3 Estimated Relative Potency[a]	4 Estimated Equivalent (kg)	5 $\frac{\text{Col 1}}{\text{Col 4}} \times 10^4$
Heroin	9.1		2		
d-Propoxyphene	2.0	71,018	0.025	1,775	11.27
Methadone	1.2		1		
Codeine	0.5	22,096	0.05	1,105	4.52
Oxycodone	0.5	929	0.5	465	10.75
Meperidine	0.4	2,259	0.1	226	17.70
Pentazocine	0.4	5,442	0.25	1,361	2.94
Morphine	0.1	239	1	239	4.18
Hydromorphone	0.1	31	9	279	3.58

[a] Relative potency compared to morphine.

Table 6. Abuse estimates of selected depressants, stimulants and narcotics

Drug	1 DAWN Nov. 1975 Percent Mentions	2 Kilograms Prescribed Jan.–Sept. 1975 (IMS America)	3 Estimated Relative Potency[a]	4 Estimated Equivalent (kg)	5 $\frac{\text{Col 1}}{\text{Col 4}} \times 10^4$
Amphetamine and *d*-Amphetamine	1.9	1,988	1	1,988	9.56
Methamphetamine	0.4	194	1	194	20.62
Methylphenidate	0.4	1,410	0.5	705	5.67
d-Propoxyphene	2.0	71,018	0.025	1,775	11.27
Codeine	0.5	22,096	0.05	1,105	4.52
Morphine	0.1	239	1	239	4.18
Diazepam	10.3	13,118	10[b]	131,180	0.79
Secobarbital	2.6	6,127	1	6,127	4.24
Pentobarbital	0.9	9,188	1	9,188	0.98
Meprobamate	0.8	189,900	0.07	13,293	0.60

[a] Relative potency compared to *d*-amphetamine, morphine, or pentobarbital as appropriate.

[b] Relative potency estimate not based on assay.

mentions for the prescription drugs of the top 35 drugs in the November 1975 DAWN list with the percentage each drug comprised of the total prescriptions of the same sample of drugs, based on IMS America total prescriptions data. That comparison yielded a high and significant correlation ($r = 0.85$; $p < 0.01$). This suggests that if a drug is related to one of the criterion drugs of the depressant, stimulant, or narcotic type in its clinical use, we could predict the prescription drugs on the DAWN data on the basis of prescribing practices. That is, in the DAWN data the most often abused drug is the drug most often prescribed.

A weakness in this analysis is that abused nonprescription drugs are not considered. That the DAWN data are more representative is suggested by another comparison. Haertzen[29] has collected the responses of post-addict prisoners in regard to the number of times of use for a large number of drugs. When his data were compared with the DAWN percent mentions data there was a substantial and significant correlation ($r = 47$; $p < 0.01$).

In sum, it appears, with minor exceptions, that for depressant drugs, testing in animals for the drug's ability to substitute for barbiturates or for its production of abstinence signs following discontinuation of chronic administration will predict the abuse liability of that drug should it become readily available. Furthermore, it appears that the frequency of abuse of a particular depressant drug will be largely a function of the frequency of its prescription.

LITERATURE CITED

1. Seevers, M. H., and Tatum, A. C. 1931. J. Pharmacol. Exp. Ther. 42:217.
2. Isbell, H., Altschul, S., Kornetsky, C. H., Eisenman, A. J., Flanary, H. G., and Fraser, H. F. 1950. Arch. Neurol. Psychiat. 64:1.
3. Fraser, H. F., Isbell, H., Eisenman, A. J., Wikler, A., and Pescor, F. T. 1954. Arch. Intern. Med. 94:34.
4. Fraser, H. F., Isbell, H., Wikler, A., and Pescor, F. 1953. Fed. Proc. 12:322.
5. Fraser, H. F., and Isbell, H. J. 1954. Pharmacol. Exp. Ther. 112:261.
6. Isbell, H., Fraser, H. F., Wikler, A., Belleville, R. E., and Eisenman, A. J. 1955. Quart. J. Stud. Alcohol 16:1.
7. Isbell, H. 1956. World Health Organization APD/75.
8. Fraser, H. F., Wikler, A., Isbell, H., and Johnson, N. K. 1957. Quart. J. Stud. Alcohol 18:541.
9. Essig, C. F., and Ainslie, J. O. 1957. J. Am. Med. Assoc. 164:1382.
10. Essig, C. F., and Fraser, H. F. 1958. EEG Clin. Neurophysiol. 10:649.

11. Fraser, H. F., Essig, C. F., and Wolbach, A. B., Jr. 1961. Bull. Narcot. 13:1.
12. Essig, C. F., and Flanary, H. G. 1961. Exp. Neurol. 3:149.
13. Essig, C. F., and Carter, W. W. 1962. Neurology 12:481.
14. Essig, C. F. 1963. Am. J. Psychiat. 119:993.
15. Jaffe, J. H., and Sharpless, S. K. 1965. J. Pharmacol. Exp. Ther. 150:140.
16. Essig, C. F., and Fraser, H. F. 1966. Clin. Pharmacol. Ther. 7:466.
17. Essig, C. F. 1966. Int. J. Neuropharmacol. 5:103.
18. Essig, C. F. 1967. Epilepsia 8:21.
19. Essig, C. F., and Lam, R. C. 1968. Arch. Neurol. 18:626.
20. Deneau, G. A., and Weiss, S. 1968. Pharmako-psychiat. Neuro-Psycho-pharmakol. 1:270.
21. Essig, C. F., Jones, B. E., and Lam, R. C. 1969. Arch. Neurol. 20:554.
22. Freund, G. 1969. Arch. Neurol. 21:315.
23. Goldstein, D. B., and Pal, N. 1971. Science 172:288.
24. Yanagita, T., and Takahashi, S. J. 1973. Pharmacol. Exp. Ther. 185:307.
25. Kohli, R. P., Singh, N., and Kulshrestha, V. K. 1974. Psychopharmacologia 35:327.
26. Jones, B. E., Prada, J. A., and Martin, W. R. 1976. Psychopharmacologia (Berl.) 47:7–15.
27. Drug Abuse Warning Network, Statistical Summary, Joint Publication Drug Enforcement Administration and National Institute on Drug Abuse. November 1975.
28. National Prescription Audit. 1975. Therapeutic Category Report. September, 1975. IMS American Ltd., Ambler, Pa. Copyright 1975.
29. Haertzen, C. A. Personal communication of unpublished data.

NOTE ADDED IN PROOF

The Himmelsbach substitution method for opiates cited on page 35 is described in Himmelsbach, C. K. 1937. Clinical Studies of Drug Addiction. II. "Rossium" Treatment of Drug Addiction. Public Health Reports, Supplement No. 125, pp. 1–18.

Methodological Considerations in Testing Physical Dependence Potential of Sedative-Hypnotics in Animals

Tomoji Yanagita

Based on past experiences with testing the dependence potentials of various types of drugs primarily in rhesus monkeys and, to a lesser extent, in beagle dogs and rats, physical dependence can be classified into two major types: 1) the morphine type, in which the withdrawal signs are always precipitable by administration of morphine antagonists such as naloxone, and 2) the barbiturate type, in which dependence is developed on those drugs that can substitute for barbital in maintaining physical dependence on barbital. Development of physical dependence on stimulants and hallucinogenic drugs is not known. Our experiences with cocaine, amphetamines, methylphenidate, phenmetrazine, pipradrol, nicotine, caffeine, mescaline, LSD-25, STP, and delta-9-THC support this. In the case of THC, however, some other investigators have demonstrated its physical dependence potential in the rhesus monkey by intravenous programmed administration of its suspensions at relatively large doses.[1] Since the scope of this publication excludes the opiates and synthetic analgesic-antitussives, and since most of the stimulants and hallucinogenic drugs are regarded to be physical dependence-free, with the exception of THC, the following discussion on testing the physical dependence potential of drugs in animals is inevitably limited to dependence of the barbiturate type.

DRUGS THAT PRODUCE PHYSICAL DEPENDENCE OF THE BARBITURATE TYPE

The major groups of drugs that produce physical dependence of the barbiturate type are the barbiturates and the diazepine derivatives.[2,3]

Several other drugs, such as alcohol, chloral hydrate, meprobamate, methyprylon, and glutethimide, are also known to produce physical dependence of this type.[3-7] There are also a number of nonbarbiturate and nondiazepine sedative-hypnotics that may possess a physical dependence potential.[8] Contrary to this, such sedative-hypnotics as perlapine and benzoctamine are known to be physical dependence-free.[3] The phenothiazine and butyrophenone derivatives also do not produce physical dependence in spite of their potent central nervous system effects. Interestingly, methaqualone, one of the principal hypnotics of nonmedical use in man, was found to be utterly physical dependence-free in a recent study.[9] Brief results of the tests on these drugs conducted in the rhesus monkey are summarized in Table 1.

BASIC METHODS FOR TESTING PHYSICAL DEPENDENCE POTENTIAL OF DRUGS

The most basic laboratory method for testing physical dependence potential of sedative-hypnotics is repeated administration of the drugs to initially drug-naive animals under sufficient dosing schedules for a certain period of time. Subsequently, upon termination of drug administration, withdrawal manifestation is observed for several days, and the extent of development of physical dependence can be assessed from the severity of the withdrawal manifestation. The test under these procedures may be called a physical dependence-producing test. In our routine procedure, drugs are manually administered for 4 weeks, 1 to 4 times daily, then withdrawn for 1 week. This cycle is then repeated once or twice according to the clarity of the results.

The precipitation test of withdrawal signs by drugs is one of the standard procedures for the observation of the development of physical dependence of the morphine type, but it is not applicable here since no barbiturate antagonist is available yet. The physical dependence-producing test alone, however, may not be sufficient for testing the physical dependence potential of drugs, because a negative-false result can be easily reached, unless a proper dosing schedule of drugs is used in this test. In order to avoid this problem, the single dose-substitution test in barbital-dependent and withdrawn animals may also be indispensable. So far as is presently known, any drug that shows cross-physical dependence to barbital in the substitution test produces physical dependence in the dependence-producing test. On the other hand, the drugs that show no cross-dependence in the substitution test rarely produce weak physical dependence in the latter test.

Table 1. Summary of physical dependence tests on sedative-hypnotics in rhesus monkeys

	Substitution Test (Barbital 75 mg/kg, p.o. × 2/day)		Physical dependence–producing test			
	Suppression	Complete suppression Dose (mg/kg)	Dose (mg/kg × times/day)	Period (weeks)	Withdrawal grade ( ): No. of monkeys	References
Barbital	+	100 p.o.	150 p.o. × 1	4	Severe(4), Intermed.(3)	2
Phenobarbital	not tested		100 p.o. × 1	6	Severe(2), Mild(1)	2
Pentobarbital	+	25 i.v.	Self-ad. 5 × 59-85	2	Severe(2)	2
Alcohol	+	4,000 p.o.	Self-ad. 1g × 5-7.5	5–10	Severe(3), Intermed.(1)	3
Meprobamate	+	200 p.o.	200–400 p.o. × 2	8	Severe(3), Intermed.(2)	3
Diazepam	+	5 p.o.	10–20 p.o. × 1	8	Severe(2), Intermed.(2)	3
Chlordiazepoxide	+	20 p.o.	75–113 p.o. × 1	12	Severe(3), Intermed.(1)	3
Lorazepam	+	10 p.o.	10–30 p.o. × 2	8	Severe(1), Intermed.(3)	18
Nitrazepam	+	2 p.o.	10–15 p.o. × 2	8	Intermed.(4)	20
Estazolam[a]	+	2 p.o.	10–15 p.o. × 2	8	Severe(1), Intermed.(3)	21
Cloxazolazepam[b]	+	20 p.o.	40–60 p.o. × 2	8	Severe(1), Intermed.(3)	22
Methaqualone	–		50 p.o. × 2	8	None(5)	9
Perlapine[c]	–		50 p.o. × 1	8	None(4)	3

[a] 8-chloro-6-phenyl-4H-s-triazolo-[4,3-a]-[1,4]benzodiazepine

[b] 10-chloro-11b-(*O*-chlorophenyl)-2,3,5,6,7,11b-hexahydrobenzo [6,7]-1,4-diazepine-[5,4-b]-oxazole-6-one

[c] 6-(4-methyl-1-piperazinyl)morphanthridine

CHOICE OF ANIMAL SPECIES

The essential factor in choosing the most appropriate animal species for predicting the physical dependence potential of sedative-hypnotics in man is a similarity of a certain animal species to man in pharmacodynamic and pharmacokinetic susceptibilities to a particular drug. For example, it was not rare to observe that while relatively potent depressant effects on animal gross behavior were shown in mice or rats, the effects were very weak in dogs or monkeys, or vice versa. Similar differences were also observable in the duration of drug effects. Such species differences may greatly influence the results of the test of the physical dependence potential of a drug because the extent of the development of physical dependence on a drug of this class is known to be parallel to the depth and duration of depressive manifestations observed in animals during the repeated administration period.[2,10] The best way to observe these species differences is through gross behavioral observation of drug effects in normal subjects at single and/or repeated dosing schedules. However, the comparative pharmacokinetic studies on the half-time of the blood concentration of a drug and the content ratio of its major metabolites in the blood or urine may provide a significant basis for choosing an appropriate animal species for the test. Presently available knowledge indicates that the nonhuman primates, particularly the maccaques, may generally be the best suited animal species for most drugs of this class, particularly for many of the benzodiazepine derivatives.

The other factors to be considered are the clarity of the withdrawal manifestations and the availability of objective methods for observing the withdrawal signs in a certain animal species. These are discussed later. From a practical viewpoint, technical ease of maintaining and handling the animals is also an important factor in the choice of animal species.

CHOICE OF PARAMETERS FOR WITHDRAWAL SIGNS

The most widely used parameters for withdrawal signs of barbiturate type dependence are such gross behavioral manifestations as hyperirritability, tremor and convulsions. An example is illustrated in Table 2. In comparing barbital withdrawal manifestations among the rhesus monkeys, beagle dog, and Sprague-Dawley rat, the monkey was found to be the best and the dog second in terms of clarity, particularly in such withdrawal signs as apprehension, hyperirritability, tremor,

Table 2. Grade of withdrawal signs in barbiturate-dependent monkeys[2]

Grade	Signs
Mild	apprehension hyperirritability mild tremor anorexia piloerection
Intermediate	aggravated tremor muscle rigidity impaired motor activities retching or vomiting weight loss (10%)
Severe	convulsions delirium (hallucinatory behavior, nystagmus, dissociation from environment) hyperthermia (> 1.5°C)

impaired motor activity, hallucinatory behavior, nystagmus, and dissociation from the environment. In addition to these animal species, the mouse and cat were often used by many other investigators.[11-16] Although the gross behavioral observation seems to fulfill the requirements as a measure of withdrawal observation, some investigators are trying more objective and quantifiable measures. These include determination of the seizure threshold by convulsants, or the electric shock and electrophysiological observation of the CNS functions. An example is shown in Figure 1.

INFLUENCE OF DOSING SCHEDULE, DEPRESSANT EFFECTS, AND TOLERANCE DEVELOPMENT ON THE DEVELOPMENT OF PHYSICAL DEPENDENCE

As mentioned previously, the development of physical dependence on sedative-hypnotics is greatly influenced by the depth and duration of drug effects that are manifested in the animals' gross behavior during the drug administration period. Development of tolerance to a drug lessens the intensity or shortens the duration of these effects, and thus reduces the development of physical dependence. Both dispositional tolerance and functional tolerance (which consists of tissue tolerance and the behavioral tolerance) may exist in such cases. Therefore the

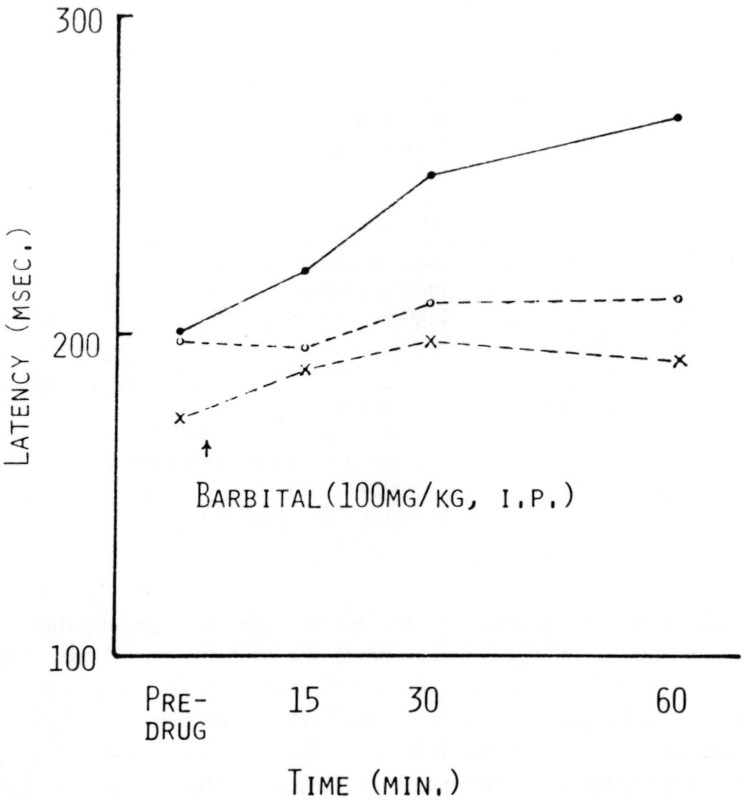

Figure 1. The figure represents the latent time of the evoked potentials in rats as stimulated at the sciatic nerve and recorded from the parietal cortex. Single dose administration of barbital prolonged the latent time in normal rats (●——●), but not in barbital-tolerant rats (*o------o*). The latent time became shorter than that of normals at the pre-drug period in barbital-tolerant and withdrawn rats (×------×) (Yanagita and Shimada, unpublished).

dosing schedule in the physical dependence-producing test has to be determined according to the gross behavioral manifestation of the drug effects, so that the intensity and duration of the effects at a certain level are maintained. In other words, it can be said that the extent of the development of physical dependence on a drug of this class is more relevant to the actual drug effects that are manifested in animals than to the absolute dose levels. This has been confirmed by our previous study.[2] Thus, when the depressant effect of a drug is relatively weak, a dosing schedule that allows the maintenance of the plateau effect level must be used; what is sought in this test is the physical dependence potential of a drug when the drug is used nonmedically, rather than when it is used medically under a doctor's auspices.

PHARMACODYNAMIC PROPERTIES AND PHYSICAL DEPENDENCE POTENTIAL

As described at the beginning of this paper, phenothiazines and butyrophenone do not produce physical dependence in spite of their potent CNS depressant effects. Contrary to this, some diazepines, which never produced anesthesia at large doses, produced obvious physical dependence of the barbiturate type. Clearly, there must exist some definite differences between the pharmacodynamic properties of these two types of drugs. One distinct difference is in the anticonvulsant effect, since the phenothiazines and butyrophenone are known to possess no, or at most, a weak effect. Contrary to this, such a drug as lorazepam possesses a significantly stronger effect than that of diazepam,[17] but the physical dependence potential of lorazepam tested in the substitution and dependence-producing tests in rhesus monkeys was lower than, or at most equal to, that of diazepam.[18] Although the anticonvulsant effect was not found to be an appropriate parameter for predicting physical dependence potential of the barbiturate type, some other pharmacodynamic properties will undoubtedly be identified as the appropriate parameters for prediction, so that at least a primary prediction can be made from the pharmacodynamic characteristics of drugs. The property of a drug that produces the marked tissue tolerance is believed to be closely related to the physical dependence–producing property, and usually the observation of tolerance development appears to be easier and more quantifiable than that of physical dependence development. Therefore, this approach should be studied as a possible method for predicting the physical dependence potentials of drugs.

DRUGS TO BE TESTED

From our past experience, it is known that the drugs that produced physical dependence of the barbiturate type always possessed a definite CNS depression of animals' gross behavior, while the drugs that had no observable depressant effects never produced dependence. Thus, the drugs that show definite CNS depressant effects and are not identifiable as the other class of the drugs should be the subjects of this test, but the drugs that are regarded to be similar, chemically and pharmacologically, to such drugs as the major phenothiazines, butyrophenone, and reserpine may be excluded. Some tricyclic anti-depressants, such as imipramine, produced weak depressant effects, but several drugs of this group, including imipramine, were found to be physical dependence–free in the tests on the rhesus monkeys.[19] Therefore, the derivatives of these drugs can be dealt with in a manner similar to the cases of the phenothiazines and other derivatives. If cases of the nonmedical uses in man of some particular sedative-hypnotics should arise, naturally the test is to be recommended for these drugs as well.

LITERATURE CITED

1. Kaymakcalan, S. 1973. Bull. Narcotics 25:39.
2. Yanagita, T., and Takahashi, S. 1970. J. Pharmacol. Exp. Ther. 172:163.
3. Yanagita, T., and Takahashi, S. 1973. J. Pharmacol. Exp. Ther. 185:307.
4. Martin, W. R. 1971. Drug dependence. In: Drill's Pharmacology in Medicine, 4th Ed. McGraw-Hill Book Co., Inc., New York.
5. Aston, R. 1973. In the technical papers of the 2nd rept. of the National Commission of Marihuana and Drug Abuse. U.S. Government Printing Office #5266-00004.
6. Essig, C. F. 1964. Clin. Pharmacol. Ther. 5:338.
7. Wld Hlth. Org. 1964. Tech. Rep. Ser. 287.
8. AMA Committee on Alcoholism and Addiction. 1965. The Journal of the American Medical Association 193:673.
9. Yanagita, T., and Miyasato, K. 1976. CIEA Preclin. Rpt. 2:57.
10. Fraser, H. F. J. 1954. Pharmacol. Exp. Ther. 112:261.
11. Okamoto, M., Rosenberg, H. C., and Boisse, N. R. 1975. J. Pharmacol. Exp. Ther. 192:555.
12. Essig, C. F., and Flanary, H. G. 1959. Exp. Neurol. 1:529.
13. Jaffe, J. H., and Sharpless, S. K. 1965. J. Pharmacol. Exp. Ther. 150:140.
14. Kaneto, H., Koida, M., Tsuchie, F., and Miyagawa, H. 1973. Folia Pharmacol. Jap. 69:729.
15. Goldstein, D. B., and Pad, N. 1971. Science 172:288.
16. Ogata, H., Ogata, F., Mendelson, J. H., and Mello, N. K. 1972. J. Pharmacol. Exp. Ther. 180:216.
17. Iizuka, H., Imamura, H., and Yanagita, T. 1975. CIEA Preclin. Rpt. 1:59.

18. Yanagita, T., Takahashi, S., and Oinuma, N. 1975. CIEA Preclin. Rpt. 1:1.
19. Yanagita, T., and Takahashi, S. 1970. J. Pharmacol. Exp. Ther. 172:163.
20. Yanagita, T., Takahashi, S., and Oinuma, N. 1975. CIEA Preclin. Rpt. 1:151.
21. Yanagita, T., Takahashi, S., and Sei, M. 1976. CIEA Preclin. Rpt. 2:35.
22. Yanagita, T., Takahashi, S., Nakanishi, H., and Oinuma, N. 1975. CIEA Preclin. Rpt. 1:223.

Physical Dependency Characteristics of a Long-Acting Barbiturate, Barbital, Compared to the Short-Acting Pentobarbital

Cat as an Experimental Physical Dependency Model System

Michiko Okamoto

Production of physical dependence can be considered a chronic drug toxicity. Accordingly, a quantifiable evaluation procedure that is based on solid pharmacological discipline is essential in order to make a meaningful assessment of physical dependence capability of a drug. Just as an acute drug effect can be characterized by its dose-response and time-action, and is quantitatively expressed against its prototype, the same quantitative disciplinary approach should be taken in the evaluation of physical dependence capability.

Present knowledge of the pharmacological determinants for physical dependence production and withdrawal produced by drugs such as CNS depressants indicates that the same functional pharmacological principle that permits quantitative characterization of acute drug action operates, and therefore can be utilized in setting rigid criteria for evaluation of physical dependence capability. These pharmacological determinants have been indicated many ways in abundant literatures;[1] however, their quantitative applications have often been neglected in overall evaluation of physical dependence.

Data presented are from the investigation supported by NIADAMHA, Research Grant DA-00591. Co-investigator, N.R. Boisee.

In this chapter I would like to illustrate some of those pharmacological determinants, some of which have already been mentioned by the other authors. For this reason, I would like to utilize our barbiturate physical dependence animal model system as an example, and utilize pentobarbital and barbital as standard prototypes of CNS depressants possessing different physicochemical properties, and further demonstrate the usefulness of the animal model system for this type of study.

As has been stated before, the production of physical dependence, in a broad sense, can be considered a chronic drug toxicity. Therefore, a meaningful comparison of the capability of each CNS depressant to produce physical dependence is more rationally derived when this toxicity is assessed against the effects usually sought in the abuse of these drugs, i.e., intoxication, CNS depression.

As a practical chronic dosing method that provides dosing conditions more similar to that of human addicts, intermittent chronic dosing has been widely utilized in producing barbiturate dependence. This approach has also been adopted in our study, as it has been used by most investigators to produce dependence in higher animal species like cat,[2-6] dog,[7,8] and monkey,[9,10] and in man.[11-14]

While it is not certain whether or not the development of physical dependence is due to the presence of the drug per se or to the pharmacological action, namely to the depression of the nervous system produced by the drug, considerable evidence favors the view that the depression of the nervous system is more important.[cf.15] Accordingly, the CNS depressants, the barbiturates, and a host of chemically dissimilar CNS depressants, including alcohol, nonbarbiturate sedative-hypnotics, and minor tranquilizers, are qualitatively similar both in their dose-related actions to depress the nervous system and their withdrawal reactions. Furthermore, these so-called general depressants require dosing sufficient to produce prolonged overt depression of the nervous system.[4,9,10,16,17,cf.18] If physical dependence production results primarily from the chronic depression of the nervous system, then the measurement of the degree of CNS depression produced during dependence production is as important as the measurement of chronic drug load in comparing physical dependence production capability of different CNS depressants. Setting criteria for the study in these circumstances, therefore, might be best achieved by an experimental design that permits production of equieffective CNS depression to different drugs during chronic treatment.

Further support for this approach to physical dependence production, i.e., setting equieffective the CNS depression produced during physical dependence production as one of the primary criteria in comparing the dependence-producing capabilities of different CNS depressants, is found in relation to the inevitable development of tolerance to drugs during chronic treatment. Because the nature and extent of tolerance development for physicochemically different CNS depressants are expected to be different,[cf. 1] the degree of CNS depression produced during chronic treatment cannot remain the same between two drugs, unless the criteria for treatment are based upon drug response rather than on drug load alone.

Therefore, the recently developed "maximally tolerable" pentobarbital dosing method in the cat[5,6] in which each animal is treated to produce equieffective CNS depression throughout chronic treatment for pentobarbital, was thought to be the ideal method for comparing the physical dependence–producing capability of different CNS depressants. This procedure requires the quantitative determination of drug response, namely degree of CNS depression produced along with the measurement of dose load.

An example of a quantitative evaluation of overall CNS depression that we have utilized in our laboratory is shown in Table 1. The degree of CNS depression in response to barbiturate doses is measured at pre-set times daily, by rating functional losses obtained in neurological response testing. This rating system consists of a depression scale of 0 to 14. A zero is assigned when no CNS depression is detectable, while a 14 is assigned to the most severe depression with impending death. The higher the score, the greater the degree of CNS depression. In addition, in order to make meaningful assessment of chronic drug load, blood concentration of the drug was correlated simultaneously against dose and response achieved during the chronic treatment and withdrawal period.

The equieffective CNS depression by barbiturates having different physico-chemical properties should be attainable by setting dosing intervals that allow for equal recoveries. This assumption would be varified by three measurable response criteria: 1) the peak CNS depression, 2) the residual depression observed at the time of the next dosing, 3) the total depression based on areas under time effect curves. For each CNS depressant tested, the criteria should be equal if equieffective dosing was achieved.

The basic data obtained for establishing so called "chronically equivalent" dosing regimens with barbital and pentobarbital are

Table 1. CNS depression rating scale for evaluation of overall CNS depression[a]

Rating	awake; +,+/0,0	arouse to consciousness; +,+/0,0	corseal reflex 0 to 3	mictitating membrane tone, 0 to 3	pain withdrawal 0 to 3	Respirations— N = normal M = mixed D = diaphragmatic N,D or N,D rate in breaths per minute	right self; +,+/0,0	stand; +,+/0,0	walk; +,+/0,0	land on feet when dropped upright from 3 ft. +,+/0,0	land on feet when dropped upsidedown from 3 ft. +,+/0,0	Comments
0	+	+	3	3	3	N	+	+	+	+	+	no CNS depression
1	+	+	3	3	3	N	+	+	+	+	+/0	
2	+	+	3	3	3	N	+	+	+	+, +/0	0	
3	+	+	3	3	3	N	+	+	+/0	0	0	
4	+	+	3	3	3	N	+	+	0	0	0	
5	+	+	3	3	3,2	N	+	+/0	0	0	0	
6	+	+	3	3	3,2	N	+	0	0	0	0	
7	+,+/0	+	3	3	3,2	N	+/0	0	0	0	0	
8	0	+,+/0	3	3	3,2	N,M	0	0	0	0	0	barely conscious, or delerious
9	0	0	3	3,2	3,2,1	N,M	0	0	0	0	0	licking, involuntary movements
10	0	0	3,2	2,1	2,1	M	0	0	0	0	0	light anesthesia, minimal respiratory depression
11	0	0	2	1,0	1,0	D, N D > 12 N, D	0	0	0	0	0	moderate respiratory depression
12	0	0	1	1,0	0	N, D D = 12	0	0	0	0	0	marked respiratory depression
13	0	0	1,0	0	0	D < 12	0	0	0	0	0	very deep anesthesia
14	0	0	0	0	0	D < 12	0	0	0	0	0	deep coma, hypothermia, cyanosis, near death

[a] On the top, the list of various subjective neurologic testing responses measured at pre-set times during chronic treatment. "Pain withdrawal of front paw" is the flexor response to a hard squeeze of the footpad of a forelimb. This stimulis is also used to determine whether the cat could be awakened. For those responses recorded +, +/0 and +/ 0 indicate responses and 0 indicates absence of the response. For those responses graded from 0 to 3, 0 indicates no response and 3 indicates normal response.

Table 2. "Maximally tolerable" dosing regimens for barbital and pentobarbital that produce CNS depression rating scale of approximately 11[a]

Dose	Barbital	Pentobarbital
Starting dose	400 mg/kg	40 mg/kg
Dose changes	50 mg/kg steps	5 mg/kg steps
Dosing interval	72 hours	12 hours
Total duration	5 weeks	5 weeks

[a] The regimens are derived through dose-response, time-action, and pharmacokinetic studies for barbital and pentobarbital.

shown in Table 2. Extensive dose-response, time-action, blood concentration measurement and pharmacokinetic studies furnished these barbital-pentobarbital relationships. Based on these data, the sequentially adjusted sodium barbiturate doses are given intragastrically to produce a chronic CNS depression of 10–11 according to our standard CNS depression rating scale.

As shown in Figure 1, an analysis of drug response based on neurologic response testing during the chronic treatment of large groups of animals has confirmed that the previously defined criteria for equivalency of chronic treatment—equivalency of peak, residual, and total depression—were satisfied for barbital and pentobarbital. Constancy and equivalency of peak effect throughout the chronic treatments ensured that the contribution of dose to CNS depression was equivalent for barbital and pentobarbital despite tolerance development. Equivalency of residual CNS depression throughout the treatments ensured that the dosing interval had been properly chosen to correct for differences in barbital and pentobarbital time action. The importance of the continuity of drug effects between doses (residual) to ensure the development of physical dependence has been emphasized by several investigators.[8-11,18,19] The use of total depression, the integral of response over time, as a measure of treatment equivalency deserves special comment. Data obtained by Jaffe and Sharpless[4] in the cat indicate that the degree of dependence produced by pentobarbital increases with the total dose administered over time. Also, Goldstein[17] found that the degree of dependence produced in mice exposed to alcohol vapor increased with the product of dose and duration (total dose), but was independent of the time over which the total dose was administered. Since total response is a function of total dose, these two findings suggest that the degree of dependence produced is independent of the shape of the time-action

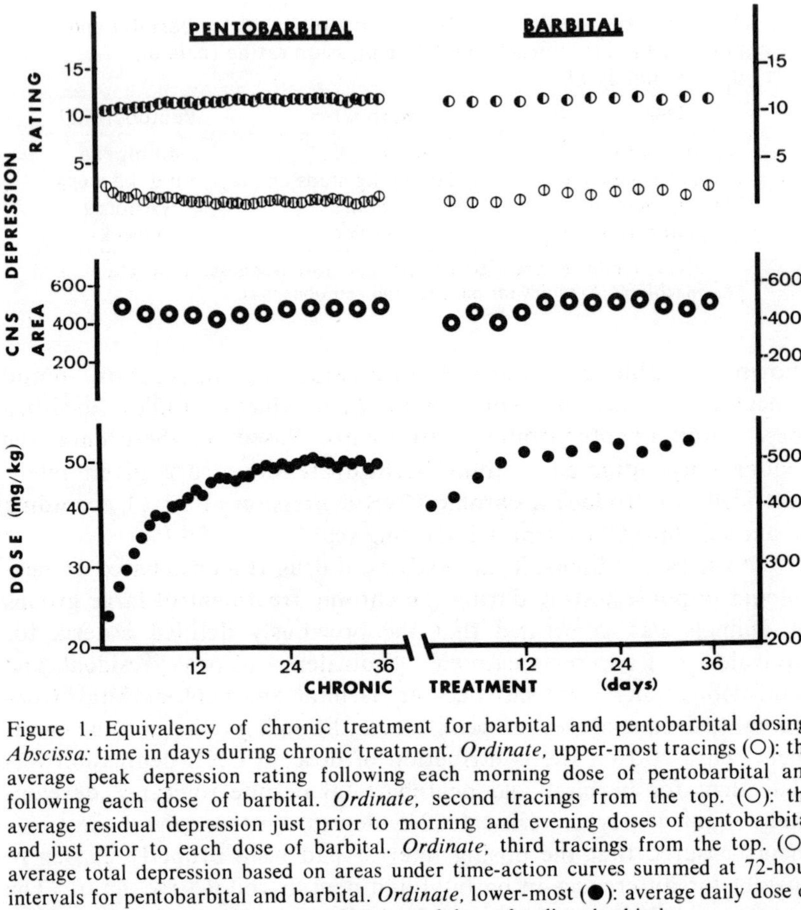

Figure 1. Equivalency of chronic treatment for barbital and pentobarbital dosing. *Abscissa:* time in days during chronic treatment. *Ordinate*, upper-most tracings (○): the average peak depression rating following each morning dose of pentobarbital and following each dose of barbital. *Ordinate*, second tracings from the top. (○): the average residual depression just prior to morning and evening doses of pentobarbital and just prior to each dose of barbital. *Ordinate*, third tracings from the top. (○): average total depression based on areas under time-action curves summed at 72-hour intervals for pentobarbital and barbital. *Ordinate*, lower-most (●): average daily dose of sodium pentobarbital and average administered dose of sodium barbital.

curve, and more related to the total effect. Thus, the constancy and equivalency of total depression obtained throughout the present experiments has provided added assurance of the equivalency of barbital and pentobarbital treatments, and confirmed the implicit assumption that the total effect produced by one barbital dose was equivalent to that produced by six equipotent pentobarbital doses.

The ideal and the importance of simultaneous monitoring of blood concentration of the drug during the chronic treatment are shown in Figure 2. The figure demonstrates the differences between barbital and pentobarbital in their capability to produce dispositional and functional tolerance by careful measurement of blood concentration and elimination kinetic study. As it is shown in the figure, the elimination kinetic for barbital does not change by chronic treatment but it does change for pentobarbital, presumably because of liver microsomal enzyme induction.[cf.20,21] Thus, dispositional tolerance occurs for pentobarbital but not for barbital. In contrast, the bottom tracings show that the extent and rate of functional tolerance developed for barbital and pentobarbital are very similar, which is indicated by the steady parallel increase in peak blood concentrations to achieve the constant level of CNS depression. This is a dramatic illustration in that the degree of functional tolerance development for two physicochemically different barbiturates is very similar when their

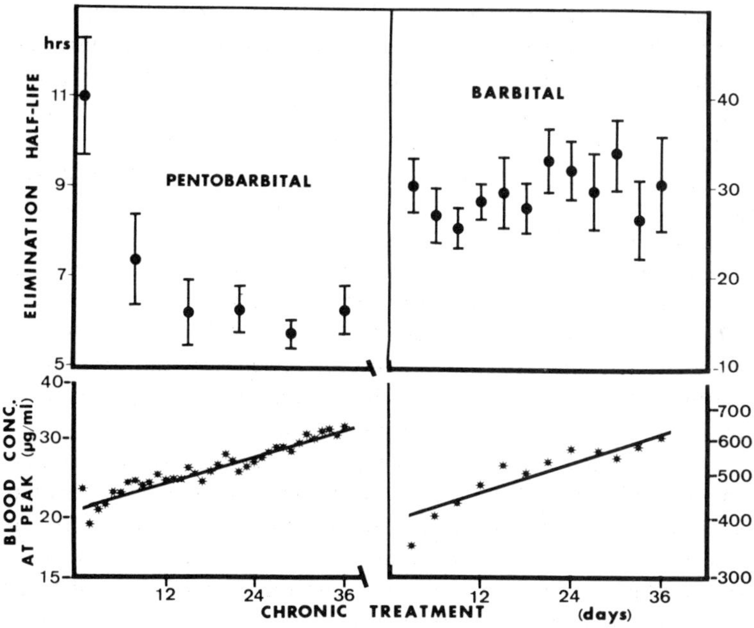

Figure 2. *Top:* Elimination half-lives for barbital and pentobarbital from blood during chronic treatment. *Abscissa:* Time in days during chronic treatment. *Ordinate:* elimination half-life in hours. Half-lives were calculated for each animal by a least squares exponential regression of blood barbiturate concentrations against time. Each point and vertical bar represents the mean and standard error. *Bottom:* Analysis of blood concentrations at the time of peak CNS depression produced (see Figure 1, Top) during chronic treatment with pentobarbital and barbital. *Abscissa:* time in days during chronic treatment. *Ordinate:* average pentobarbital concentration in blood sampled 1–1 ¼ hours after the morning dose of pentobarbital and the average barbital concentration in blood sampled 6–6 ½ hours after each dose of barbital.

chronic dosing regimens are adjusted to be equal. Because this functional tolerance would ultimately determine the degree of physical dependency production, the results are important. Again, it points out the importance of quantitative approach to the study of the drug-dependence problem.

If the severity of the abstinence syndrome depends upon the chronic drug load, as it is illustrated in man,[cf.22] it follows from the dose-response principle that the withdrawal responses would appear in graded fashion. Pari passu this would reflect the degree of dependence. Accordingly, a measurement of the manifested withdrawal signs should also be quantitative if one is to make a meaningful assessment of the intensity of physical dependence in relation to chronic drug load.

The abstinence signs produced in animal model systems, the cat, for example, resemble those in the human. These signs include resting and intention tremors, muscle twitches, nystagmus, weakness, impaired motor coordination, increased muscle tone, disturbances of gait and posture, grand mal type convulsion, cessation of eating and sleeping, piloerection, mydriasis, hyperthermia, increased startle response, and behavioral alteration, including behavior suggesting hallucination.

Although there have been many methods used in evaluating withdrawal intensity, we have elected to follow the procedure similar to the "abstinence score" method initially established by Kolb and Himmelsbach[23] and Himmelsbach[24] for narcotic withdrawal in man. The application of this method has been refined and extended by Martin[25], Fraser[26], Jasinski[27], and many others.

Figure 3 shows a list of withdrawal signs and the grading system we have used for evaluation of withdrawal intensity. The evaluation was carried out at pre-set times, three times a day during the entire course of withdrawal. Since there have been no quantitative evaluations on relativity of the appearance and intensity of each sign during the withdrawal in the literature, use of one or a few signs, whether subjectively or objectively measured, cannot be assumed to give a true assessment of the actual degree of physical dependence until the influence of dose and treatment chronicity on the intensity and time-course of all withdrawal signs is quantitatively evaluated.

Table 3 shows an example of the intensity scoring system for graded signs that we have devised for evaluation of overall intensity of withdrawal. Each grade number assigned at peak intensity was multiplied by the corresponding percent of incidence and summed for all

BARBITURATE ABSTINENCE EVALUATION

I.	MOTOR	
	Ear & Facial Twitches	0,1,2,3
	Resting Tremors	
	Head	0,1,2,3
	Body & Limbs	0,1,2,3
	Intention Tremors	
	Forepaw	0,1,2,3
	Weakness	0,1,2,3
	Motor Functions	
	Muscle Tone	N = normal W = weak S&R = spastic & rigid
	Posture	N = normal standing posture HP = high posture; stands with limbs fully extended & arched back LP = low posture; stands with limbs partially flexed or extended CP = crouched posture; unable to stand SE = spread eagle posture; unable to stand; lies flat on chest with limbs fully extended & spread apart
	Motor Coordination	
	Quantitative	0 = stands, walks & lands; normal 1 = stands & walks; cannot land 2 = stands; cannot walk or land 3 = cannot stand, walk or land
	Movements	
	Qualitative	N = normal Ak = akinetic At = ataxic HS = high-stepping gait
	Patellar Tendon Reflex	N, ↑, or ↓
	Overall Motor Activity	N, ↑, or ↓
	Myoclonic Jerks	0,1,2,3
	Seizures	
	#Recorded	______
	Characteristic Type	C = clonic TC = tonic-clonic BC = brief clonic CC = continuous clonic
	Body Shakes (wet dog)	0,1.5,3
II.	AUTONOMIC	
	Piloerection	0,1,2,3
	Body Temperature	______ °C.
	Respiratory Pattern	N = normal P = panting
	Pupillary Dilatation	0 = normal 1.5 = dilated 3 = near maximally dilated
	Pupillary Light Reflex	0 = normal 1.5 = diminished 3 = absent
	Eating	0 = none 1 = little 2 = some 3 = well
III.	BEHAVIORAL	
	Gen'l Behavior	N = normal Ap = apprehensive Ag = aggressive P = passive OA = overly affectionate Bz = bizarre
	Startle Response	
	Auditory	0,1,2,3
	Tactile	0,1,2,3
	Drowsing	+ or 0
IV.	MISC.	
	Body Weight	______ Kg.
	Death	+ or 0

Graded Evaluations:

0 = normal
3 = maximal change

Figure 3. List of barbiturate abstinence signs evaluated at pre-set times during the withdrawal. Many signs were graded subjectively from 0 to 3; 3 denotes the greatest magnitude of change observed. Other signs, not readily quantifiable, were recorded as present or absent (+ or 0), or by an arrow indicating the direction of change (↑ or ↓). Posture, motor movements, and behavior were also noted and recorded in the protocol as one of several distinct categories that best characterized the condition of the animal at the time of observation. Continuous monitoring of each cat's motor activity was accomplished by using activity monitoring cages that have been shown to record the grand mal type convulsions quite clearly.

Table 3. "Total intensity scores" $\sum$ [intensity $\times$ (%) incidence] for each graded sign[a]

Abstinence Sign	Barbital	Pentobarbital Control	Ratio (B/P)
Motor			
Twitches	133.4	193.7	0.689
Resting tremors:			
Head	158.5	247.6	0.640
Body and limbs	133.3	208.2	0.640
Intention tremors	99.9	214.9	0.465
Motor incoordination	91.6	211.4	0.433
Myoclonic jerks	50.0	168.3	0.297
Autonomic			
Piloerection	133.3	212.9	0.626
Pupillary dilation	0.0	269.0	—
Diminished light reflex	0.0	147.0	—
Behavioral			
Increased startle responses:			
Auditory stimuli	75.1	98.4	0.763
Tactile stimuli	91.7	161.8	0.567
GRAND TOTAL	966.8	2133.2	0.453

[a] "Total intensity scores" calculated for each graded withdrawal sign for barbital (B) and pentobarbital (P). Each grade number assigned (see Figure 3) was multiplied by the corresponding percent incidence of total animals studied at the peak intensity and summed for all grades for each individual sign. These values are termed "total intensity scores" for graded signs. Ratios of "total intensity scores" of barbital to pentobarbital are also listed on the table.

grades for each individual sign. These values, called "total intensity scores" for graded signs, are found useful in quantitative comparison of withdrawal intensities produced by the different CNS depressants, for comparison of barbital and pentobarbital.

All the experimental observations of withdrawal made on animals treated with the "chronically equivalent" dose of barbital and pentobarbital supported the generally accepted notion that the long-acting barbiturate, barbital, is less liable to produce physical dependence than the short-acting barbiturate, pentobarbital.[cf.28] However, whether or not this difference in withdrawal intensities between barbital and pentobarbital truly reflected a difference in the degree of underlying physical dependence between these two drugs had to be further explored in order to rationally evaluate the physical dependence–producing capability.

The first general recognition of the importance of the drug elimination rate in the overt expression of withdrawal was made by Wulff.[28] In his major monograph on the barbiturate abstinence syndrome in humans, he established a correlation between the rate of barbiturate elimination from the blood and the appearance of withdrawal phenomena during the abstinence period in patients addicted to various barbiturates. No withdrawal signs were observed following chronic intoxication with barbital or pentobarbital. However, convulsions and delirium were very frequent after long-term exposure to the short-acting barbiturates. The importance of elimination kinetics on the study of physical dependence has been similarly commented on by Schuster and Johanson[29] LeBlanc[30], and also by others in this book. Therefore, the influence of barbiturate elimination kinetics upon the expression of withdrawal signs was explored by manipulating the rate of barbiturate elimination following chronic treatment with a long- and short-acting barbiturate.

To determine if the slow rate of barbital elimination would attenuate the severity of withdrawal for dependence developed to pentobarbital, the barbiturate elimination rate following chronic pentobarbital treatment was slowed by substituting barbital for pentobarbital at the end of the chronic treatment. Also, the pentobarbital elimination rate was directly reduced without a change in drug by readministering pentobarbital intravenously at hourly intervals according to a computer-based calculation of first order dose reduction to mimic barbital elimination kinetics.

Both procedures—barbital substitution and first order pentobarbital dose reduction—effectively reduced the rate of barbiturate elimination to mimic barbital control, which was confirmed by the blood kinetic study. The influence of the reduced rate of barbiturate elimination upon the expression of pentobarbital physical dependence in withdrawal signs is shown in Table 4. For all quantitative measures indicative of severity of abstinence—the average number of signs appeared per animal, the incidence and mean frequency of convulsions, the incidence of death and the "total intensity scores" for graded signs—the withdrawal was less intense than pentobarbital control when the elimination rate was slowed.

More convincing evidence for the key role of the elimination rate in the expression of withdrawal signs derives from experiments in which the barbiturate elimination rate was increased to mimic pentobarbital, following dependence production of barbital. An increase

Table 4. Effect of decreasing barbiturate elimination rate[a]

Procedure	t 1/2	*N*	Number of Signs per Animal	Incidence of Convulsions	Incidence of Death	"Total Intensity Scores" Grand Total	"Total Intensity Scores" Ratio (altered/control)
Pentobarbital Control	5.37 (±0.48 SE)	63	18.3 (±0.3 SE)	100.0% (15.4 ± 1.4 SE)	41.3%	2133.2	1
Barbital Substitution	24.5[b] (±2.3 SE)	8	8.3[b] (±1.1 SE)	25.0%[b] (0.75 ± 0.53 SE)	0%	687.7	0.322
First Order Dose Reduction	26.9[b] (±2.0 SE)	7	9.9[b] (±1.5 SE)	71.4%[b] (2.0 ± 0.6 SE)	0%	835.8	0.392

[a] Effects of decreasing pentobarbital elimination rate to that of barbital by barbital substitution or first order dose reduction on withdrawal intensity. t 1/2 indicates the blood elimination half-life measured. Number of signs per animal indicates average number of withdrawal signs out of 21 signs measured per animal tested. Numbers in the parentheses under convulsions indicate the average number of grand mal type convulsions (status-type convulsions are counted as one) recorded per animal studied. "Total Intensity Scores," see Table 3.

[b] Significantly different from pentobarbital control. ($p < 0.05$). SE = standard error.

in elimination rate was achieved by substituting pentobarbital for one "chronically equivalent" dose of barbital. Also, the barbital elimination rate was directly increased by peritoneal dialysis following the last dose of chronic treatment. The effectiveness of the peritoneal dialysis procedure in increasing the rate of barbital elimination was confirmed by careful blood barbiturate kinetic study.

The effect of increasing the rate of barbiturate elimination by these procedures on the intensity of barbital physical dependence, expressed in withdrawal signs, is shown in Table 5. The greater number of signs that appeared per animal, the greater incidence and frequency of convulsions, the greater incidence of death, and the greater "total intensity scores" for graded signs compared to barbital control indicate that "chronically equivalent" dose of barbital is indeed capable of inducing a severe state of physical dependence, which is only evidenced by eliminating the drug faster from the body.

These pharmacokinetic manipulations during barbiturate withdrawal demonstrate the key role of the elimination rate in determining the severity and time-course characteristics of withdrawal signs, once physical dependence has been developed. No longer can the severity of the withdrawal reaction be equated to the degree of underlying physical dependence. These two expressions—"withdrawal" and "physical dependence"—should be dissociated in their meaning and in their use. As is indicated by others in this book, in the absence of a specific antagonist to most rapidly displace the CNS depressants from their site of action, it may not be possible to fully disclose the degree of underlying physical dependence in a withdrawal reaction. Accordingly, the results of the study strongly urge the need to monitor the rate of drug elimination during withdrawal, as it is a major determinant of the overt expression of "physical dependence."

In the present study, the kinetic manipulations sought were to mimic the barbital elimination rate following chronic pentobarbital dosing, and to mimic the pentobarbital elimination rate following "chronically equivalent" barbital dosing. In this way, the influence of pharmacokinetic differences between barbital and pentobarbital were equated and the relative capability of these long- and short-acting barbiturates to induce physical dependence were able to be compared at a "chronically equivalent" CNS depression. Accordingly, the results of the study indicate that if barbital and pentobarbital do differ in their relative capability to induce physical dependence, these differences are indeed small in relation to the contribution of elimination kinetics to the expression of withdrawal signs. Furthermore, the

Table 5. Effect of increasing barbiturate elimination rate[a]

Procedure	t 1/2	*N*	Number of Signs per Animal	Incidence of Convulsions	Incidence of Death	"Total Intensity Scores" Grand Total	"Total Intensity Scores" Ratio (altered/control)
Barbital Control	28.6 (±3.1 SE)	12	11.5 (±0.6 SE)	8.3% (2.75 ± 2.75 SE)	0%	966.8	1
Pentobarbital Substitution	3.75[b] (±0.82 SE)	12	18.3[b] (±0.6 SE)	100.0%[b] (10.8 ± 2.2 SE)	8.3%	2337.7	2.42
Peritoneal Dialysis	7.93[b] (±0.73 SE)	5	18.8[b] (±1.0 SE)	80.0%[b] (10.2 ± 4.2 SE)	80.0%[b]	2040.0	2.11

[a] Effect of increase in barbital elimination to that of pentobarbital by "chronically equivalent" pentobarbital substitution or peritoneal dyalysis. See Table 4 for detail.

[b] Significantly different from barbital control. ($p < 0.05$). SE = standard error.

results indicate that the "CNS depression" may likely be the primary determinant of barbiturate dependence production. The implication of these findings is that the capability of all sedative-hypnotic drugs to produce physical dependence may indeed be inseparable from their CNS depressant property. If this is so, it then becomes important to design dosing regimens to minimize the risk of physical dependence production in humans. In this respect, the findings of Goldstein[19] on the production of alcohol dependence in mice might be very important. Goldstein found that the carry-over of physical dependence, as identified by withdrawal scores, increased as the interval between three-day bouts of exposure to an alcohol vapor chamber was reduced; when complete recovery from withdrawal was allowed between cycles, no cumulation of physical dependence occurred. The implication of her findings is that regimens that permit discontinuity of CNS depression between doses, i.e., widening the interval between doses or selecting hypnotics with short time-action and rapid elimination, may permit the safer use of these agents. Accordingly, Shelton and Hollister[31] and Colmore and Moore[32] were unable to produce physical dependence in man to a sedative, tybamate, which has an elimination half-life of about 4 hours.

In summary, I believe that only through a careful quantitative approach, based on basic pharmacological discipline in evaluation of physical dependence–producing capability of drugs, with the example demonstrated by barbiturates in this chapter, can we gain a rational understanding of physical dependence production. Furthermore, this kind of quantitative approach is essential if the physical dependence liability of a drug is to be accurately determined. Finally, the usefulness of the animal model system for the study of physical dependence production was illustrated.

LITERATURE CITED

1. Kalant, H., LeBlanc, A. E., and Gibbins, R. J. 1971. Tolerance to and dependence on, some non-opiate psychotropic drugs. Pharmacol. Rev. 23:135–191.
2. Essig, C. F., and Flanary, H. G. 1959. Convulsions in cats following withdrawal of barbital sodium. Exp. Neurol. 1:529–533.
3. Essig, C. F., and Flanary, H. G. 1961. Convulsive aspects of barbital sodium withdrawal in the cat. Exp. Neurol. 3:149–159.
4. Jaffe, J. H., and Sharpless, S. K. 1965. The rapid development of physical dependence on barbiturates. J. Pharmacol. Exp. Ther. 150:140–145.

5. Rosenberg, H., and Okamoto, M. 1974. A method for producing maximal pentobarbital dependence in cats: dependency characteristics. In: J. M. Singh (ed.), Drug Addiction: Experimental Pharmacology, Vol. 3, pp. 89–103. Miami Symposium Specialist, Miami.
6. Okamoto, M., Rosenberg, H. C., and Boisse, N. R. 1975. Tolerance characteristics produced during the maximally tolerable chronic pentobarbital dosing in the cat. J. Pharmacol. Exp. Ther. 192:555–569.
7. Seevers, M. H., and Tatum, A. L. 1931. Chronic experimental barbital poisoning. J. Pharmacol. Exp. Ther. 42:217–231.
8. Fraser, H. F., and Isbell, H. 1954. Abstinence syndrome in dogs after chronic barbiturate medication. J. Pharmacol. Exp. Ther. 112:261–267.
9. Yanagita, T., and Takahashi, S. 1970. Development of tolerance to and physical dependence on barbiturates in rhesus monkeys. J. Pharmacol. Exp. Ther. 172:163–169.
10. Yanagita, T., and Takahashi, S. 1973. Dependence liability of several sedative-hypnotic agents evaluated in monkeys. J. Pharmacol. Exp. Ther. 185:307–316.
11. Isbell, H., Altschul, S., Kornetsky, C. H., Eisenman, A. J., Flanary, H. G., and Fraser, H. F. 1950. Chronic barbiturate intoxication: an experimental study. Arch. Neurol. Psychiat. 64:1–28.
12. Fraser, H. F., Isbell, H., Eisenman, A. J., and Wikler, A. 1954: Chronic barbiturate intoxication, further studies. Arch. Intern. Med. 94:34–41.
13. Fraser, H. F., Wikler, A., Essig, C. F., and Isbell, H. 1958. Degree of physical dependence induced by secobarbital or pentobarbital. JAMA 166:126–129.
14. Essig, C. F., and Fraser, H. F. 1958. Electroencephalographic changes in man during use and withdrawal of barbiturates in moderate dosage. Electroencephalogr. Clin. Neurophysiol. 10:649–656.
15. Seevers, M. H., and Deneau, G. A. 1963. Physiological aspects of tolerance and physical dependence. In: F. G. Hofmann and W. S. Root (eds.), Physiological Pharmacology, Vol. 1, pp. 565–640.
16. Freund, G. 1971. Alcohol, barbiturate, and bromide withdrawal syndrome in mice. In: Recent Advances in Studies of Alcoholism, pp. 453–471. U.S. Government Printing Office, Washington.
17. Goldstein, D. B. 1972. Relationship of alcohol dose to intensity of withdrawal signs in mice. J. Pharmacol. Exp. Ther. 180:203–215.
18. Essig, C. F. 1972. Drug Withdrawal Convulsions in Animals. In: D. P. Purpura, J. K. Penry, D. B. Tower, D. M. Woodbury, and R. D. Walter (eds.), Experimental Models of Epilepsy, pp. 495–508. Raven Press, New York.
19. Goldstein, D. B. 1974. Rates of onset and decay of alcohol physical dependence in mice. J. Pharmacol. Exp. Ther. 190:377–383.
20. Bush, M. T., and Sanders, E. 1967. Metabolic fate of drugs: barbiturates and closely related compounds. Ann. Rev. Pharmacol. 7:57–76.
21. Conney, A. H. 1967. Pharmacological implications of microsomal enzyme induction. Pharmacol. Rev. 19:317–366.

22. Wikler, A. 1970. Diagnosis and treatment of drug dependence of the barbiturate type. In: P. H. Blockly and C. A. Thomas (eds.), Drug Abuse, Data and Debate. pp. 283–295. Charles C Thomas, Springfield.
23. Kolb, L., and Himmelsbach, C. K. 1938. Clinical studies of drug addiction. III. A critical review of the withdrawal treatments with method for evaluating abstinence syndromes. Amer. J. Psychiatr. 94:759–797.
24. Himmelsbach, C. K. 1939. Studies of certain addiction characteristics of (a) dihydromorphine ("paramorphan"), (b) dihydrodesoxymorphine-*d* ("despmorphine"), (c) dihydrodesoxycodeine-*d* ("desocodeine"), and (d) methyldihydromorphine ("Metopon"). J. Pharmacol. 67:239–249.
25. Martin, W. R. 1966. Assessment of the Dependence Producing Potentiality of Narcotic Analgesics, In: L. Lasagna and C. Radouco-Thomas (eds.), International Encyclopedia of Pharmacology and Therapeutics, Vol. 1. pp. 155–180. Pergamon Press, Glasgow.
26. Fraser, H. F. 1972. Criteria for Evaluating Physical Dependence and Overall Abuse Potential of Drugs in Man. In: H. Brill and S. J. Mule (eds.), Chemical and Biological Aspects of Drug Dependence, pp. 85–95. CRC Press, Cleveland.
27. Jasinski, D. R. 1973. Assessment of the dependence liability of opiates and sedative-hypnotics. Bayer-Symposium IV, Psychic Dependence, pp. 160–170. Springer-Verlag.
28. Wulff, M. H., 1959. The barbiturate withdrawal syndrome. A clinical and electroencephalographic study. Electroencephalogr. Clin. Neurophysiol. (suppl.) 14:1–173.
29. Schuster, C. R., and Johanson, C. E. 1974. The use of animal models for the study of drug abuse. In: R. J. Gibbins et al. (eds.), Research Advances in Alcohol and Drug Problems. Volume I, pp. 1–31. John Wiley and Sons, New York.
30. LeBlanc, A. E. 1975. Perspectives in Drug Abuse with Particular Reference to Sedative Hypnotics. In: F. Kagan, T. Harwood, K. Rickels, A. D. Rudzik, and H. Sorer (eds.), Hypnotics—Methods of Development and Evaluation, pp. 201–212. Spectrum Publications, Inc., New York.
31. Shelton, J., and Hollister, L. E. 1967. Simulated abuse of tybamate in man. Failure to demonstrate withdrawal reactions. JAMA 199:338–340.
32. Colmore, J. P., and Moore, J. D. 1967. Lack of dependence and withdrawal symptoms in healthy volunteers given high doses of tybamate. J. Clin. Pharmacol. J. New Drugs 7:319–323.

[illegible] drug [illegible]
[illegible] (eds.), [illegible]
[illegible]
[illegible]
[illegible]

Remarks

Peter Dews

The evil effects of gross drug abuse on an individual are so obvious to observers that to the first serious investigators it seemed self-evident that the taking of the drug must be exquisitely pleasurable to persuade and compel the addict to go on hurting himself. In the calculus of hedonism, the quantity of pleasure had to exceed by a substantial margin the quantity of pain. A new word was coined to described the pleasure, euphoria, and it was supposed that the prediction of addiction liability was essentially equivalent to prediction of euphorgenic power. As with most self-evident ideas, the mere matter of their being essentially no evidence in favor of it, and much against it, had little effect on its acceptance. Addicts did not talk much of exquisite pleasure, even when words were put in their mouths; mostly they talk of no more than a transient thrill. The types of effects caused by heroin, alcohol, amphetamines, and tobacco smoking are so grossly different that no one has ever identified a common factor in the effects of all the drugs, euphoria, that causes them all to be abused. The effects of tobacco smoking are ordinarily so subtle that a CNS effect is not detectable, yet smoking is as compulsive a habit as any.

The euphoria notion has been disposed of many times and few here today would subscribe explicitly to a simple euphoria theory of drug abuse. We know too much about the enormous role of external circumstances in determining whether an individual will take drugs or not, and if so, which drugs, for us to try to pin all the responsibility for abuse on an intrinsic euphoriant property of the drug. Nevertheless, it is my thesis in these few lines that the aftermath of the euphoria theory is still subtly influencing research in the field and, in particular, influencing the choice of methods to predict abuse liability. It is causing us to overlook other aspects of the pharmacology of the drugs that may be highly important in determining their abuse liability. I shall try to make the point that some otherwise trivial aspects of the pharmacology of a drug may be quite important in influencing its abuse liability.

Consider now a more contemporary question: Can abuse liability be predicted from studies on self-administration of drugs by animal subjects? Is prediction of abuse liability equivalent to prediction of reinforcing power? The answer here appears to be a hesitant "yes," at any rate in a qualitative sense. It is impossible not to be impressed by the fact that just those drugs that are conspicuously *not* abused in society—notably, chlorpromazine-like phenothiazines and nalorphine and related morphine antagonists—are the drugs that do not ordinarily maintain self-administration behavior. The ability of self-administration studies to distinguish clearly between morphine and chlorpromazine is all the more dramatic when it is remembered that in most studies that have been made on the behavioral pharmacology of morphine and chlorpromazine they have been found to be very much alike in most of their effects. True, they can be distinguished by certain analgesia tests, but these tests are ad hoc, and specifically contrived to make the distinction. On the quantitative side, self-administration is less clearly predictive of abuse liability: e.g., morphine and heroin maintain less vigorous self-administration responding than their reputation as drugs of abuse would lead one to expect. Some of the discrepancies can be accounted for in terms of other, direct, effects of the drug. In most studies of self-administration, the drugs are given repeatedly during the session, so that responding is influenced by the direct effect of the presence of the drug as well as by its reinforcing power. Morphine tends to suppress most types of responding with little regard to what is maintaining the responding. It is not surprising, therefore, that it seems to suppress responding maintained by administration of morphine itself. When the schedule of administration is changed to a second-order schedule, with the drug given only once at the end of the daily session, so that the responding maintained by the reinforcing efficacy is not subjected to the direct suppressing effects of the drug, the reinforcing effects of morphine appear much more impressive.[1]

But let us not be lulled into a false sense of security in our predictive tests. The list of drugs that have been abused is very long, and so is the list of drugs that are self-administered, while the list of drugs that are not abused and not self-administered is short. Such bias greatly weakens our ability to validate the predictors. Indeed, a little over 20 years ago it seemed that any drug with a significant, prompt impact on the CNS would be abused, from glue solvents to V2 rocket-fuel to chloroform to heroin to amphetamine. Chlorpromazine (CPZ) came along and spoiled that generalization, but it is important to remember that among powerful CNS drugs, CPZ-type drugs, nonreinforcers, are the exception. As I have suggested before, it may be more profitable to look for the specific property of CPZ that leads to CPZ *not* being abused than to seek in the effects of the generality of CNS drugs for a specific property that leads them to be abused. Also, food is abused and not only or even usually by the sensual gourmet who derives the greatest pleasure from eating; but rather by the indiscriminate, unappreciative eater who crams anything down regardless of quality. Also, fingernails are abused by being bitten and even skeletal muscles in tics. It appears that many things can reinforce and many things can be maintained by reinforcement; which is fine, of course, provided that we do not come to suppose that in demonstrating that an event is a reinforcer we have demonstrated something more than that the event is a reinforcer. Let me explain. Any worker studying behavioral phenomena knows that a reinforcer is defined and recognized through its effects on behavior; the sole criteria are behavioral. But any impartial observer of the same workers will see that teleology, like hope, springs eternal in even a scientific worker's breast. He will see that not merely reinforcers are discussed but positive and negative reinforcers. Further, positive reinforcers will be instanced by presentation of food to a food-deprived subject or water to a water-deprived subject. True, such presentations can usually be used effectively as reinforcers. Food to a food-deprived subject and water to a water-deprived subject also function as physiological restoratives; they are "good" for the subject in the sense of promoting survival of the individual and it makes sense, evolutionarily, that they should have become reinforcers. But it does not follow that food to a food-deprived subject and water to a water-deprived subject are reinforcing *because* they are physiologically restorative. The thousands of pages on need-relation hypotheses of reinforcement need no increment here. Fortunately, the question of whether a reinforcer must reduce a need is no longer subject to debate. It has been shown, confirmed, and reconfirmed many times that severe electric shocks can function as a "positive" reinforcer. In one of the original experiments,[2] a squirrel monkey pressed a lever some 700,000 times in a series of sessions over a period approaching a year; the only consequence of pressing the lever was occasional delivery of 12.6 ma shock to the tail. Some 1,900 total shocks were delivered. (Can a drug do better?) In no credible sense can a severe electric shock be considered to reduce a need.

The point about electric shock is not only that it cannot effect physiological restoration but also that it has no evolutionary history.

Species cannot have evolved their responses to electric shocks. Michael Faraday lived not much more than 100 years ago, and the systematic application of electric shocks to subjects is very much more recent, excepting perhaps shocks to human subjects in the electric chair, which can have had little evolutionary impact. We can appeal to neither physiological nor evolutionary reasons for electric shock functioning as a reinforcer. When the shocks are functioning as a reinforcer, the electric shocks are delivered promptly at a response, and the shocks certainly have saliency, but there are no other obvious properties of electric shocks to which may be attributed their power to reinforce.

Returning to the original discussion of the lingering effects of having once thought of abuse liability as being dependent on euphorigenic potential of drugs, is it not true that most workers on self-administration think of the drugs as reinforcing in the same manner as food and water reinforce: in a good, pleasurable way so far as the subject is concerned. They do not think of the drugs reinforcing after the manner of electric shocks. Yet surely drugs have much more in common with electric shocks than they do with food and water. Neither drugs nor shocks, in contrast to food and water, have any physiological restorative power, and both may be harmful. Drugs and shocks, as opposed to food and water, have no evolutionary history. In seeking to understand more about drugs as reinforcers surely we can learn more from shock-maintained responding than we can from the food and water-maintained responding, to which our latent teleology and the anamnesis of euphoria guide us.

What practical consequences does the reorientation have? It was suggested above that the only obvious properties that shock had that could make it a reinforcer were promptness (on the response) and saliency. Perhaps we should add brevity. If drugs as reinforcers are analogized to shocks as reinforcers, then we are lead to consider promptness and saliency of the drug effect as potentially important properties in determining reinforcing ability. Differences that are trivial for therapeutic purposes, such as differences in rate of passage through the blood-brain barrier, as between morphine and heroin, might occasion significant differences in abuse liability. Certainly, intravenous drug-taking would be expected to be more strongly maintained than oral or intramuscular injecting. If we accept brevity of electric shock as an attribute helping it function as a reinforcer, then the shortness of the salient effect of intravenous heroin, as described by the addict, may help rather than hinder the reinforcing power of the drug. Even the strength of tobacco smoking behavior becomes more understandable. The deep drag on a cigarette leads to immediate stimulation of the mucosa of the respiratory tract. In terms of immediacy, the effect of a cigarette makes the effect of even intravenous heroin relatively slow. In tobacco smoking, nicotine is also very rapidly absorbed and goes straight to the left side of the heart and is in the brain faster than morphine in opium smoking. The immediacy of the conditioned reinforcer (stimulation of the respiratory tract) and the promptness of the pharmacological effect of nicotine, are able to parlay the relatively slight pharmacological effect of nicotine in smoking tobacco into a powerful reinforcer. It follows from the importance of route of administration in determining time effects that in predicting abuse liability we must closely match experimentally the possible routes a drug may be taken by an abuser.

One last sobering thought. If time factors are as important in influencing reinforcing power as suggested, may we not be spending too much money and effort in, for example, choice studies in monkeys measuring effects that depend largely on the relative lipid solubility of a series of agents, a determination that certainly could be done more cheaply and quickly by other means.

LITERATURE CITED

1. Goldberg, S. R. 1975. Stimuli associated with drug injections as events that control behavior. Pharmacol. Rev. 27:325–340.
2. Kelleher, R. T., and Morse, W. H. 1968. Schedules using noxious stimuli. III. Responding maintained with response-produced electric shocks. J. Exp. Anal. Behav. 11:819–838.

Stimulant Abuse in Man

The Use of Animal Models to Assess and Predict Behavioral Toxicity

Everett Ellinwood
and
M. Marlyne Kilbey

The main purpose of this report is to outline the acute, chronic, and residual behavioral effects of stimulant (amphetamine-like compounds and cocaine) administration in rats, cats, monkeys, and man in order to identify possible detrimental effects in man from use of these drugs. We will be concerned not only with reviewing the evidence of behavioral toxicity, but also in assessing the reliability and predictiveness of measures used to determine behavioral toxicity. For the purposes of this text, the central questions are: 1) What are the physical and behavioral toxic effects of acute and chronic administration of stimulants in man? 2) After cessation of stimulant use, are there residual effects? 3) Do animal models using observational methods demonstrate similar acute, chronic, and residual changes? 4) Are observational behavioral toxicity measures in animals reliable?

Evidence obtained over the past few years relevant to the long-term consequence of chronic stimulant administration demonstrates an evolving and complex pattern of behavioral alteration. The relationship of the biological and/or behavioral alteration with chronic use to parameters of relevant environment, subject, and drug factors is

---

Research supported by NIDA Grant DA 00057.

largely unknown or based on anecdotal or unsystematic evaluation. It has been within this decade, in fact, that multiple and quantitative behavioral measures and rating scales have been developed allowing systematic investigation of the behavioral effects of stimulants. Much of the work on the effects of stimulants has been flawed by the use of a single data point describing the peak drug effect, thus overlooking all information relevant to the time course of the drug effect. Common behavioral paradigms have measured only a single dependent variable. Despite these limitations, we have attempted to summarize the following:

1) The drugs that have been shown to produce abnormal behaviors similar to those produced by amphetamine (taken as the prototypic drug) in four species and their characteristic effects.
2) Our conceptualization of: a) the acute peak effects, b) the effects seen with chronic administration, and c) the residual effects of prior, chronic use of psychomotor stimulants. For the rat and cat, the process outlined describes the results of several investigations completed in our laboratory. In primates the process of an evolving pathological state with sustained stimulant use has not been investigated as systematically. In man the evidence rests largely upon clinical appraisal, and is subject, therefore, to all the cautions that must be exercised in interpreting data that are often retrospective and subjective, and in which important variables may be unidentified.

ACUTE EFFECTS OF STIMULANTS IN MAN

The acute effects of stimulants in man are, of course, determined by multiple drug, subjective, and environmental factors. Two major drug factors are dose and route of administration. The major initial effect of a moderate oral dose of amphetamine is the induction of a sustained elevation of mood, or euphoria, most often associated with an energizing arousal. Intravenous use of high doses of amphetamine or cocaine produces an immediate ecstasy, the "flash," at times described as an orgiastic experience. However, as early as 1938 there was experimental evidence that euphoric reactions were not universal. Bahnsen and co-workers[1] reported that while 28 of 46 volunteer normal subjects reported pleasurable subjective effects of oral administration of amphetamine, 18 reported the opposite. Dysphoric reactions are reported to be more common in women than in men.[2] The contribution of these initial reactions to amphetamine abuse potential is currently unassessed.

While there are no systematic investigations of the effect of dose of amphetamine-like compounds or cocaine on mood in humans, adverse responses to initial use may occur. Low doses have been reported to exacerbate psychotic symptomatology in individuals with borderline personalities[3] and schizophrenia.[4] Acute toxic hallucinatory states also may occur with high doses.[5] Moreover, single large doses have been reported to induce psychosis.[6,7] However, it would appear important to carefully reevaluate these findings, focusing on the distinction between toxic hallucinatory state and psychosis and evaluating the presence of predisposing factors.

CHRONIC EFFECTS OF STIMULANTS IN MAN

Perhaps the best-known effect of chronic stimulant administration is psychosis. Psychosis has been associated with chronic use of several stimulants; e.g., *d*- and *l*-amphetamine, methylphenidate, phenmetrazine, and cocaine. As extensive descriptions have been made of amphetamine psychosis, this section will focus on these drugs. Clinical details of the cocaine psychosis have not been reported since the early 1900s,[8,9] and even though one would expect differences between the cocaine and amphetamine syndromes, secondary to the strong local anesthetic effect of cocaine, these have not been documented.

Amphetamine psychosis mimics paranoid schizophrenia, or paranoia, so closely that it has been misdiagnosed as such by knowledgeable clinicians many times. Usually the psychosis develops over time and is associated with the user's increasing amphetamine intake to over 150 mg/day; reaching, at times, 600 to 3,000 mg/day. Although there appear to be individual differences in sensitivity to development of the amphetamine psychosis,[10] when it develops there are characteristic symptoms: delusions of persecution, ideas of reference, visual, auditory, and olfactory hallucinations, changes in body image, hyperactivity, and excitation. Although the amphetamine syndrome presents many faces, including hypomanic-like reactions, usually there is no disorientation or clouding of memory, as occurs in toxic hallucinatory psychoses.

In our studies,[10,11] clinical descriptions of the effects of chronic amphetamine were derived from a standardized interview with patients. Clinical and psychological assessments were made to identify differences between those persons ($N = 10$) who clearly developed a psychosis, and those who clearly had not ($N = 8$). There were an additional seven individuals who displayed some symptoms of psychosis but could not be categorized. Behaviors that appeared in both those individuals who became psychotic and those who did not included bruxism and stereotyped touching and picking of the face and extremities. Feelings of an acute sense of novelty and a distorted time sense were reported also. Ninety percent of the patients who became psychotic, compared to 25% of those who did not, described the compulsion to disassemble, to analyze, to sort, and on rare occasions, to reassemble objects. These activities were accompanied by an intense and "pleasurable" sense of curiosity. Rylander,[12] Kramer, Fischman and Littlefield[13] as well as Smith (unpublished)[14] have reported similar observations.

Symptoms tending to increase progressively with the development of psychosis included fearfulness, suspiciousness, and a feeling of being watched. Mild suspiciousness was a prevailing symptom in all patients who became psychotic, and in 50% of the nonpsychotic group. However, as psychosis developed, increased suspiciousness became associated with heightened awareness and overreaction to stimuli, especially to slight movements in the peripheral visual field. Fellow amphetamine abusers were described as having a constant side-to-side looking behavior. The well-formed delusions of persecution, characteristic of later stages of amphetamine psychosis, often were described by abusers as more intense and concrete expressions of the earlier suspiciousness and feelings of being watched. Another symptom that appeared to increase as the patients became psychotic was the intensity of thought processes and the feelings associated with thoughts. "Revelations" and "eureka" experiences of a delusional nature were frequent.

Two symptoms noted primarily in the group who experienced psychosis were olfactory and tactile hallucinations. The latter often developed into delusions of parasitosis. The delusions of parasitosis were preceded by periods of repetitious stereotyped grooming behavior, primarily manifested as a picking and probing of the skin, leaving small punctate lesions. Similar delusions of parasitosis and dermatological excoriations are seen in cocaine psychosis.

Finally, as the psychosis progressed many individuals described intense fear and terror. It is these feelings of fear and terror that cause many persons suffering amphetamine psychosis to seek treatment, and when seen in the emergency room these individuals are often extremely reactive to extraneous stimuli.

In addition to the effects just outlined, several authors[10,13,15,16] have described various dyskinetic and dystonic reactions. Tatetsu, Goto, and Fijiwara[17] described cases of frozen, bizarre, catatonic-like postures, and Kramer[18] described an aphasic, paralyzed condition, "overamping," which may last for hours or days following high i.v. doses. Abusers describe this as a state of "suspended animation" in which they are aware of people and the environment around them. Their mind is racing. Yet, their own movement is not part of their consciousness and they remain immobile.

Amphetamine addicts report a variety of tics, especially facial tics, dyskinesias of the mouth and tongue not unlike tardive dyskinesias, as well as choreiform movements.[19] While these effects are thought to result from chronic administration of high doses, the dose and duration of use in addicts is uncertain, at best. However, Mattson and Calverley[20] reported various kinds of dyskinesias after therapeutic doses of amphetamine, a finding indicating that there are individuals with an idosyncratic supersensitivity to these amphetamine effects. These motor disorders do not show a relationship to the development of amphetamine psychosis because they develop both in individuals who become psychotic as well as in those who do not (63% of the nonpsychotic versus 70% of the psychotic individuals developed bruxism and repetitious mouthing movements).[10]

RESIDUAL EFFECTS OF STIMULANTS IN MAN

The possibility of residual effects from chronic amphetamine intoxication in man remains one of the most important questions concerning stimulant use. The absence of systematic data on this point, however, requires that one marshal clinical observations in order to provide an initial assessment of the question. In humans, amphetamine abuse may at times precipitate brain damage in the form of cerebral-vascular accidents.[21-24]

Frequently, post-amphetamine users describe an apathetic "spaced out" condition characterized by a rather emotionally colorless life with little or no desire.[19,25] At times they may lose their train of thought and in some there appears to be a deficit in emotional memory. Documentary evidence of these clinical impressions is lacking (most I.Q. scores are in the normal range, but Rylander[16] reports that 14 of 50 advanced addicts demonstrated impairment on memory tests).

When delusions are established during chronic amphetamine intoxication,[26,27] or with cocaine,[28] they may persist tenaciously during abstinence for periods of over a year. Evidence of possible residual psychological effects is noted in Minnesota Multiphasic Personality

Inventory profiles of former chronic amphetamine abusers that differ significantly from those of former narcotic addicts, especially on the Schizophrenia and Psychasthenia Scales.[10]

When considering chronic residual effects of amphetamine intoxication, one must always be aware that studies of amphetamine psychosis include individuals who, to greater or lesser degrees, manifested schizophrenic and/or schizoid characteristics prior to drug use, and that, in part, residual effects may reflect changes in the processes underlying these. There are some indications, in fact, that these individuals may be prone to stimulant use.[10] However, many individuals with persistent belief in their amphetamine-induced delusional experiences are otherwise clear of psychotic manifestations.[26] This finding suggests that a persistence of delusional thinking may not be solely a matter of predisposing personality factors, but may, in part, represent a residue from the amphetamine-induced psychosis.

In our clinical experience, once an individual has developed an amphetamine psychosis, it is readily reinitiated, even following a long period of abstinence, by moderately high doses of stimulants. Similar observations have been made by Kramer.[27] Utena[29,30] has emphasized an increased potential for psychotic reactions due to physical and psychological stress as well as subsequent exposure to amphetamine. Analogous findings are noted in animal studies, as will be discussed. The reemergence of an amphetamine psychosis is illustrated by Bell[31] who documented the response of an abstinent amphetamine abuser given 120 mg i.v. in an interview setting: "Oh not this again. I'm starting to get the wrong idea about people again. I feel that they are all against me. All the questions in my mind—going through my mind. This is it all over again." This episode presaged a short-lived psychosis of two days that included auditory hallucinations and frankly paranoid delusions. In the early stage of reintoxication, the patient apparently recognized the precipitation of the previously manifested delusional ideas; although later more overtly psychotic behavior developed. Finally, it should be mentioned that various facial tics and mouthing movements are also noted to increase under psychological stress in the abstinent amphetamine abuser.

The drugs that have been reported to induce symptoms of psychosis or to exacerbate psychotic symptoms in humans in experimental settings are presented in Table 1. Our conceptualization of the major manifestations of the process that evolves with sustained stimulant abuse is shown in Table 2.

ANIMAL STUDIES

In assessing behavioral testing of acute and chronic stimulant intoxication we have been concerned with: 1) identifying the phenomenologically similar behaviors of man and other animals that develop with chronic intoxication; 2) establishing the detailed set of behaviors associated with full expression of the chronic stimulant-induced syndrome; 3) evaluation of the inter- and intra-rater reliability of the behavioral observations; and 4) assessment of quantifiable measures or sets of dependent variables that change as a function of dose as well as with chronic administration of a constant dose.

We have chosen to review three experimental species, each of which provides a special emphasis on some aspect of behavioral testing. The rhesus monkey permits sensitive identification of phenomena that are analogous to clinical syndromes.[32] In the cat the relatively complete expression of the chronic stimulant syndrome can be documented with reasonably quantifiable measures, using the BRIDGE scale.[33] These measures appear sensitive to the general progression of changes seen in chronic stimulant administration, including motor disorders. The rat is, of course, the experimental animal "par excellence" for establishing quantifiable measures that can be evaluated in large samples, and, as will be discussed, our scale[34] provides a good dose-response measure for the amphetamine-induced syndrome as well as certain chronic-induced changes.

ACUTE EFFECTS OF STIMULANTS IN MONKEYS

Although detailed observations of the effects of stimulants in monkeys have been made, neither we nor other researchers have established the reliability of the systems used to make these observations, nor determined whether or not these systems are sensitive to dose effects. Multiple, but spaced, injections have been a common paradigm in investigating stimulant effects in this species. Ellinwood[35] and Randrup and Munkvad[36] reported staring, eye-hand examining behaviors, and side-to-side head movements with doses from 1.0 to 2.6 mg/kg i.m. Cocaine (10 mg/kg i.p.) produced hyperactivity.[37]

CHRONIC EFFECTS OF STIMULANTS IN MONKEYS

Chronic administration of methamphetamine increasing from 1 to 20 mg/kg over a 4–6 month period resulted in several progressive

Table 1. Drugs inducing or increasing stereotypy or symptoms of psychosis in man in experimental setting

Drug	Dose	Treatment Duration	Behavior	Post-Treatment Retest Interval	Behavior	Investigator
Amphetamine	55–640 mg i.v.	Single Injection	Paranoid Psychosis with Auditory and/or Visual Hallucinations but no Thought Disorder	3 Days to 6 Months after Last Self-Prescribed Dose No Psychosis in Two Nonabusers Given 10 and 50 mg/kg Respectively		Bell, 1973
d and *l* Amphetamine	*d*: $\overline{X} = 418$ *l*: $\overline{X} = 510$ mg	Cumulative Oral Dose at 50 mg/hr	Psychosis in 3/3 Patients whose Drug History is not Described			Angrist, Shopsin, Gershon, 1971
Methylphenidate	0.5 mg/kg i.v.	Single injection	Increase in Pathology in Schizophrenic Patients; No Psychosis in Non-schizophrenic Patients			Janowsky, Huly, and Storms, In press
L-Dopa	3–6 g Daily	11–29 Days	Increased Conceptual Disorganization, Emotional Withdrawal, and Agitation; 1/6 Depressed Alcoholic Patients Developed Paranoid Psychosis			Angrist, Sathananthan, Shopsin, and Gershon, In press

ET-495	205 mg Daily	6–18 Days	4/7 Schizophrenic Patients Show Deterioration; 1 Developed Choreo-athetotic Syndrome 1/3 Nonschizophrenic Patients Developed Psychosis	Angrist, Sathananthan, Shopsin, and Gershon, In press
d- and *l*-Amphetamine; Methylphenidate	*d*: 4, 10, and 20 mg *l*: 4 mg *m*: 29 mg i.v.	1 Injection Each Dose and Drug Interval Not Specified	Intensification of Preexisting Symptoms of Schizophrenia in 17 Schizophrenic Patients Methylphenidate *d*-Amphetamine *l*-Amphetamine	Janowsky and Davis, 1974
Fenfluramine	20–240 mg	Multiple Injections 7 Days	Hallucinatory States in 3 *Ss* Characterized by Visual and Olfactory Hallucinations, Rapid and Polar Mood Changes and Paranoia	Griffith, In press

Table 2. Characteristic acute, chronic, and residual effects of high-dose stimulant administration suggested by clinical reports in man and long-term investigations in monkeys

Man	Monkey
EARLY CHRONIC EFFECTS	ACUTE PEAK EFFECTS
—Exploratory, repetitious behaviors or perceptuomotor compulsions —Visual scanning, Side-to-side —Beginning states of suspiciousness	—Stereotyped: eye-hand examination; Visual scanning, tracking, checking —Investigatory attitude
PROGRESSIVE EFFECTS	PROGRESSIVE EFFECTS
—Paranoid schizophrenic-like psychosis with delusional experiences; Auditory, visual, tactile and olfactory hallucinations —Delusions of parasitosis prominent with dermatological excoriation —Reactive behavior —Oral dyskinesias and bruxism; facial tics —Choreiform movements —Frozen, immobile, "catatonic-like" behavior (overamping)	—More constricted bizarre stereotyped components —Dyskinesias, especially oral —Dystonic movements —Reactive attitude —Excoriating self-grooming behavior —Failure to maintain normal social, sexual, and maternal behavior
RESIDUAL EFFECTS	RESIDUAL EFFECTS
—Moderate dose threshold for induction of psychosis dyskinesias —Persistent delusions	—1–2 doses reinitiate chronic end stage behavior

changes.[35] By far the most common cluster of stereotypies involved the motor and postural components of perceptuo-motor activity. Among the most frequent stereotypies developing were the "examining stereotypies," consisting of picking and probing objects in the cage, or picking and probing of the self in a grooming-like manner, patterns of looking and checking and/or visual avoidance, and oral or biting stereotypies. A number of monkeys groomed themselves to the point of inducing chronic excoriated lesions. Over the months the parts of the stereotyped behaviors became disassociated and then components would be repeated in a stereotyped fashion. Gradually the movements took on an athetoid quality. Mouthing and chewing movements and mouth examination patterns evolved into oral dyskinesias. Various dystonic neck movements appeared to evolve from side-to-side looking or avoidance movements. Prolonged writhing and, at times, opisthotonic movements appeared. Repetitious myoclonic movements of the neck and shoulders were often noted along with fine tremors of the head and upper extremities. Even the biting-examining stereotypies took on a sudden impulsive myoclonic quality; for example, the biting would consist of a sustained clonic grip on the cage wire.[35]

Schiørring[15] and Utena[29] have reported disrupted social behaviors that encompass withdrawal and failure to maintain normal maternal and sexual behaviors in chronically treated animals. Post[37] has demonstrated an evolution of behavior following cocaine administration in doses increasing from 10–17 mg/kg i.p. Behavior was characterized by a transition during the first six weeks from hyperactivity, gnawing, and stereotyped behaviors involving the trunk, limbs, and/or head to a withdrawal and cataleptic-like behavior during the six- to twenty-week period.

RESIDUAL EFFECTS OF STIMULANTS IN MONKEYS

Unfortunately, most investigations of stimulant effects in monkeys have not focused on the possible residual effects, so these have rarely been assessed. Utena[29] described reaction of behaviors that had originally evolved over a four- to six-month period of intoxication. In his experience, one or two days of amphetamine, or even saline, administration is sufficient to reintroduce the chronic symptoms. Finally, the drugs that produce abnormal behaviors in monkeys are demonstrated in Table 3, and our conceptualization of the evolving behavioral process in stimulant intoxication is shown in Table 2.

ACUTE EFFECTS OF STIMULANTS IN CATS

Drugs that have been demonstrated to produce abnormal behavior in cats are presented in Table 4. Table 5 is our conceptualization of the evolution of behaviors found with chronic stimulant intoxication. While the effects of chronic administration of amphetamine are well documented in this species, there appears to be no study of acute effects as a function of dose in the cat. Most studies have used multiple injections, usually spaced at weekly or greater intervals. Using this paradigm, Wallach and Gershon[38] demonstrated increasing stereotypy in cats at doses ranging from 0.75 to 2.0 mg/kg for *d*-amphetamine; 1.0 to 4.0 mg/kg for *l*-amphetamine; and 1.0 to 4.0 mg/kg for cocaine. Stereotyped behavior in this study was described as either continuous head turning or continuous sniffing. However, the

Table 3. Drugs inducing abnormal behaviors in monkeys

Drug	Dose	Treatment Duration	Behavior	Post-Treatment Retest Interval	Behavior	Investigator
Amphetamine	1.7 mg/kg and 2.6 mg/kg i.m.	2 Injections Separated by 4 Months	Individual Stereotypy Patterns Involving Opening and Closing Hands, Continuous Side-to-Side Movements, and Staring			Randrup and Munkvad, 1967
Amphetamine	.05 mg/kg to .37 mg/kg s.c.	Multiple Injections	Reduced Social Interaction in Pairs of Monkeys; Stereotyped Self-Grooming Seen at .15 mg/kg			Kjellberg and Randrup, 1973
Apomorphine	1 mg/kg s.c.	Multiple Injections at 7-day, or more, Intervals	Licking, Biting, Repetitive Movements of the Hands, Head and Body			Shintomi and Yamamura, 1975
Cocaine	10–17 mg/kg, i.p. daily or 2/Day for 5 Day/Week	20 Weeks	Hyperactivity, and Limb, Trunk, and Head Stereotypies and Gnawing During 0–6 Week period; Cataleptic-like Behavior During Latter Period			Post, In press
Methadone Administration and Subsequent Methamphetamine	1 to 3 mg/kg Methadone Daily for 10 to 22 Months			2 to 17 Months Later Injected 2–7.5 mg/kg Methamphetamine 4 Days Week/up to 12 Weeks	Oral Dyskinesia Developed Earlier in Former Methadone Ss than Control Ss	Eibergen and Carlson, 1975
Methamphetamine	1 Increasing to 20 mg/kg per day	4–6 MON. (4 Days/Week)	Eye-Hand Probing and Examining Movements; Bucco-Lingual Dyskinesias, Dystonias, Grooming Stereotypies	*Several Months	*Reinstitution of Final Stereotypy Pattern	Ellinwood, 1971 *Ellinwood observation
Methamphetamine		3–6 Months	Stereotypies and Residual Symptoms	4–6 Months	Exaggeration of Residual Symptoms; Reinstitution of Chronic Symptoms	Utena, 1974

basis for determination of the change in behavior and the statistical evaluation of altered response stereotypies was not presented. We have demonstrated[39] stimulant-induced motor alterations in cats with initial treatment of 15 mg/kg of methamphetamine. These consisted of stereotyped movements of the head, motor dysjunction, and an investigatory attitude often characterized by sniffing and minutia search patterns involving head movements.

CHRONIC EFFECTS OF STIMULANTS IN CATS

The system of behavioral observations we have used to characterize the effects of chronic escalating doses of methamphetamine in cats is the BRIDGE scale; that is, the Duke University Behavioral Rating Inventory for Drug-Generated Effects.[33,40] The presence of various classes of behavior with multiple subtypes is scored for 10-second epochs from video tapes, and the frequency of occurrence over 18 samples of 10 seconds each is calculated. The behavioral rating chart and definitions for behaviors scored are included in the appendix of this chapter. Whereas most studies of amphetamine intoxication have focused on hyperactivity and stereotypy, we have attempted to develop a comprehensive phenomenological characterization of disorders that may be of clinical significance and may provide information relevant to the pathology associated with chronic abuse of stimulants. For example, attitude is critically important in clinical descriptions of amphetamine psychosis and our operational definitions attempt to define the attentional mode and involvement of the animal as manifested by his postural appearance and motor activity in relation to his surroundings. Similarly, measurement of ataxia, dystonia, and dysjunctive movement and posture reflects our concern for clinically relevant motor disorders. Obviously, a scale as complex as the BRIDGE scale cannot be utilized in routine assessment or by untrained personnel. In our studies, cat behavior was rated by a clinician who was familiar with neurological and psychiatric disorders in humans and who had participated in developing the rating system. The intra-rater reliability of this observer was quite good, as noted in Table 6 both with immediate rerating and rerating approximately 3 months later. Table 7 presents the items rated in this reliability sample. All experimental behavioral samples are recorded on TV tape with 10-second timing markers. The rater reliability is assessed from blind samples presented randomly to the rater. Communicating this scale to personnel who were not trained clinicians was relatively dif-

Table 4. Drugs inducing abnormal behaviors in cats

Drug	Dose	Treatment Duration	Behavior	Post-Treatment Retest Interval	Behavior	Investigator
Amphetamine	13 mg/kg i.p.	Single Injection	Stereotyped Head Movements, Hissing and Spitting			Randrup and Munkvad, 1967
Cocaine	4–10 mg/kg i.p.	Multiple Drugs at 1-Week Intervals	Stereotyped Head and Eye Movements at 4 mg/kg; Preconvulsive Clonic State After 10 mg/kg			Wallach and Gershon, 1971
Cocaine	10 mg/kg i.m.	Daily 465 Days	Evolution From Stereotyped Sniffing to Stalking, Searching Behavior to Extremely Reactive, Hyperstartle Behavior, Leaping Behavior; Dyskinesias and Dystonias			Ellinwood and Kilbey, Unpublished data
Cocaine	5 mg/kg i.v.	12 Injections with Various CA agonist and antiagonists/1 per week	Stereotyped Ataxic, Head Movements which Became More Constricted over Weeks, Bizarre Dystonic Limbs and Body Postures			Castellani et al., Unpublished data
L-Dopa	50–100 mg/kg i.p.	Multiple Injections of Multiple Drugs	Stereotyped Head Movements			Wallach and Gershon, 1971
Methamphetamine	15 Increasing to 35 mg/kg in 2 i.p. Injections Daily	Daily for 5 Days; 2 Days Off; Daily for 4 Days	Increasing Stereotypy over Days 1–3; Increasingly Severe Disjunction Behaviors over Remaining Days; Hyperactive	6 and 12 Months	Reinstitution of Behavior Characteristic of Chronic Intoxication with Single Moderate Dose	Ellinwood and Escalante, 1970

Methylphenidate	40 mg/kg i.p.	Multiple Drugs at Weekly Intervals	Stereotyped Sniffing and Head Movements	Wallach and Gershon, 1972
Pemoline mg (OH)	50–100 mg/kg i.p.	Multiple Drugs at Weekly Intervals	Stereotyped Sniffing and Head Movements	Wallach and Gershon, 1972
Phenmetrazine	2–25 mg/kg i.p.	Multiple Drugs at 2-Week Intervals	Weak to Pronounced, Stereotyped Head Movement	Wallach, Rotrosen, and Gershon, 1973
-Proplyl- -Leucyl- Glycinamidl (PLG)	.1 to 50 mg/kg i.p.	Injection Schedule not Specified	Side-to-Side Movement, Sniffing, Licking; More Intense with Higher Doses	North, Harik, and Snyder, 1973
LSD	95 μg/kg i.p.	Multiple Drugs, 1 Injection each, at 10-Day Intervals	Repetitious Pronounced Visual Tracking Head Movement, Rigid Postures	Winters et al., 1969
Mescaline	30 mg/kg i.p.	Multiple Drugs, 1 Injection Each, at 10-Day Intervals	Repetitious Pronounced Visual Tracking Head Movements, Rigid Posture	Winters, et al., 1969
Phencycidine	4 mg/kg i.p.	Multiple Drugs, 1 Injection Each, at 10-Day Intervals	Repetitious Pronounced Visual Tracking Head Movements	Winters et al., 1969

Table 5. Characteristic acute, chronic, and residual effects of stimulant administration as determined by long-term investigations in cats and rats

CAT	RAT
ACUTE PEAK EFFECTS	ACUTE PEAK EFFECTS
—Stereotyped perceptuomotor movements of head —Investigatory attitude —Dysjunctive movements —Postural fixation	—Restricted locomotion and exploration —Stereotyped sniffing licking, gnawing
PROGRESSIVE EFFECTS	PROGRESSIVE EFFECTS
—Reactive attitude with hyperstartle —Akathisia —Pivoting movements —Camel back posture —Ataxia	—Increased restrictiveness or intensity of stereotypy with same dose of stimulant or apomorphine —Dyskinetic movements —Backward walking and jumping —More reactive
RESIDUAL EFFECTS	RESIDUAL EFFECTS
—Conditioned behavior to injection and/or setting —Moderate dose of stimulants produce endstage behavior	—Persistent augmented response to same stimulant dose or apomorphine

Table 6. Percent agreement for several comparisons of selected categories in the modified BRIDGE rating system

	Intra-Rater		Inter-Rater		
Category	Proximal (N1:NN1)[a] 648[b]	Blind (B1:N1)[a] 180[b]	Student 1: Consensus (N2:Consensus)[a] 216[b]	Student 2: Consensus (N3:Consensus)[a] 216[b]	Student 1: Student 2 (N2:N3)[a] 216[b]
Attitude	94.6	86.1	63.0	53.2	65.3
Arousal	98.9	98.9	83.8	100.0	91.7
Movement Speed	92.7	89.4	40.7	48.6	83.8
Head Movement	95.8	99.2	83.1	63.0	69.2
Head Stereotypy[c]					
Presence	98.8	96.7	89.8	83.8	89.6
Type	98.8	96.7	89.1	83.8	85.2
Sniffing Involvement	94.6	98.9	82.9	84.7	90.7
Dystonia	99.8	98.9	89.4	63.0	56.9
Disjunction	93.5	87.8	60.7	54.6	60.7
Ataxia	97.4	99.4	63.0	70.4	92.6

From Sudilovsky et al., 1975.[33]

[a] Mnemonic.

[b] Number of intervals.

[c] Derived from head movement category. Presence: agreement on the presence of head stereotypy, regardless of type. Type: Agreement on both the presence and type of head stereotypy.

Table 7. Precis of behaviors included in the selected representative subset of categories from the original rating system

Attitude	Arousal	Sniffing Involvement
Asleep (A)	Asleep (1)	Discrete (D)
Indifferent (I)	Somnolent (2)	Throughout (T)[a]
Interested, Normal (INN)	Normal (3)	*Head Pattern Modality*
Interested, Abnormal (INA)	Aroused (4)	Sniffing (Sn)
Interested, Focused (INF)[a]	Hyperaroused (5)	Looking (L)
Investigative, Normal (IVN)	*Movement Speed*	*Dystonia and Disjunction*
Investigative, Abnormal (IVA)	No Movement (1)	Postural (P) None (N)
Reactive,	Slow (2)	Motor (M)[a]
Reactive, Focused (RF)[a]	Normal (3)	Ataxia
Unaware (U)	Fast (4)	Level 1 (1) None (N)
Head Movement	Sudden, Reactive (5)	Level 2 (2)
(Unstereotyped)	(Stereotyped)	(Incorporated into Stereotypy)
Tremor (Tm)[a]	Minutia Search (M)	Look (l)[a]
Stagger (St)[a]	Balinese (B)	Pause (p)[a]
Shake (Sh)[a]	Up-and-Down (U)	Dip (d)[a]
Recoil (R)[a]	Side-to-Side (Si)	Recoil (r)[a]
Look (L)[a]		
Transient (T)		

From Sudilovsky et al., 1975.[33]

[a] Items consolidated with other behaviors or dropped from the system.

ficult, even when several aspects of the behavior were redefined to require less discrimination. Inter-rater reliability for technicians with this simplified scale is shown in Table 6. However, the levels of reliability are sufficient to assess several major aspects of stimulant-induced behavior in the cat. Furthermore, reliability was demonstrated to increase with experience, especially if the number of behaviors rated was reduced. A discussion of these and other points can be found in Sudilovsky et al.[33]

Using the BRIDGE scale we have demonstrated that over a period of increasing daily doses head movement stereotypies initially increase and become constricted but then decline in frequency. Akathesia develops, as does pivoting and various paw-shaking reactive movements. Dystonias also are noted to increase over the period of chronic intoxication.[39,40] Several aspects of these relationships are demonstrated in Table 8. Figure 1 demonstrates the change in

Table 8. Some amphetamine-induced motor alterations[a]

Motor alteration	C[b] N = 876	Day 1 n = 1260				Day 3 N = 1169				Days 6 and 7	Day 8 N = 504				Day 11 N = 960				Day 12 N = 270		Day 25 N = 108	
		Pre	00	10–30	90	Pre	00	10–30	90		Pre	00	10–30	90	Pre	00	10–30	90	Pre	00	Pre	00
Hyperkinesia																						
head stereotyped mvts.																						
Minutia-search pattern	0.3	0.5	7.6	22.3	33.8	0.0	0.0	16.0	13.7	No Drug ADMINISTRATION	0.9	15.8	49.5	55.6	3.3	10.5	31.8	43.7	11.2	32.5	0.0	13.0
up-and-down pattern	0.0	0.0	0.0	23.3	18.7	0.0	7.2	12.1	7.1		0.0	6.5	31.7	50.0	8.9	9.3	19.5	6.9	7.4	13.9	0.0	0.0
side-to-side pattern	0.0	0.0	0.0	36.7	21.2	9.6	11.6	20.2	9.6		0.7	16.6	43.5	0.0	0.0	0.0	4.1	7.6	0.0	0.0	1.9	1.9
balinese pattern	0.0	0.0	0.0	0.0	9.1	0.0	0.0	7.4	0.0		0.0	0.0	0.0	0.0	0.0	0.0	0.0	0.0	0.0	0.0	0.0	0.0
other	0.0	0.0	0.0	8.3	9.1	0.0	0.0	0.0	0.0		0.0	0.0	0.0	0.0	0.0	0.0	0.0	0.0	0.0	0.0	0.0	0.0
pivoting mvts.	0.1	0.0	0.0	0.0	7.6	0.0	0.6	9.9	11.2		0.9	0.0	19.2	22.3	0.6	0.0	19.1	18.1	0.0	0.0	0.0	3.7
paw-shaking mvts	0.0	0.0	0.0	0.0	0.0	0.0	0.0	0.2	0.0		0.0	0.0	0.0	0.0	0.6	0.6	1.5	4.2	0.0	0.0	0.0	0.0
akathisia	0.0	0.0	0.0	0.0	0.0	0.0	0.0	25.1	25.9		0.0	0.0	23.6	0.0	23.5	20.4	43.4	50.2	4.9	33.3	0.0	0.0
Dyatonia																						
camel-back phenomenon	10.0	8.3	13.6	55.5	54.5	11.1	39.4	67.0	70.6		5.9	60.2	66.6	97.2	54.7	77.2	82.2	97.2	54.9	84.3	33.3	100.0
hunching-back mvts.	0.0	0.0	0.0	2.6	38.9	0.0	0.0	12.9	8.6		0.0	0.0	25.9	30.6	4.5	0.0	4.6	9.0	0.0	0.0	0.0	0.0
leg extensor posturing	0.1	0.0	3.0	2.8	0.0	0.0	1.1	1.1	1.0		0.9	0.0	0.0		1.2	0.0	0.4	2.1	0.0	2.8	0.0	0.0
Motor disjunction	0.0	0.0	0.0	16.0	45.5	0.0	4.4	27.8	24.9		3.7	4.6	41.7	36.1	12.8	14.8	1.7	12.5	0.0	27.8	0.0	0.0
Ataxia	0.0	0.0	0.0	2.8	18.2	0.0	0.0	30.8	60.4		0.0	14.8	40.3	75.0	30.2	35.2	71.3	87.5	33.3	50.0	0.0	0.0

From Sudilovsky et al., 1974.[39]

[a] Entries in the table represent the rate of occurrence of the indicated items as a percentage of all intervals included under the given condition.

[b] Saline injection

C (Control) = all conditions on day 0; pre = preinjection condition, 00 = immediate post-injection condition; 10–30 = all intervals in the 10-, 20-, 30-minute post-injection conditions; 90 = the 90-minute post-injection conditions.

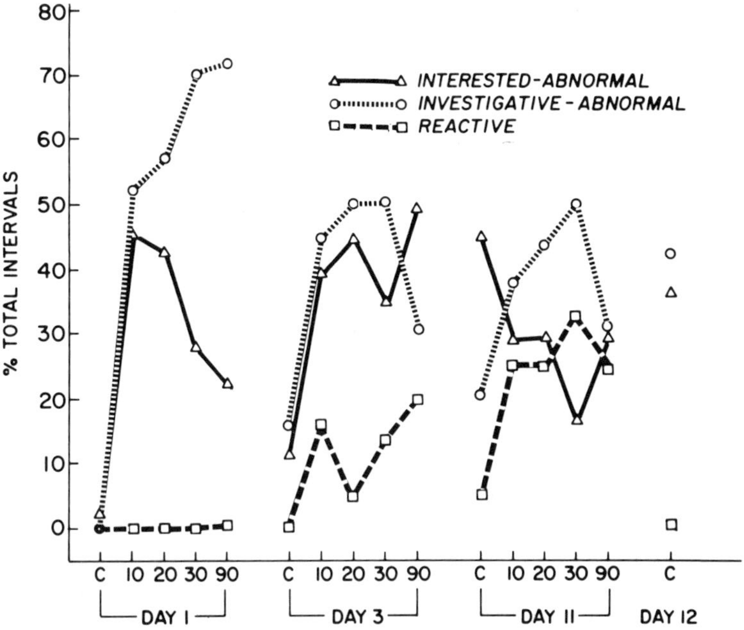

Figure 1. Mean occurrence of abnormal attitudes across days. *Ordinate:* percent of intervals in which attitude was observed. *Abscissa:* observation periods. (C = preinjection, 10 = 10 min post-injection, 20 = 20 min post-injection, etc.) From Ellinwood et al., 1972.[40]

attitudes noted over days. Investigatory attitude was pronounced on the initial day, and a reactive attitude was found increasingly toward the end of the intoxication period. Reactive attitudes refers to a jittery apprehensive attitude associated with hyperstartle responses—many times to stimuli that are not appreciated by the investigator.

Detailed behavioral inventories like the BRIDGE inventory allow for specific documentation of the correlated physiological changes. The cat, of course, is an ideal animal for electrophysiological measurement, and in our studies we have recorded subcortical electrophysiological signals on analog tape for correlation with the recorded behavior. This has provided a preliminary demonstration that hyperstartle reactive behaviors are frequently preceded by high voltage spindles and/or discharges in the mesolimbic system, including the amygdala olfactory tubercle and accumbens.[41]

We have yet to systematically analyze behavior with chronic cocaine administration, but it appears that dystonic postures are more intense and stereotypies are comprised mainly of focused looking patterns that are even more constricted than those seen with amphetamine administration. In a pilot animal that was given cocaine for over a year (10 mg/kg daily), extreme forms of hyperstartle reactivity, which appear to be correlated with mesolimbic spindle activity, and discharges have evolved to a degree never seen with the amphetamine intoxication paradigms. It should be pointed out, however, that we know of no observational study in which amphetamine was administered for a comparable period. Because the hyperstartle response may reflect processes similar to the hyperreactivity noted in chronic stimulant abusers, we have focused on it in our current investigations.

RESIDUAL EFFECTS OF STIMULANTS IN CATS

In cats, two major indexes of residual effects have been found. Conditioned behavior is manifested by behavioral and autonomic responses characteristically associated with drug. These are noted when the cats are given saline injections or placed in the experimental situation following cessation of daily drug administration.[42,43] In addition, acute readministration of stimulants at moderate doses elicits behavior characteristic of the animal's response during former chronic high-dose treatment, suggesting a lowered threshold for elicitation of the abnormal end stage behaviors. The mechanism underlying this effect may underlie similar observations noted in man and monkey.

ACUTE EFFECTS OF STIMULANTS IN RATS

The acute administration of *d*- and *l*-amphetamine and cocaine in rats results in a dose-dependent behavior pattern that can be described as a continuum from hyperactivity through restricted stereotypy. Table 9 is a rating scale developed in our laboratory. The inter-rater reliability of the system is excellent. At five and ten minutes post-drug, when behavior is changing rapidly, the correlation coefficients were 0.54 and 0.70 respectively, but at all other times they were 0.93 or above. Using the scale we have shown statistically significant dose response curves of *d*- and *l*-amphetamine (Figure 2) and cocaine. With initial administration of cocaine of 15 and 40 mg/kg the dose function is expressed primarily as a prolonged duration of effect with 40 mg/kg, rather than as a significantly more intense response. Thus, the assess-

Table 9. Rating scale for the behavioral effects of psychomotor stimulants in rats[a]

Score		Definition
1	Asleep	Lying down, eyes closed
2	Inactive	Lying down, eyes open
3	Inplace activities (grooming, consummatory)	Normal grooming, chewing cage Litter, eating or drinking
4	Normal, alert, active	Moving about cage, sniffing, rearing
5	Hyperactive	Running movement characterized by rapid changes in position (jerky)
6	Slow patterned	Repetitive exploration of the cage at normal levels of activity
7	Fast patterned	Repetitive exploration of the cage with hyperactivity
8	Restricted	Remaining in same place in cage with fast repetitive head and/or foreleg movement (includes licking, chewing, and gnawing stereotypies)
9	Dyskinetic-Reactive	Backing up, jumping, seizures, abnormally maintained postures, dyskinetic movements

From Ellinwood and Balster, 1974.[34]

[a] Score represents activity which predominates in 20-min interval, except for 8, which is scored only when observed for entire 20-min interval.

ment of stimulant-induced abnormal behaviors in rats is reliable, and the measure reflects dose differences in a reasonably linear manner.[34]

CHRONIC EFFECTS OF STIMULANTS IN RATS

The chronic effects of stimulant administration in rats appear to be somewhat different for *d*-amphetamine and cocaine. During chronic administration of *d*-amphetamine (11–14 days) no augmentation of the maximum stereotyped response is seen, either with a constant dose regime or one in which escalating doses are used, although the temporal characteristics are altered, a finding most consistently seen as a more rapid onset of maximum stereotyped behavior.

During chronic administration of cocaine, both the maximum stereotyped response and speed of onset are enhanced. These data show that chronic administration of amphetamine results in an altered temporal response pattern that suggests modification of pharmacokinetic process, while chronic administration of cocaine results in temporal and intensity alterations that suggest modification of both

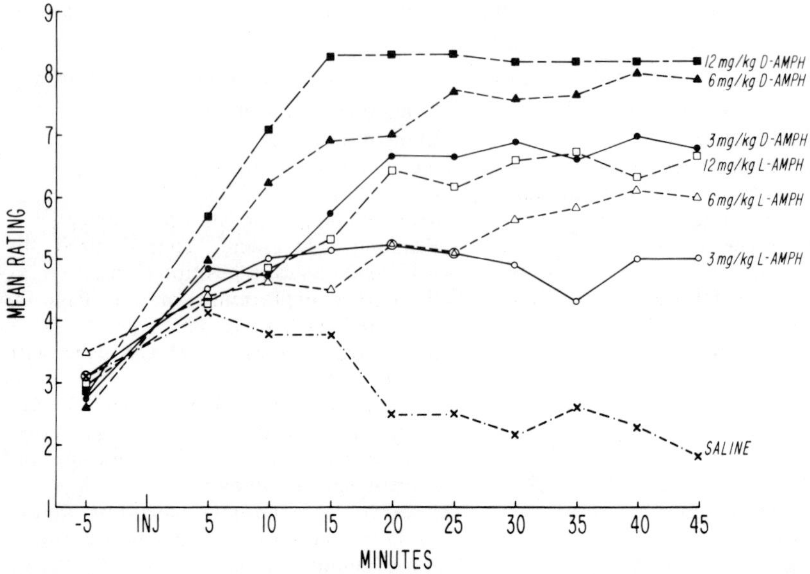

Figure 2. Behavior ratings after saline, *d*- or *l*-amphetamine. Each *data line* represents the mean of six animals except saline, where $N = 12$. From Ellinwood and Balster, 1974.[34]

pharmacokinetic and receptor functions. Possible mechanisms underlying this will be discussed after a description of the residual effects in rats of stimulant administration.

RESIDUAL EFFECTS OF STIMULANTS IN RATS

Following cessation of two weeks of daily administration of amphetamine and cocaine, readministration of drug at post-treatment periods of from 5 to 54 days elicits both augmented stereotyped behavior and a more rapid onset.[44] This augmentation is demonstrated for two doses of cocaine in Figure 3. Similar augmentation of maximum stereotyped behavior by apomorphine has been noted following cocaine treatment, indicating that the altered response reflects modified dopamine (DA) receptor function (Kilbey and Ellinwood, unpublished data). Additional evidence for the importance of DA receptor function in residual effects comes from work that has shown augmented response to apomorphine in guinea pigs up to ten days following cessation of chronic amphetamine treatment.[45]

Table 10 shows the drugs that have been reported to induce abnormal behavior in rats. In Table 5 we have outlined the behavioral sequence that evolves in rats with sustained stimulant administration.

In summary, in rats abnormal behaviors elicited by acute administration of psychomotor stimulants are a positive function of the dose, and range from hyperactivity to restricted stereotypy. Dyskinetic-reactive behaviors, with the possible exception of seizures, are not produced reliably by acute administration of psychomotor stimulants in the rat. Acute stimulant-induced abnormal behaviors are antagonized in a dose-dependent manner by agents that block DA receptor function,[34,46,47] indicating the importance of this neurotransmitter system for expression of these behaviors. During chronic administration of cocaine response, augmentation is observed. Likewise, during chronic administration of amphetamine and cocaine significantly faster onset of abnormal behaviors is seen. For both stimulants, accelerated onset and augmented responding are found

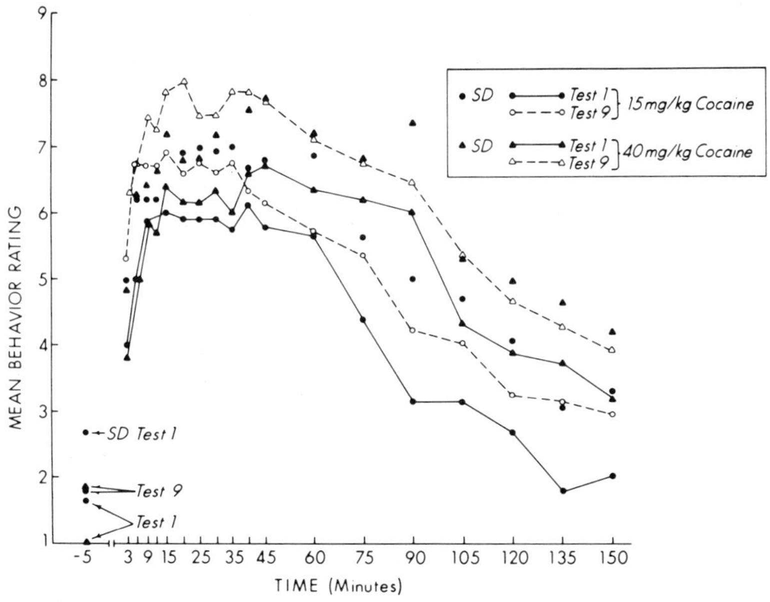

Figure 3. Mean standard deviation of behavior rating for two groups of rats ($N = 14$, $N = 11$) administered cocaine. Test one follows the initial administration and test nine is 54 days following the cessation of 14 daily administrations. From Kilbey and Ellinwood.[44]

Table 10. Drugs inducing abnormal behaviors in rats

Drug	Dose	Treatment Duration	Behavior	Post-Treatment Retest Interval	Behavior	Investigator
d-Amphetamine	3–12 mg/kg i.p.	3 Injections/72 hr. Intervals i.p.	Stereotyped Exploration to Inplace Stereotypy			Ellinwood and Balster, 1974
l-Amphetamine	3–12 mg/kg i.p.	3 Injections/72 hr. Intervals i.p.	Hyperactivity to Stereotyped Exploration			Ellinwood and Balster, 1974
d-Amphetamine	7 mg/kg	14 Daily Injections i.p.	Decreased Latency of Inplace Stereotypy at Day 14	5 Days	Inplace Stereotypy Maintaining Decreased Latency of Onset	Kilbey and Ellinwood, Unpublished data
d-Amphetamine	0.5 to 7.5 mg/kg	36 Daily Injec- i.p.	Progressive Augmentation of Activity in 0.5 mg/kg Group, Decreased Latency of Stereotypy Measured by Absence of Locomotion and Prolongation of Activity in Higher Dose Groups	7 Days	Potentiation of Activity with 1.0 mg/kg	Segal and Mandell, 1974
Apomorphine (−)*N*-*N*-Propyl-norapomorphine	0.125 to 4.0 S.C. 0.006 to 0.2 S.C.	2 Injections (Interval Unspecified)	Periodic to Continuous Gnawing or Licking			Costall, Naylir Neumeyer, 1975
(+)*N*-*N*-Propyl-norapomorphine	0.01 to 1.0 S.C.	Same for all	Same for all			
p-Chloroamphetamine	5–20 mg/kg	Single Injection S.C.	Weak Rearing, Moderate Locomotion at all Doses, Stereotyped Sniffing at 20 mg/kg only	7 to 54 Days	Maintenance of Decreased onset Latency and Augmented Stereotypy	Scheel-Kruger, 1972
Cocaine	15–40 mg/kg	14 Daily Injections i.p.	Decreased Onset Latency by Day 7, Augmentation of Maximum Stereotypy	7 to 54 Days	Maintenance of Decreased Onset Latency and Augmented Stereotypy	Kilbey and Ellinwood, In press
L-Dopa	1200 mg/kg S.C.	Single Injection	Sniffing, Licking, Biting			
(−)-Ephedrine	40 to 140 mg/kg i.p.	Single Injection	Periodic to Continuous Sniffing, Licking, and Biting			Langwinski, 1970
Fencamfamine	50 mg/kg S.C.	Single Injection	Continuous Biting, Sniffing, and Licking			Fog, 1969

LSD-25	10 mg/kg S.C.	Single Injection	Continuous Biting, and Sniffing	Fog, 1969
Methamphetamine	10 mg/kg S.C.	Single Injection	Continuous Sniffing, Biting, and Licking	Fog, 1969
Methylphenidate	100 mg/kg S.C.	Single Injection	Continuous Sniffing, Biting, and Licking	Fog, 1969
α-Methyltryptamine	10–80 mg/kg S.C.	Single Injection	40 mg/kg Produced Constant, Inplace Sniffing	Randrup, Munkvad, and Usden, 1963
Phentermine	50 mg/kg S.C.	Not Stated	Licking and Biting	Scheel-Kruger et al., In press
Morphine	50 mg/kg S.C. 100 mg/kg S.C.	2 × Day, 2 Days 2 × Day, 3 Weeks	Stereotyped Biting Beginning on Day 3, Constant Biting, Licking, Gnawing after 7 Days	Fog, 1970
Nialimide + 5-HTP	100 mg/kg 24 hr prior to 100 mg/kg S.C. 5-HTP	Single Injection Each Drug	Continuous Sniffing, Licking, or Biting	Randrup and Munivad, 1966
Nialimide + Tryptamine	100 mg/kg S.C. 24 hr prior to 350 mg/kg Tryptamine S.C.	Single Injection Each Drug	Continuous Sniffing, Biting, and Licking	Randrup and Munkvad, 1966
Nomifensine	30 mg/kg S.C.	Not Stated	Sniffing and Licking	Scheel-Kruger et al., In press
Pemoline	200 mg/kg S.C.	Single Injection	Constant Sniffing, Biting, and Licking	Fog, 1969
Phenmetrazine	50 mg/kg S.C.	Single Injection	Constant Sniffing, Biting, and Licking	Fog, 1969
B-Phenylethylamine	60 mg/kg i.v.	Single Injection	Continuous Sniffing, Licking, or Biting	Randrup and Munkvad, 1966
Pipradrol	100 mg/kg S.C.	Single Injection	Constant Sniffing, Licking, Biting	Fog, 1969
Piribedil (EI-495)	12.5 to 100 mg/kg i.p.	Single Injection	Continuous Sniffing, Periodic Biting or Chewing for 12.5 mg/kg	Costall & Naylor, 1973

STUDY_____ SUBJECT_____ DAY_____ CONDITION_____ DATES _____ recorded _____ rated

INTERVAL	1	2	3	4	5	6	7	8	9	10	11	12	13	14	15	16	17	18
ORIENTATION																		
ATTITUDE																		
AROUSAL																		
MOVEMENT SPEED																		
HEAD POSITION																		
HEAD MOVEMENT																		
LOOKING CHARACTER																		
LOOKING LOCATION																		
SNIFFING INVOLVEMENT																		
BODY POSITION																		
BODY MOVEMENT																		
FORELEG POSITION																		
FORELEG MOVEMENT																		
HINDLEG POSITION																		
HINDLEG MOVEMENT																		
TAIL POST / TAIL MVT																		
GROOMING CHARACTER																		
GROOMING LOCATION																		
ST MODAL / ST RELAT																		
DYSTONIA																		
DISJUNCTION																		
ATAXIA																		
AUTONOMIC RESP																		
MISCELLANEA																		

Figure 4. Rating form used to encode one 3-minute segment of behavior.

during post-treatment intervals, and appear to represent an alteration of DA receptor function because similar response alterations are seen when apomorphine is administered.

We have noted that the reliable demonstration of dyskinetic-reactive behavior in the rat is difficult to achieve, with the possible exception of seizures. Downs and Eddy[48] and Post[37] have shown that daily administration of an originally subconvulsive dose of cocaine eventually induces convulsions. Stripling and Ellinwood[49] have shown a sensitizing effect of a subconvulsive dose of cocaine in that daily treatment with this dose lowered the convulsive threshold compared to that in animals who had not been given the subconvulsive dose.

DISCUSSION

A review of the clinical and experimental behavioral toxicity observations following chronic stimulant intoxication impresses one with two major categories of behavior: 1) the development of the amphetamine psychosis in humans and the behavioral abnormalities in experimental animals, and 2) the development of motor disorders in humans, as well as in experimental animals. These behavioral categories have important implications for stimulant abuse liability, as well as for our understanding of the underlying mechanisms of psychosis and movement disorders. The data reviewed also indicate that components of these abnormal behavioral categories are manifested as residual effects of chronic stimulant intoxication, primarily in an increased sensitivity to their induction.

In research applications the amphetamine psychosis has served to generate two major positions: 1) amphetamine-induced abnormal behavior in man and animals serves as a heuristic model of the psychotic process,[10,36,50-57] and 2) investigations of the biochemical actions of amphetamine's catecholamine-releasing and block of reuptake properties[55-57] have further suggested the "CA hypothesis of psychosis," i.e., the notion that dysfunction in the NE and DA systems underlies, at least in part, the ontogeny of psychosis. Furthermore, human investigations have shown that amphetamine, L-dopa, methylphenidate, and other agents that increase DA availability exacerbate schizophrenic symptoms in borderline and schizophrenic individuals.[3,4,58,59] At the very least, these studies indicate that schizophrenia and amphetamine-induced psychosis share a common dopaminergic final pathway for the expression of a variety of abnormal behaviors. Mechanisms underlying the sensitivity of schizophrenics and persons who previously abused amphetamine to induction of stimulant psychosis may be further elucidated by investigations using animal models, since "analogous" processes appear to take place following chronic amphetamine intoxication in experimental animals.

A possible stimulant abuse liability in man that has been neglected is the development of motor dyskinesias and dystonias.[10,13,15,16] The experimental evidence reviewed in this paper shows that dystonia and dyskinesias develop in cats and monkeys administered stimulants.[35,39,40] In experimental animals the mechanisms underlying the dyskinesias have not been differentiated from those underlying stereotyped behavioral patterns.[45] Observations of the evolution of dyskinesias suggest that they may be remnants of the original stereotyped motor patterns. In our observations of monkeys developing oral dyskinesias,[35] we initially noted—even on Day 1—dainty, repetitious chewing and mouthing movements. Originally these appear to be an increased frequency of normal chewing and chatter movements. These movements also appeared as a part of hand-mouth examination pattern over weeks and months of chronic intoxication. During this period the muscle movements became increasingly pronounced and consisted of open-mouth rotation and excursions of the jaw with protrusion of the tongue. The tongue would frequently rotate and turn to one side. The jaw movements increasingly became gyrating, lateral displacements. The tongue and jaw movements were similar to the oral dyskinesias noted in humans. Similarly, eye-hand examination patterns not infrequently would deteriorate over time. Originally, the stereotype would involve handling of objects; later, there was no object involvement in the stereotypy and the hand movements appeared to be remnants of the original well-coordinated stereotyped pattern. The fingering movements were not unlike parakinesias noted in some schizophrenics. Biting-oral examination stereotypies deteriorated in the final months into dystonic biting of the cage wire. Thus, in summary, behavioral data seems to indicate that severe dyskinesias may evolve from what was originally a component of the stereotyped pattern. The concern with the evolution of dyskinesias with stimulants takes on an additional relevance when one considers that many stimulant abusers also abuse narcotics. Recently, Eibergen and Carlson[60] have demonstrated that chronic methadone maintenance pretreatment in monkeys can potentiate a dyskinetic response to stimulants for as long as 17 months. The mechanism underlying this effect may in part represent a supersensitivity induced by previous narcotic blockade of dopamine receptors.[60-63]

We have reviewed the data demonstrating that following long-term stimulant intoxication subsequent doses of stimulants frequently induce a qualitatively different behavior than that originally noted. These end stage behaviors included constricted stereotypies, hyper-reactive behaviors, postural abnormalities, and dyskinesias, and have been noted in monkeys, cats, rats, and guinea pigs.[35,45,64] Even with short periods of chronic stimulant intoxication (10 to 14 days), one finds there is an augmentation of stimulant-induced locomotor activity[65] and stereotypy[44,49] to the same unit dose as well as increased sensitivity to apomorphine[45] (Kilbey and Ellinwood, unpublished data). In addition to the behavioral findings, cocaine also induces an augmentation of electrical activity in the amygdala and a lowered behavioral seizure threshold that persists following cessation of chronic cocaine treatment,[49] possibly indicating a neurophysiological reorganization.[66,67] The importance of the augmented behavioral response may relate not only to the induction of movement disorders that are found in chronic amphetamine addicts,[10,68] but also to the lowered threshold for psychotic disorders in abstinent amphetamine addicts reported to follow only moderately high doses of amphetamine.[18,27] A receptor supersensitivity in the DA neuronal systems is one explanation that may partially account for these phenomena.[67] Chronic localized and/or generalized residual CA depletion may set the stage for the supersensitive response. In cats undergoing chronic amphetamine intoxication we have previously demonstrated[69,70] a neutonal chromatolysis in areas with marked neuronal CA depletion. Gunne and Lewander[71] originally reported that administration of amphetamine for six days reduced brain NE to 75% and DA to 50% of control levels in rats. More recently, Seiden, Fischman, and Schuster[72] have demonstrated that there is a striking depletion of DA in the caudate nucleus (70% reduction) and a marked depletion of NE in the mid-brain and frontal cortex that persisted for three to six months after cessation of chronic methamphetamine administration in monkeys. Thus, there is evidence suggesting either persistent CA depletion or neuronal death. This could establish, at least in animals chronically intoxicated with high doses of stimulants, the setting for a functional deficit and/or a post-synaptic super-sensitivity.

In summary, the development of motor disorders and psychosis, the persistence of delusional ideation, and the sensitivity to reactivation of psychosis following moderately high doses may comprise a series of abuse liabilities with chronic use of stimulant compounds. Existing experimental animal evidence indicates there are evolving chronic effects and residual effects, and warrants, in our opinion, continued investigation using behavioral observational methods. While in no case are current rating schemes completely satisfactory, methods of rating cat and rat behavior offer sensitive indexes of sensitization to drug effects, residual effects, and development of motor disorders. With continued refinement, observational methods for evaluating abuse liability should take their place as a major technique, and, in addition, should provide an experimental paradigm in which the contribution of physiological, psychological, and experimental factors in the development of abnormal behavior can be identified and assessed.

Appendix

THE INVENTORY

In the following Catalogue of Definitions for the BRIDGE system, all categories have been grouped in three main areas of interest (Animal-Environment Relationship, Motor Profile, and Autonomic and Reflex Responses), and Miscellanea, which comprise the less frequently observed behaviors.

I. Animal-Environment Relationship
  A. Physical relationship
    1. Place (2)*

Refers to the actual location of the animal within the cage, as determined by the relation of his trunk to several theoretically separate zones of the floor of the cage; may be designated as *Front* (*F*), *Back* (*B*), *Right* (*R*), or *Left* (*L*) half of the cage. When appropriate, the more specific designation of *Front-right* (*Fr*), *Back-right* (*Br*), *Front-left* (*Fl*), or *Back-left* (*Bl*) should be used. If the animal occupies two diagonally opposite quadrants or the boundary zone between two halves, the ratings are *Diagonal* (*D*) or *Midline* (*M*) location, respectively. Ratings reflect the order of occurrence of location and are made on the basis of time spent by the animal at specific cage locations. If possible, two entries should be made indicating the two

* To convert the ratings to computer-readable format, it was necessary to limit the number of behaviors coded in each category for each 10-second interval. The number in parentheses indicates the entries allowed.

locations that account for the largest part of the 10-second interval. If the animal uses the major part of the 10-second interval for translative movements, so that no specific location is occupied, the appropriate score is *Changing* (*Ch*).

2. Orientation (2)

Describes the orientation of the animal's body within the cage, as determined by the direction of his longitudinal axis (represented by the spine); may be rated as *Front* (*F*), *Back* (*B*), *Right* (*R*), *Left* (*L*), or as *Front-right* (*Fr*), *Front-left* (*Fl*), *Back-right* (*Br*), and *Back-left* (*Bl*). Alternatively, if the animal is moving, the corresponding score will be *Changing* (*Ch*). Rating of this category follows the rules indicated for the previous one (*Place*) with respect to number and order of entries.

B. Psychomotor relationship

1. Arousal (1)

Refers to the degree of readiness or alertness of the animal, as indicated by his static and kinetic configurations and the conjunction of several features contributing to these. Such features are useful in defining the five levels of arousal described below, but should be regarded merely as indicators for the recognition of each rateable level. Arousal, as we consider it, conceptualizes the intensity of the relationship between the animal and his environment. Thus, knowledge of his habitual behavior in the experimental setting is necessary to discriminate the various possible states. *Level 1* represents the sleeping state, generally characterized by closed eyes, dropped head, muscular relaxation, and relative unresponsiveness. *Level 2* corresponds to a somnolent state usually manifested by slow, progressive, and nonsustained closing of the eyes, decreased muscle tone (head nodding), slow postural readjustments, and decreased sensorial availability (receptivity and responsiveness) to environmental stimuli. *Level 3* indicates the syntonic state (baseline behavior of a normal awake animal) characterized by adequate but selective sensorimotor availability to environmental stimuli in the absence of muscular tension greater than the minimum necessary to maintain posture. *Level 4* is equivalent to the aroused state, characterized by increased muscular tension indicative of readiness to move, moderate apprehension or curiosity toward the environment, and restricted distractibility. *Level 5* represents the hyperaroused state, usually manifested by marked apprehensiveness, hypersensitivity to external stimuli, and exaggerated muscular tension with disproportionate reactions and/or restlessness.

2. Attitude (1)

Defined by the attentional mode and involvement of the animal, as manifested by his postural appearance and motor activity in relation to his surroundings and his own body (environment). Whereas posture represents the end point of a movement or action, attitude reflects the quality of the animal-environment relationship. Classifications are *Asleep* (*A*): Self-explanatory; *Indifferent* (*I*): Lack of manifest attentional involvement with the environment; *Interested* (*IN*): Directed attentional contact with the environment or a part of it as selected stimulus, but without definite physical approach; *Investigative* (*IV*): Selected attentional contact and active reaching out or approaching and examining of one or more parts of the environment. In the *IN* attitude, the animal may single out aspects of the environment, but in the *IV* attitude an active interaction with those aspects is achieved through a selected response; *Reactive* (*R*): An abnormal attitude characterized by shifting attentional contact manifested in increased peering about the environment, frequent postural readjustments, and sudden inadequate or apparently unmotivated movements with a tense and jumpy quality; *Unaware* (*U*): An abnormal attitude in which detachment from the environment is detected through a lack of sensorial availability (analogous to that seen in stuporous states).

The *IN* and *IV* attitudes may present a nervous, tense, or apprehensive quality after administration of a psychostimulant drug in relatively large doses. In that case, they are termed *Interested Abnormal* (*INA*) or *Investigative Abnormal* (*IVA*), respectively. On occasion, a given attentional mode (directed, selected, or shifting) can persist even as the animal changes his posture or level of activity. In that case, a focused quality is indicated by scoring either *Interested Focused* (*INF*), *Investigative Focused* (*IVF*), or *Reactive Focused* (*RF*).

3. Looking Activity (2 for each aspect)

Two aspects are rated. The first is the character of the animal's looking activity. *Vacant* (*V*): Eyes open, with no specific or appreciable visual placing. *Casual* (*C*): Transient glancing or visual placing on the environment in general. *Observant* (*O*): Attentive visual contact and/or looking movements in relation to one or a few specific aspects of the environment. *Staring* (*S*): Intense and/or relatively sustained observant looking activity. *Frozen staring* (*F*): Persistent staring with no head movement or during a "pure" stereotypy of the head (see II.A.3., *Head Movements*).

The second aspect is the location of the animal's gaze. *Close* (*CL*): Localized in the immediate surroundings, that is, within the space limited by the cage walls. *Image* (*I*): Visual placing on the animal's own reflection on any of the cage walls: *Ceiling* (*C*): Visual placing on or through the roof of the cage. *Distant* (*D*): Visual placing on either the immediate or distant area outside the Plexiglas sides of the cage.

If the animal's eyes are closed, the corresponding score for both aspects of this category is *None* (*N*).

4. Sniffing Activity (1)

Discrete (*D*) or *Throughout* (*T*), depending on its duration within the 10-second interval.

5. Grooming Activity (2 for each aspect)

Two aspects are rated. The character of any grooming is indicated as *Paw-wiping* (*P*), *Licking* (*L*), *Biting* (*B*), or *Scratching* (*S*). An *Abortive* (*A*) character is scored if one of the motor components of a grooming pattern occurs without consummation of the grooming activity. This phenomenon frequently appears as a tonic leg posturing, with the leg either flexed or extended and occasionally showing sudden phasic flexor or extensor movements.

The bodily location of the grooming is designated as *Face* (*F*), *Ear* (*E*), *Back* (*B*), *Chest* (*Ch*), *Abdomen* (*A*), *Groin* (*G*), *Foreleg* (*Fo*), *Hindleg* (*H*), or *Tail* (*T*).

II. Motor Profile

A. Motor output

1. Movement Speed (1)

A five-point scale is used to evaluate speed of movement. *Level 1* is complete immobility, that is, no movement in any region of the body. *Level 2* is a state of slow mobility, as in a drowsy, relaxed, or stuporous condition. *Level 3* is the usual moving speed of an awake and normally aroused animal. *Level 4* is a state of fast mobility, but with maintenance of the flowing harmony of the movements. *Level 5* is a state of nonharmonic, fast mobility in which reactive movements are predominant. Thus, levels 2, 3, and 4 represent the range of movement speed under normal conditions with levels 2 and 4 being extremes of that range.

Familiarity with the animal's range of movement speed in the experimental setting will facilitate accuracy. Occasionally, in order to decide on the score for a given 10-second interval, it may be helpful to observe the ongoing movements for a longer period.

2. Head Position (2)

Head position is determined by the angle formed by the intersection of the cervico-occipital region of the head with the spine. *Upright* (*U*): Whenever the angle so formed is less than 180°. *Lowered* (*L*): Whenever the angle so formed is equal to or larger than 180°. If either *U* or *L* is accompanied by definite neck extension, the corresponding scores will be *Upright-extended* (*Ue*) and *Lowered-extended* (*Le*). In any case, if the head is turned relative to the animal's body, this is specified by scoring, in addition, either *Facing-side* (*S*) or *Facing-back* (*B*), depending on the extent of the turn. *Dropped* (*D*): A position in which the head is not completely supported by the neck. *Changing* (*Ch*): Scored if no clear position is adopted.

3. Head Movements (2)

Transient (*T*): Transitory movements without sequential relationship to those preceding or following. It may be a single displacement (horizontal or vertical) or a composed one (bobbing, dipping, casual scanning, etc.). *Tremor* (*Tm*): Small rhythmic oscillatory movement. *Stagger* (*Sg*): Coarse and nonrhythmic movements of the head-neck ensemble suggestive of lack of stability. If this movement appears in more than a few consecutive 10-second intervals, it can be taken as indicative of ataxia. *Shake* (*Sh*): Sudden and more or less violent consecutive movements. *Recoil* (*R*): Sudden retreating movement usually associated with unexpected stimuli and occasionally incorporated into a stereotypy pattern (see below). *Look* (*L*): A head movement clearly directed for visual placing on a specific object or in a specific direction.

Stereotyped (*S*): Any movement repeated sequentially and describing a path of displacements recognizable as a kinetic configuration is rated as stereotyped by placing an *S* before the symbol. The most frequently observed stereotypy configurations have been given specific names. These are *Minutia-search* (*M*): Pecking-like movements executed by rotation of the head around the interauricular axis; *Side-to-side* (*Si*): Horizontal head-neck movement around the base of the neck or rotational movement of the head around the occipito-atlantoid articulation; *Balinese* (*B*): Circumduction head-neck movement around the base of the neck by which the tip of the animal's nose describes a more or less irregular ovoid or circular path.

The stereotypy may be "pure" or, if contaminated by other nonsequential movements, "impure." Thus, scoring of two codes is indicative of interrupted ("impure") stereotypy. The stereotypy configurations may also, in the course of their evolution, incorporate a transitory movement or pause, thereby acquiring a distinctive characteristic. This incorporation is represented by adding to the stereotypy code a symbol for the incorporated element (*look,* (*l*), *pause* (*p*), *dip* (*d*), or *recoil* (*r*)), using the lower case to differentiate it from nonincorporated interruptive occurrences of the same behavior. Finally, if no movement occurs during the 10-second interval, this will be indicated by scoring *None* (*N*).

4. Body Posture (2)

Lying (*L*): Either side of the animal is supported on the floor of the cage. No signs of active body support or of an effort to maintain such posture should be detectable. *Sphinxing* (*Sp*): Support is provided by the animal's abdomen on the floor with hindlegs completely flexed and forelegs either flexed or extended forward. *Crouching* (*Cr*): The animal is supported on all four flexed legs while the abdomen is close to, but not in contact with, the floor of the cage. This posture is similar to that of an animal preparing to spring or shrinking with fear, but not necessarily as tense. *Sitting* (*Si*): Support is shared by extended or partially flexed forelegs and completely flexed hindlegs, with the hindquarters in contact with the floor. *Standing* (*S*): Support is given by all four extended or slightly flexed legs. *Standing-on-hindlegs* (*Sh*): Forelegs are off the ground, body is vertical and rests on the hindquarters; it is similar to the rearing posture in the rat. *Pushed-up hindquarters* (*Ph*): Forelegs are flexed or extended forward, abdomen is off the ground, and hindlegs are relatively extended, elevating the hindquarters; it may look similar to an estrous-crouch. *Camelback* (*c*): The back is arched at the dorsal-lumbar level and looks like a hump. In a sitting cat, this is seen as an exaggeration of the normal curvature of the back.

5. Body Movements (2)

Tremor (*Tm*), *Staggering* (*Sg*): Coarse, irregular, vacillating body movements, usually indicative of ataxia. *Swaying* (*Sw*): Relatively large oscillatory movements to the sides, most easily detectable when the animal is standing quietly. *Stretching* (*Sx*): Slow deliberate elongation of the forelegs, hindlegs, or trunk with a tensing of the muscles in the elongated region of the body. *Twitching* (*Tw*): Sudden and instantaneous contraction of a muscle or of a restricted group of muscles. *Jerking* (*Je*): Similar to twitching, but resulting in sudden displacement of a body region. *Hunching* (*H*): Transitory elevation of the back forming a momentary camelback or exaggerating an existing one. If dependent on the execution of an ongoing stereotyped motor response at the head-neck region, this should be indicated by scoring *Hunching-associated* (*Ha*). *Falling* (*F*): Loss of any body posture resulting from absence of gravitational equilibrium. *Jumping* (*J*): Rapid upward displacement, leaving no part of the body in contact with the floor. *Standing on hindlegs* (*Sh*): Moving from a quadrupedal to a bipedal stance. *Push-up forequarters* (*Pf*): Change from flexion to extension of the forelegs with maintenance of the hindquarters posture. *Push-up hindquarters* (*Ph*): The same movement as push-up forequarters but occurring in the hindquarters and having a slight repositioning quality (see II.A.7., *Leg Movements*). *Pumping* (*P*): Up and down displacement due to successive flexion and extension of all four legs simultaneously, without their being lifted from the floor. *Advancing* (*A*): Moving forward or in a forward direction. *Retreating* (*R*): Moving backwards. These last two movements imply displacement of the body (change of place and/or orientation) and may involve stepping with all four legs or with only the forelegs or hindlegs if a large enough single step is taken. *Pivoting* (*Pi*): Oscillating movements around a fixed point, usually the hindquarters. Most frequently, the forelegs step alternately to the right and left of the relatively fixed hindlegs. *Turning* (*T*): Changing direction while moving. *Circling-cage* (*Cc*): Locomotor displacement that almost uninterruptedly follows a path around the perimeter of the cage. *Circling-self* (*Cs*): Continuous or almost continuous turning in a single direction, bringing the animal to his original orientation. *Spinning* (*Sn*): Fast circling-self.

In the case of turning, circling, and spinning movements, direction should be indicated by adding the codes (*r*) for *right* or (*l*) for *left* after the symbol. Some of the body movements described above may become stereotyped; *P, Pi,* and the combination *A* and *R* are usually apparent stereotypy configurations. In any case, an *S* should be placed before the corresponding mnemonic symbol.

6. Leg Posture (2)

Flexed (*F*) and *Extended* (*E*) have the accepted anatomical definitions based on the angle of the leg joints. The rabbit attribute, indicated by following the symbol with an *r,* refers to a peculiar leg posture in which support is maintained by the paws and also by placing the first segment of the leg in contact with the floor. *Wide-base* (*W*): Greater than normal separation between fore- or hindlimbs while supporting the body.

7. Leg Movements (2)

Twitching (*T*) and *Jerking* (*J*) are defined as in Body Movement above, but are here confined to the legs. *Claw-extending*

(*C*): Spreading of the toes to expose the claws. *Sliding* (*Sl*): Movement of the legs while maintaining continuous contact with the floor. Sliding usually occurs while the animal is leaning against a wall of the cage or is in a wide-based stance; it is indicative of dystonia. *Shaking* (*Sh*): Rapid movement of the leg, as if trying to get rid of something sticky and, especially in the hindlimbs, having a fast, clonic quality. *Raising* (*Ra*): A pulling-up movement, usually differentiated from Repositioning by its slowness of execution and by maintenance of the raised position for a short period. *Reaching-out* (*Re*): a foreleg movement directed toward a specific point in the environment, although the foreleg does not necessarily make contact with that point. *Treading* (*Tr*): Alternating pushing movements of forelegs or hindlegs. *Pushing* (*Pu*): As in the Push-up or Pumping body movements or pushing against the walls of the cage when the animal is in a lying position. *Repositioning* (*R*): Placement and removal of one or more legs on the cage floor, with or without shifting the body weight and without modifying place and orientation. *Stepping* (*St*): Placement of one or more legs on the cage floor with shift in body weight and modification of place and/or orientation. *Walking* (*W*): Sequential stepping with displacement of the animal in the cage.

If any of these leg movements becomes stereotyped, an *S* should be placed before the corresponding mnemonic symbol.

8. Tail Posture and Tail Movements (2 for each item)

Raised (*R*): Forming an angle greater than 45° with the hindlimbs. *Lowered* (*L*): Forming an angle equal to or less than 45° with the hindlimbs. *Dropped* (*D*): Hanging and apparently not being included in the animal's behavioral state, or resting entirely on the floor.

Transient (*T*): Any movement of the tail aside from *Squirrel* (*Sq*): A fast, repetitive, flowing twitch.

Waxy (*w*): A plastic quality to any tail posture or movement.

9. Stereotyped Activity (1 for each aspect)

Two aspects of the stereotyped activity displayed by the animals are rated. The first is the nature of Modality of the head stereotypy, which includes *Sniffing* (*Sn*), *Looking* (*L*), and the combination of *Sniffing and Looking* (*Snl*). Execution of the head stereotypies always involves groups of muscles normally subserving either orientation (*L*) or exploration (*Sn*) activities. The identification of the stereotypies as being of the *Sn* and/or *L* modalities implies only an activation of the motor components of those behaviors.

The second aspect is the Relatedness, by virtue of alternation, simultaneity, or opposition, of concomitant regional stereotypies.

Such relatedness is indicated by listing the body regions seen to be related: *Head-Body* (*Hb*), *Head-Legs* (*Hl*), *Body-Legs* (*Bl*), or *Head-Body-Legs* (*Hbl*).

B. Motor Function

1. Dystonia (1)

Recognizable in either abnormal *postures* (*P*) or abnormal *movements* (*M*). If both are present, *PM* is scored. Dystonia is characterized by hyperflexion or hyperextension of body regions with awkward appearance.

2. Disjunction (1)

Identified by lack of proper relationship among *posture* (*P*) or *movements* (*M*) in two or more body regions, resulting in a fragmentation of the static or kinetic configuration of the body. *PM* indicates disjunction of both the postural and movement types.

3. Ataxia (1)

Characterized by inadequate control of the range and precision of movements and/or by quivering of flexed and/or extended regions of the body; it refers to kinetic or static manifestations, or both. Thus, if an animal keeps a certain posture, staggering or swaying movements are indicative of this motor alteration. *Level 1* indicates a moderate degree of ataxia. If marked incoordination is present, so that the animal tends to fall or is grossly unable to coordinate all four legs in order to walk or to maintain a standing posture, *Level 2* should be scored. Absence of ataxia is indicated by scoring *None* (*N*).

III. Autonomic and Reflex Responses (3)

Pupil dilation: Equal bilateral dilation (*Pe*) is differentiated from *unequal or unilateral dilation,* (*Pl*) if left is larger, or (*Pr*) if right is larger. *Eyes-wide* (*E*): Increased palpebral opening. *Sneeze* (*Sn*), *Salivation* (*Sa*), *Panting* (*P*), *Yawning* (*Y*), *Gagging* (*G*), *Vomiting* (*V*), *Pilorection* (*Pi*), and *Defecation* (*D*) can also be indicated. If none of these responses is present, *None* (*N*) is entered.

IV. Miscellanea (3)

Response to stimulus: Clear and sudden postural shifting or movement activity corresponding to a *visual* (*Rv*), *auditory* (*Ra*), or *undetermined* (*Ru*) source or event. If a normally stimulating event does not provoke a response, *a failure to respond* (*Rf*) is scored. *Claw-Sharpening* (*Cl*), *Meowing* (*M*), *Hissing* (*H*), *Face-twitch* (*Tw*), and *Ear-twitch* (*E*) are self-explanatory. *Licking* (*L*): Actual licking of an object in the environment (Plexiglas, cage floor, etc.) not related to a grooming activity. *Biting* (*B*): Actual biting (not related to grooming) of an object in the environment (EEG cable, cage wires, etc.) *Chewing* (*Ch*): Suggested masticatory movement not associated with eating. *Fly-catching* (*F*): A fast sudden turning or swinging head movement with opening and closing of the mouth and, on occasion, protrusion of the tongue. It may be accompanied by other body movements, such as pawing, head-shaking, etc. *Nose-wiping* (*Nw*): Slow swinging head movement, usually describing an arc tangential to the floor and almost rubbing the nose against it. *Wet lips* (*W*): Wetting of the lips with the tongue. This often precedes gagging and vomiting. It may be associated with increased salivation. *Hallucinating* (*H*): Rated by analogy with the human phenomenon on the basis of hissing, motor reactions (such as striking at nonexistent objects in the air, sudden retreating movements, or eluding jumps apparently related to "internal" cues), character of looking activity (most frequently staring gaze), and facial expression. *Akathisia* (*A*): Restlessness and/or repeated weight-shifting movements of the legs (generally repositioning or stepping movements), with or without changing of place or orientation. *Obstinate progression* (*O*): Persistent, propulsive pushing against an immoveable obstacle.

LITERATURE CITED

1. Bahnsen, P., Jacobsen, E., and Thesliff, H. 1938. The subjective effect of beta-phenyliso-propylaminsulfate on normal adults. Acta Med. Scand. 97:1–3.
2. Flory, C. D., and Gilbert, J. 1943. The effects of benzadrine sulphate and caffeine citrate on the efficiency of college students. J. Appl. Psychol. 27:121–134.
3. Sargant, W., and Slater, E. 1963. An Introduction to Physical Methods of Treatment in Psychiatry. Livingstone, Edinburg.
4. Janowsky, D. S., and Davis, J. M. 1974. Dopamine, psychomotor stimulants, and schizophrenia: Effects of methylphenidate in schizophrenia. In: E. Usdin (ed.), Neuropsychopharmacology of Monoamines and Their Regulatory Enzymes, pp. 317–323. Raven Press, New York.
5. Griffith, J. W., Fann, W. E., and Oates, J. A. 1972. The amphetamine psychosis: Experimental manifestation. In: E. H. Ellinwood and S. Cohen (eds.), Current Concepts on Amphetamine Abuse, pp. 185–192. U.S. Government Printing Office (DHEW Pub. HSM-72-9085), Washington.
6. Rickman, E. E., Williams, E. Y., and Brown, R. K. 1961. Acute toxic psychiatric reaction related to amphetamine medication. Med. Ann. D.C. 30:209.
7. Connell, P. H. 1958. Amphetamine psychosis. (Maudsley Monographs No. 5), Oxford University Press, New York.

8. Maier, H. W. 1926. Der Kakainismus, Georg Thieme, Verlag, Leipzig.
9. Bleuler, E.: 1924. Textbook of Psychiatry. MacMillan, New York.
10. Ellinwood, E. H. 1967. Amphetamine psychosis I. Description of the individuals and process. J. Nerv. Ment. Dis. 144:273–283.
11. Ellinwood, E. H. 1972. Amphetamine psychosis: Individual settings and sequences. In.: E. H. Ellinwood and S. Cohen (eds.), Current Concepts on Amphetamine Abuse, pp. 185–192. U.S. Government Printing Office, Washington.
12. Rylander, G. 1966. Preludin-narkomanes fran klinisk och medicinsk-kriminologisk synpankt. Svensko Lakartidn. 63:4973.
13. Kramer, J. C., Fischman, V. S., and Littlefield, D. C. 1967. Amphetamine abuse—pattern and effect of high doses taken intravenously. JAMA 201:305–309.
14. Smith, R. The marketplace of speed: Violence and compulsive methamphetamine abuse. Unpublished manuscript.
15. Schiørring, E. 1977. Changes in individual and social behavior induced by amphetamine and related compounds in monkey and man. In E. H. Ellinwood and M. M. Kilbey (eds.), Cocaine and Other Stimulants, pp. 481–522. Plenum Press, New York.
16. Ryland, G. 1969. Clinical and medical criminal aspects of addiction to central stimulating drugs. In: F. Sjoqvist and M. Tottie (eds.), Abuse of Central Stimulants, Sjoqvist, pp. 251–274. Raven Press, New York.
17. Tatetsu, S., Goto, A., and Fujiwara, T. 1956. The Awakening Drug Intoxication. Igaku Shoin Ltd., Tokyo.
18. Kramer, J. C. 1969. Introduction to amphetamine abuse. J. Psychedelic Drugs. 2:1–6.
19. Ellinwood, E. H. 1973. Amphetamine and stimulant drugs. In: Drug Use in America: Problem in Perspective, pp. 140–157. U.S. Government Printing Office, Washington.
20. Mattson, R. H., and Calverley, J. R. 1968. Detroamphetamine-sulfate-induced dyskinesias. JAMA 204:400–402.
21. Rumbaugh, C. L. 1977. Small vessel cerebral vascular changes following chronic amphetamine intoxication. In: E. H. Ellinwood and M. M. Kilbey (eds.), Cocaine and Other Stimulants, pp. 241–252. Plenum Press, New York.
22. Rumbaugh, C. L., Bergeson, R. T., Fang, F. C. H. F., and McCormick, R. 1971. Cerebral angiographic changes in the drug abuse patient. Radiology 101:335–344.
23. Goodman, S. J., and Beker, D. P. 1970. Intercranial hemorrhage associated with amphetamine abuse. JAMA 212:480.
24. Kane, E. F. J., Keller, M. F., and Reifler, C. B. 1969. Neurological crises following amphetamine. JAMA 210:556–557.
25. Tatesu, S. 1963. Methamphetamine psychosis. Folia Psychiat. Neurol. Jap. Suppl. 7:337–380.
26. Ellinwood, E. H. 1971. Assault and homocide associated with amphetamine abuse. Am. J. Psychiatr. 127:1170–1175.
27. Kramer, J. C. 1972. Introduction to amphetamine abuse. In: E. H. Ellinwood and S. Cohen (eds.), Current Concepts on Amphetamine

Abuse, pp. 177–184. U.S. Government Printing Office (DHEW Pub. HMS-72-9085), Washington.
28. Eddy, N. B., Halbach, H., Isbell, H., and Seevers, M. H. 1965. Drug dependence: Its significance and characteristics. Bull. WHO 32:729.
29. Utena, H. 1974. On relapse-liability: Schizophrenia amphetamine and animal model. In: H. Mitsuda and T. Fukuda (eds.), Biological Mechanisms of Schizophrenia and Schizophrenia-like Psychosis, pp. 285–287. Igaku Shoin Ltd., Tokyo.
30. Utena, H. 1966. Behavioral observations in methamphetamine intoxicated animals and chemical correlates in the brain. Prog. Brain Res. 21B, 1902.
31. Bell, D. S. 1973. The experimental reproduction of amphetamine psychosis. Arch. Gen. Psychiat. 29:35–40.
32. Ellinwood, E. H., and Escalante, O. 1972. Chronic methamphetamine intoxication in three species of experimental animals. In: E. H. Ellinwood and S. Cohen (eds.), Current Concepts on Amphetamine Abuse, pp. 59–68. U.S. Government Printing Office, Washington.
33. Sudilovsky, A., Ellinwood, E. H., Dorsey, F., and Nelson, L. 1975. Evaluation of the Duke University Behavioral Rating Inventory for Drug-Generated Effects (BRIDGE). In: A. Sudilovsky, S. Gershon, and B. Beer (eds.), Predictability in Psychopharmacology: Preclinical and Clinical Correlations, pp. 189–212. Raven Press, New York.
34. Ellinwood, E. H., and Balster, R. L. 1974. Rating the behavioral effects of amphetamine. Eur. J. Pharmacol. 28:35–41.
35. Ellinwood, E. H. 1971. Effects of chronic methamphetamine intoxication in rhesus monkeys. Biol. Psychiat. 3:25–32.
36. Randrup, A., and Munkvad, I. 1967. Stereotyped activities produced by amphetamine in several animal species and man. Psychopharmacologia 11:300–310.
37. Post, R. M. Progressive changes in behavior and seizures following chronic cocaine administration: Relationship to kindling and psychosis. In: E. H. Ellinwood and M. M. Kilbey (eds.), Cocaine and Other Stimulants, pp. 353–372. Plenum Press, New York. (In press).
38. Wallach, M. B., and Gershon, S. 1972. The induction and antagonism of central nervous system stimulant-induced stereotyped behavior in the cat. Eur. J. Pharmac. 18:22–26.
39. Sudilovsky, A., Nelson, L., and Ellinwood, E. H. 1974. Amphetamine dyskinesias: A direct observational study in cats. In: J. M. Singh and H. Lal (eds.), Drug Addiction, pp. 17–37. Stratton Intercontinental Medical Book Co., New York.
40. Ellinwood, E. H., Sudilovsky, A., and Nelson, L. 1972. Behavioral analysis of chronic amphetamine intoxication. Biol. Psychiatr. 4:215–230.
41. Ellinwood, E. H. 1974. Behavioral and EEG changes in the amphetamine model of psychosis. In: E. Usdin (ed.), Neuropsychopharmacology of Monoamines and Their Regulatory Enzymes, pp. 281–297. Raven Press, New York.
42. Ellinwood, E. H. 1971. Accidental conditioning with chronic metham-

phetamine intoxication: Implications for a theory of drug habituation. Psychopharmacologia 21:131–138.

43. Ellinwood, E. H., and Escalante, O. 1970. Chronic amphetamine effect on the olfactory forebrain. Biol. Psychiatr. 2:189–203.
44. Kilbey, M. M., and Ellinwood, E. H. 1977. Chronic administration of stimulant drugs: Response modification. In: E. H. Ellinwood and M. M. Kilbey (eds.), Cocaine and Other Stimulants, pp. 409–430. Plenum Press, New York.
45. Klawans, H. L., and Margolin, D. I. 1975. Amphetamine-induced dopaminergic hypersensitivity in guinea pigs. Arch. Gen. Psychiat. 32:725–732.
46. Del Rio, J., and Fuentes, J. A. 1969. Further studies on the antagonism of stereotyped behaviour induced by amphetamine. Eur. J. Pharmacol. 8:73–78.
47. Randrup, A., and Munkvad, I. 1968. Behavioural stereotypies induced by pharmacological agents. Pharmako-psychiatrie-Neuro-Psychopharmakologie. 1:18–26.
48. Downs, A. W., and Eddy, N. B. 1932. The effect of repeated doses of cocaine on the rat. J. Pharmac. Exp. Ther. 46:199–200.
49. Stripling, J. S., and Ellinwood, E. H., Jr. 1977. Sensitization to cocaine following chronic administration in the rat. In: E. H. Ellinwood and M. M. Kilbey (eds.), Cocaine and Other Stimulants, pp. 327–352. Plenum Press, New York.
50. Matthysse, S. 1974. Implications of catecholamine systems of the brain in schizophrenia, In: F. Plum (ed.), Brain Dysfunction in Metabolic Disorders, pp. 305–315. Raven Press, New York.
51. Snyder, S. H. 1973. Amphetamine psychoses: A "model" schizophrenia mediated by catecholamines. Amer. J. Psychiat. 130:61–67.
52. Angrist, B. M., Shopin, B., and Gershon, S. 1971. Comparative psychotomimetic effects of stereoisomers of amphetamine. Nature 234:689–704.
53. Ellinwood, E. H., Jr. 1969. Amphetamine Psychosis: A Multidimensional Process. Seminars in Psychiatry. 1:208–226.
54. Kety, S. S. 1960. Recent biochemical theories of schizophrenia. In: D. D. Jackson (ed.), The Etiology of Schizophrenia, pp. 137–138. Basic Books, New York.
55. Carlsson, A. 1974. Amphetamine and brain catecholamines. In: E. Usden (ed.), Neuropsychopharmacology of Monoamines and Their Regulating Enzymes, pp. 289–300. Raven Press, New York.
56. Anden, N. E., and Svensson, T. H. 1973. Release of dopamine from central noradrenaline nerves after treatment with reserpine plus amphetamine. J. Neurol. Trans. 34:23–30.
57. Glowinski, J., and Axelrod, G. 1964. Inhibition of uptake of tritiated noradrenaline in the intact rat brain by imipramine and structurally related compounds. Nature 204:1318–1319.
58. Angrist, B. M., Sathananthan, G., Shopsin, B., and Gershon, S. The comparative psychotogenic effects of L-DOPA and ET-495. In: E. H. Ellinwood and M. M. Kilbey (eds.), Cocaine and Other Stimulants, Plenum Press, New York. (In press.)
59. Janowsky, D. S., Huey, L., and Storms, L. 1977. Psychologic test

responses to methylphenidate. In: E. H. Ellinwood and M. M. Kilbey (eds.), Cocaine and Other Stimulants, pp. 675–688. Plenum Press, New York.
60. Eibergen, R. D., and Carlson, K. R. 1975. Dyskinesias elicited by methamphetamine: Susceptibility of former methadone-consuming monkeys. Science 190:588–590.
61. Eidelberg, E., and Erspamer, R. 1975. Dopaminergic mechanisms of opiate actions in brain. J. Pharmacol. Exp. Ther. 192:50–57.
62. Gianutsos, G., Hynes, M. D., Puri, S. K., Drawbaugh, R. B., and Lal, H. 1974. Effects of apomorphine and nigrostriatal lesions on aggression and striatal dopamine turnover during morphine withdrawal: Evidence for dopaminergic supersensitivity in protracted abstinence. Psychlpharmacologia 34:37–44.
63. Vasquez, B. J., Overstreet, D. H., and Russel, R. W. 1974. Psychological evidence for increase in receptor sensitivity following chronic morphine treatment. Psychopharmacologia 38:287–302.
64. Ellinwood, E. H., and Kilbey, M. M. 1975. Amphetamine stereotypy: The influence of environmental factors and prepotent behavioral patterns on its topography and development. Biol. Psychiat. 10:3–16.
65. Segal, D. S., and Mandell, A. J. 1974. Long-term administration of *d*-amphetamine: Progressive augmentation of motor activity and stereotypy. Pharm. Biochem. Behav. 2:249–255.
66. Ellinwood, E. H., Kilbey, M. M., Castellani, S., and Khoury, C. 1977. Amygdala hyperspindling and seizures induced by cocaine. In: E. H. Ellinwood and M. M. Kilbey (eds.), Cocaine and Other Stimulants. Plenum Press, New York.
67. Ellinwood, E. H., Stripling, J., and Kilbey, M. M. Chronic changes with amphetamine intoxication: Underlying processes. In: E. Usdin and J. Barchas (eds.), Neuroregulators and Hypotheses of Psychiatric Disorders. Oxford University Press, London. (In press.)
68. Rylander, G. 1972. Psychosis and the punding in choreiform syndromes in addition to central stimulant drugs. Psychiatr. Neurol. Neurochir. 75:203–313.
69. Escalante, O. D., and Ellinwood, E. H. 1970. Central nervous system cytopathological changes in cat with chronic methedrine intoxication. Brain Res. 21:555.
70. Escalante, O. D., and Ellinwood, E. H. 1972. Effects of chronic amphetamine intoxication on adrenergic and cholinergic structures in the central nervous system: Histochemical observation in cats and monkeys. In: E. H. Ellinwood and S. Cohen (eds.), Current Concepts on Amphetamine Abuse, pp. 97–106. U.S. Government Printing Office, Washington.
71. Gunne, L., and Lewander, T. 1967. Long term effects of some dependence-producing drugs on the brain monoamines. In: O. Wahaas (ed.), Molecular Basis of Some Aspects of Mental Activity, pp. 75–81. Academic Press, New York.
72. Seiden, L. S., Fischman, M. W., and Schuster, C. R. 1977. Changes in brain catecholamines induced by long-term methamphetamine administration in rhesus monkeys. In: E. H. Ellinwood and M. M. Kilbey (eds.), Cocaine and Other Stimulants. Plenum Press, New York.

Relationship Between Abuse Liability of Drugs and Their Degree of Discriminability in the Rat

Donald A. Overton

and

Satish K. Batta

ABSTRACT

An experiment was performed to test whether or not the discriminability of a drug would predict its liability for abuse. Rats were trained to discriminate drug versus no drug in a T-maze; they were required to turn left when undrugged and right when drugged. The number of training sessions required to establish discriminative responding in this task was used as an index of discriminability. This index was established for eighty-seven drugs at the maximum usable dosage of each drug. Although the amount of training required to establish differential responding varied considerably with different drugs, virtually all centrally acting drugs were eventually discriminated. The results indicate that discriminability measurements of this type are not predictive of abuse liability to a useful degree.

INTRODUCTION

Most centrally acting drugs have effects that are called "discriminable." This is shown by the fact that rats can learn to respond differentially depending on whether or not they are injected with a drug. Although the specific basis of such drug discriminations is unknown,

---

Supported by DA00301 and MH25136, and by Eastern Pennsylvania Psychiatric Institute, Office of Mental Health, Department of Public Welfare, Commonwealth of Pennsylvania.

they are commonly assumed to reflect interceptive stimulus consequences of drug action, perhaps including events that might also be called changes in mood or affect. Some drugs are said to be more discriminable than others, referring to the fact that drug discriminations are much more readily acquired with these drugs than with others. In addition to these quantitative differences between drugs, discriminable effects of two drugs are said to be similar or dissimilar, depending on whether the drugs can substitute for one another in a drug discrimination procedure.

Various hypotheses have been put forth relating drug discriminations to drug abuse and to the perceived consequences of drug action in human subjects.[1,2] For example, it has been suggested that the etiology of abuse might involve acquisition of specific repertoires of "drug state" behavior, contingent upon drugs for their occurrence.[3] As another example, it has been suggested that drugs with similar discriminable effects in rats might have similar effects in human subjects—a plausible if unproven hypothesis.[4]

Some time ago, data regarding the relative discriminability of different classes of drugs began to suggest that the ease with which a drug was discriminated might provide a predictor of its abuse liability.[5] A priori, this relationship appeared unlikely, as a high correlation between discriminability and abuse liability implies that only positively reinforcing drug effects are discriminable. Nonetheless, the data available when the present study was undertaken strongly suggested a correlation between abuse liability and discriminability.[2]

The specific purpose of the present study was to test whether or not a high correlation exists between the degree of discriminability of drugs in rats and the abuse liability of the same drugs by humans; i.e., to determine whether a measurement of the discriminability of a drug would predict its abuse liability. To test this hypothesis, we measured the discriminability of a wide variety of abused and nonabused drugs in a standardized drug discrimination paradigm. The resulting indices of discriminability were compared with the abuse potential of the same drugs as determined by clinical experience and animal self-administration studies.

GENERAL METHODS

Subjects

Experimentally naive Long Evans hooded rats were purchased from Blue Spruce Farms and were maintained with food and water continuously available during testing. All rats weighed 200–300 g at the beginning of training and were males, except where specified. Prior to training, they were allowed to explore the T-maze for twenty minutes.

Apparatus

A T-maze was constructed with wire grid floor and gray plywood walls. The usual T-shape was modified by placing a 90° angle in each side arm so that the goal boxes were not visible from the choice point. A barrier door could be placed in front of each goal box to prevent entry. The choice point was the 6-inch square area where the three alleys converged. A 150 watt spotlight was placed 36 inches above the choice point to illuminate the maze. A Grason-Stadler Scrambler (E1064GSN) provided 1.6–2.5 ma electric shock which was applied to the grid floor everywhere except in the goal boxes. Rats were retained in a wastebasket between trials.

Training Procedure

On each individual trial, the rat was dropped from a height of 6 inches onto the floor of the start box facing the choice point. The shock was already turned on. The rat was allowed to run freely in the maze until it reached, and remained in, the accessible goal box. The rat's "choice" was defined as the direction in which it first departed from the choice point. A training session consisted of 10 training trials spaced at about one minute apart, with the same choice (either right or left) required on all trials.

For each rat, a drug state and the no drug state were selected to act as discriminative conditions. During successive daily sessions, the imposed drug condition alternated, as did the required choice. Hence a right turn was always required when the rat was drugged and a left turn when undrugged.

Analysis of Data

Performance on the first trial of each training session was analysed to provide measurements of discriminability.[6] Criterion performance was eight correct first trial choices during ten consecutive sessions. The number of sessions to begin criterion performances (STC) was computed for each rat; STC was 60 for rats that failed to achieve criterion with 70 sessions.

Drugs

A drug state (D) was defined as the condition existing at a specified delay after intraperitoneal injection of a specified drug and dosage.

The delay interval was chosen so that drug effects would be maximal at the time of testing. The "no drug" condition (N) signified no injection (saline was sometimes injected to demonstrate that behavior was not influenced by the injection procedure per se). Throughout this paper, stated doses include the weight of salt and are expressed in mg/kg. Drugs were dissolved in water or saline except where otherwise specified, and administered in a volume of 1 mg/cc whenever possible. Many drugs were very generously contributed by the companies mentioned below.*

The following compounds and doses were used: Acetaminophen 600 (mg/kg) suspended in 1% carboxy-methyl-cellulose solution (in CMC); alphaprodine HCl 10[11], dl-alpha-methyl-p-tyrosine, methyl ester HCL 140, amyl nitrite 90 (suspended in sesame oil), *d*-amphetamine 8, antipyrine 250, arecoline 20, artane 100[13], asperin 250 (in CMC), atropine sulfate 50–100 (data pooled for this range of doses), Na barbital 100–150, bemegride 7.5, benactyzine HCl 5–50, benadryl HCl 30[17], caffeine 100, carbacol 0.4–0.6, carisprodol 75[27] (in CMC), chlordiazepoxide HCl 30[11], chlorpromazine HCL 4[24], cocaine HCl 50, codeine phosphate 50, cogentin mesylate 40[16], cyclazocine 25[25] (in CMC), cyproheptadine HCl 50[16] (in CMC), dextromethorphan HBr 50[11], diazepam 60–80[11] (in CMC), ditran 7–60[12], doxepin HCl 20[18], dramine 75[23], ethoheptazine citrate 100[29], ethosuximide 300–400[17], ethylalcohol 3000, fentanyl citrate 0.1[15], fluphenazine HCl 2[22], flurazepam dihydrochloride 100[11], flutethimide 100[26] (in CMC), haloperidol HCl 2.5[15] (in 0.1 tartaric acid), heroin HCl 20, histamine phosphate 200[14], imipramine HCl 40[9], isoproterenol HCl 75[25], ketamine 40–60[17], levallorphan tartarate 75[11], levorphanol tartarate 10[11], lidocaine HCl 60,[6], lithium citrate 80, lobeline sulphate 30, mecamylamine 30[16], meperidine HCl 40[25], meprobamate 200[27] (in CMC), mesantoin 120[21] (in CMC), mescaline HCl 50, methadone HCl 10[14], methaqualone HCl 20[30] (in CMC), methocarbamol 300[19] (in CMC), methylphenidate HCl 40[9], methyprylon 75[11], methysergide maleate 50[21], metrazol 30, morphine sulfate 32, naloxone HCl 25[10], naltrexone HCl 25–100[10], nicotine 4, nikethamide 200[9], noradrenalin bitartarate 2[25], parnate sulfate 10[24], pentazocine HCl 40[25], Na pentobarbital 20;

---

* Drugs were very generously contributed by the following companies: Abbott Laboratories; Astra Pharmaceutical Products; Bio-Ceutics; Endo Labs; Lakeside Labs; Eli Lilly & Company; Merck, Sharpe, & Dohme; Pfizer; Wm. H. Rorer; Schering Labs; Smith, Kline & French; USV Pharmaceutical Corp.; Warner Lambert; Orgamol S. A.; Aldrich Chemical Company; Ayerst Labs; CIBA-GEIGY: Hoffmann-La Roche, Inc.; Lederle Labs; McNeil Labs; Parke, Davis & Company; A. H. Robins; Sandoz-Wander; G. D. Searle; Sterling Winthrop; Wallace Labs; Wyeth Labs.

perphenazine 50[22] (in CMC), phencyclidine HCl 10–20, phenelzine sulfate 75[28], Na phenobarbital 80, phenoxybenzamine HCl 10[24], phentolamine HCl 50[9], physostigmine sulphate 1, picrotoxin 1, piminodine ethanesulphonate 20[25], piperidine HCl 200, procaine HCl 50[4], profadol HCl 40[17], propoxyphene 30[14], propranolol HCl 35[7], pyrilamine maleate 50, scopolamine HBr 4–100, strychnine sulphate 0.8, trimethadione 300[4], urethane 750.

DOSE-RESPONSE STUDIES

Procedure

Complete dose effect curves for discriminability were obtained with some drugs. For each of these drugs, a dosage was initially determined above which training was not feasible due to toxic effects. Dose effect determinations were started immediately below this dose, and continued down to lower doses. A variety of drugs and doses were tested, with at least three rats per dose. Each individual rat was trained to discriminate a particular drug and dosage (D) from the no drug condition (N). Training continued for 70 sessions, or until criterion performance was achieved.

Results

Figure 1 shows dose-response curves for several drugs. For each drug, as dosage increased, the discrimination was formed more and more readily, as indicated by the decreasing number of training sessions required to reach criterion performance. The curves appear generally linear, except that with very high doses of some drugs, discriminability tends to asymptote. In most instances, this departure from linearity appears to reflect the intrusion of behaviorally toxic drug effects that prevent increasingly rapid acquisition of discriminative performance as dosage is raised.

Discussion

In all cases, the value of STC obtained with the highest tested dose was the lowest value obtained, or very near to the lowest value obtained. Based on this property of the dose response curves, it was decided that for the present study, data would be collected at only one lower dosage in cases where this appeared necessary to verify the general shape of the dose effect curve.

Since discriminability is so strongly influenced by dosage, it might be argued that a comparison of discriminability across drugs is

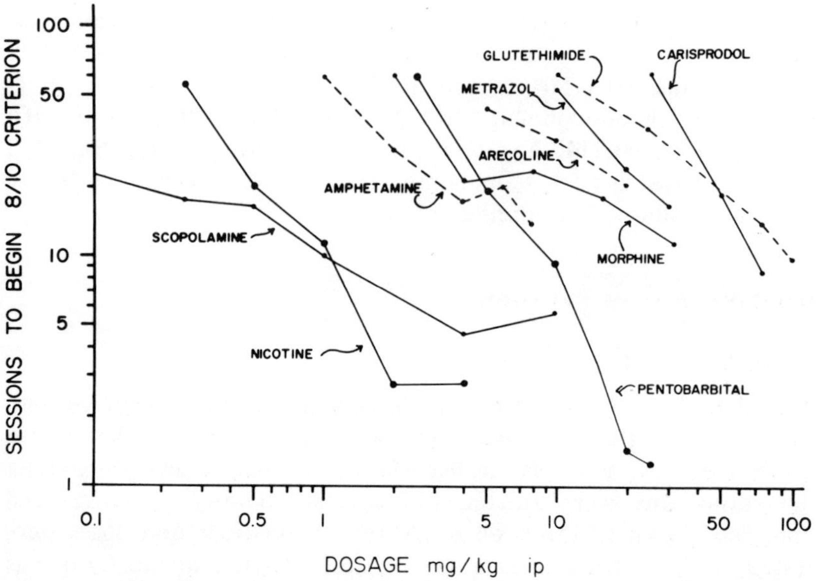

Figure 1. Dose response curves obtained by training rats to discriminate drugs versus no drug with various doses of several drugs. *X axis* is injected dosage. *Y axis* is sessions to begin criterion performance of the drug discrimination. Smaller STC values indicate more rapid acquisition of the discrimination.

meaningless. However, this did not appear to be the case, because with some drugs it was not possible to obtain a high level of discriminability with any usable dose, whereas other drugs were readily discriminable at moderate doses. Hence it appeared meaningful to compare the relative discriminabilities of different drugs.

The specific drug effect that prevented use of a higher dose and hence determined maximum measurable discriminability was different for different types of drugs. Depending on the drug selected, dosage might be limited by convulsions, anesthesia, chronic physical toxicity, cardiovascular effects, or behavioral toxicity secondary to CNS effects. One of the serious and unsolved questions regarding the present concerns the degree to which these dose-limiting toxic effects may differ in man and in rat, thus leading to species differences in the relative maximal discriminability of various drugs.

MAXIMUM DISCRIMINABILITY OF VARIOUS DRUGS

Procedure

For 87 drugs, the maximum usable dose was determined, and 3 or more (usually 6) rats were trained in the T-maze to discriminate this

Table 1. Number of training sessions before discriminative performance was learned with maximal doses of various drugs[a]

Class Drug	Dose	*N*	STC	"Dose-limiting effects"
Depressants				
Barbital	100–150	9	3.7	Anesthesia
Glutethimide	100	6	9.5	Anesthesia
Methaqualone	20	3	9.6	Anesthesia
Pentobarbital	20	16	1.4	Anesthesia
Phenobarbital	80	6	1.3	Anesthesia
Stimulants				
d-Amphetamine	8	5	13.4	Acute toxic effects
Caffeine	125	5	12.7	Acute toxic effects
Cocaine	50	8	10.8	Convulsions
Methylphenidate	40	3	9.1	Acute toxic effects
Narcotics				
Cyclazocine	25	6	19.9	Behavioral disorganization
Dextromethorphan (female)	40	12	4.5	Convulsions
Dextromethorphan (male)	50	9	9.8	Convulsions
Heroin	20	6	6.8	Convulsions or "Catatonia"
Levallorphan	75	8	17.1	Acute toxic effects
Morphine (male)	32	3	11.1	Convulsions
Morphine (female)	25	9	12.2	Convulsions
Antihistamines				
Benadryl	40	3	17.8	Convulsions
Dramamine	75	7	18.6	Convulsions
Pyrilamine	50	9	19.7	Convulsions
Antimuscarinics				
Atropine	50–100	12	3.4	none-STC asymptotes
Benactyzine	5–50	25	7.1	none-STC asymptotes
Scopolamine	4–100	21	5.8	none-STC asymptotes
Tricyclic Antidepressants				
Amitryptyline	20	4	21	Chronic toxic effects
Doxepin	20	8	15	Convulsions
Imipramine	40	9	13.8	Convulsions
Antipsychotics				
Chlorpromazine	4	3	41.6	Behavioral unresponsiveness
Fluphenazine	2	3	41.5	Behavioral unresponsiveness
Perphenazine	50	3	27.0	Behavioral unresponsiveness
Thioridazine	30–50	6	11.1	Chronic toxic effects
Organic Solvents				
Acetone	2000	6	3.6	Anesthesia
Ethyl Alcohol	3000	6	3	Anesthesia
Amyl Nitrite	90	6	38	Acute toxic effects
Ethyl Acetate	1000	2	29	Acute toxic effects

[a] Dose is in mg/kg, i.p. *N* is number of rats trained. STC is sessions to begin criterion performance.

dosage of drug versus no drug. Drug names and dosages are listed above in the Methods section. Additional rats were trained to discriminate lower dosages in some cases.

Results

Table 1 presents the results obtained with selected drugs. For each drug, the table shows the dose discriminated, the number of rats trained, the geometric mean of the observed values of STC, and the drug action that prevented use of a higher dosage. Various comparisons between the discriminability of abuse and nonabused compounds can be made in the table, both within and between pharmacological classes.

Figure 2 presents data for all drugs tested in the present study. The figure shows the relationship between measured discriminability (STC) and one indicator of abuse liability (the current schedule status assigned to each drug by the Drug Enforcement Agency). Each data point in the figure indicates the geometric mean STC obtained with one drug at its maximal dosage, and the schedule status of this same drug. The dotted line in Figure 2 is a least squares regression line. The correlation coefficient between natural logarithm of STC and DEA schedule number was 0.33, which is statistically significant with $p <$

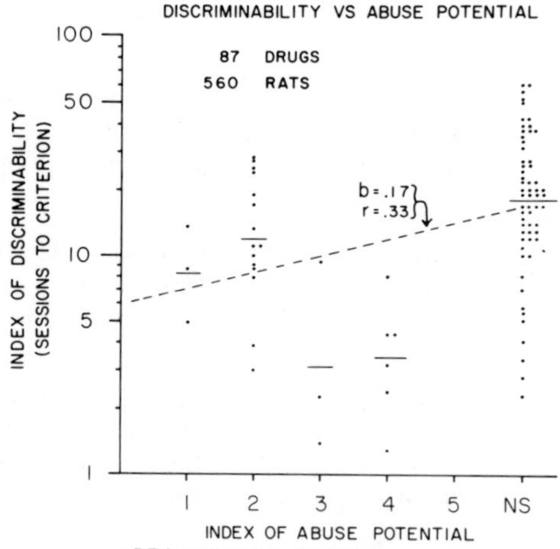

Figure 2. Discriminability as a function of abuse liability. For each *data point*, discriminability is sessions to criterion obtained with maximum usable dose of a drug (*Y axis*). Abuse liability is indicated by current DEA schedule assignment of the drug (*X axis*). NS = nonscheduled.

0.01. However, the validity of these computations is suspect due to the apparently curvilinear relationship between the STC and DEA schedule.

Discussion

Despite the significant correlation between STC and schedule status in Figure 2, examination of individual data points shows that the distribution of measured STCs for Class 2 Compounds (primarily narcotics) overlapped extensively with the distribution of measured STC values for unscheduled compounds (most of which do not have serious abuse liability). Hence Figure 2 strongly suggests that there is not a usefully high correlation between abuse liability and discriminability as measured by our procedures.

Several within-class comparisons in Table 1 also lead to the same conclusion. In the depressant class, the slow-acting barbital and phenobarbital were discriminated as readily as was pentobarbital, even though the former two are relatively nonabused. In the narcotic class, morphine was only slightly more discriminable than cyclazocine, and heroin was no more discriminable than dextromethorphan (Romilar), which is relatively nonabused. In the stimulant class, the differing abuse patterns produced by caffeine and cocaine were not reflected in their measured discriminabilities. Among organic solvents, amyl nitrite is abused but relatively nondiscriminable by comparison to acetone or alcohol. Between-class comparisons are also informative. The antimuscarinic drugs, although seldom abused, are considerably more discriminable than are the stimulant drugs. Narcotics, stimulants, tricyclic antidepressants, and antihistamine compounds all have roughly similar discriminability, although these classes differ widely from one another in their liability for abuse. Overall, Table 1 provides moderately convincing support for the null hypothesis that no correlation exists between abuse liability and the measured ease of discriminability.

GENERAL DISCUSSION

The results show very convincingly that discriminability, as measured in the T-maze task, does not predict abuse liability in humans to a useful degree. This negative finding is unfortunate, but very convincingly supported by the data.

The possibility of task differences must be considered. Our data show, for example, that pentobarbital 5 mg/kg is more discriminable than is amphetamine 1 mg/kg. However Harris and Balster,[7] using an operant drug discrimination task, reported that amphetamine acquired discriminative control as rapidly as pentobarbital ($N = 1$ rat). Hence task differences may exist, and it is conceivable that in a different task we would have obtained a very different pattern of discriminability results more predictive of abuse liability. However, this appears relatively unlikely because the bulk of available evidence points to the conclusion that basically similar drug discrimination results are obtained in most tasks.

Monkeys will self-administer several compounds not frequently abused by humans, including antihistamines and chlordiazepoxide. Although the available data are limited, our drug discrimination findings do seem to predict abuse liability in monkeys better than they predict abuse liability in man. However, this may simply illustrate a weakness in the monkey self-administration preparation, rather than any particular strength of our procedure.

If the present study had started with a theory, instead of departing from empirical findings, that theory would have postulated a virtual isomorphism between discriminable and reinforcing drug effects, such that the drug discrimination and self-administration procedures in effect measured the same drug effects. This hypothesis is clearly disproven by the data.

However, our results should not be interpreted as showing that drug abuse is totally unrelated to the discriminable effects of drugs. Rather, our findings are basically uninformative with regard to a number of possible roles of discriminability in drug abuse. For example, the data provides no information regarding the possible parallels between discriminable effects in rats and subjective drug effects in man. Similarly, the data provide no information regarding the possible role of "drug state response repertoires" in the etiology of abuse. If such repertoires are important, it may be that drugs must have discriminable effects as a necessary but not sufficient condition in order to be abused. However, these speculations remain to be proved, and in view of our negative results some rather explicit experimental verification of their significance is necessary before they can be seriously considered.

LITERATURE CITED

1. Harris, R. T., and Balster, R. L. 1970. An analysis of psychological dependence. In: R. T. Harris, W. N. McIsaac, and C. R. Shuster, Jr.

(eds.), Advances in Mental Science II: Drug Dependence, pp. 214–226. Univ. of Texas Press, Austin.

2. Overton, D. A. State-dependent learning produced by addicting drugs. 1973. In: S. Fisher and A. M. Freedman (eds.), Opiate addiction: Origins and treatment, pp. 61–75. V. H. Winston and Sons, Washington, D.C.
3. Overton, D. A. 1972. State-dependent learning produced by alcohol and its relevance to alcoholism. In: B. Kissen and H. Begleiter (eds.), The Biology of Alcoholism. Vol. II: Physiology and Behavior, pp. 193–217. Plenum Press, New York.
4. Winter, J. C. 1973. Comparison of the stimulus properties of mescaline and 2,3,4-Trimethoxyphenylethylamine. J. Pharmacol. Exp. Ther. 185:101–107.
5. Overton, D. A. 1971. Discriminative control of behavior by drug states. In: T. Thompson and R. Pickens (eds.), Stimulus Properties of Drugs, pp. 87–110. Appleton-Century-Crofts, New York.
6. Overton, D. A. 1974. Experimental methods for the study of state dependent learning. Fed. Proc. 33:1800–1813.
7. Harris, R. T., and Balster, R. L. 1971. An analysis of the function of drugs in the stimulus control of operant behavior. In: T. Thompson and R. Pickens (eds.), Stimulus Properties of Drugs, pp. 111–132. Appleton-Century-Crofts, New York.

Stimulant and Depressant Drugs and Learning in Great Apes

A Progress Report

Walter A. Pieper

The primary goal of this research program is the development of methods for evaluating the effects of psychoactive drugs on learning in great ape subjects, and to utilize this methodology for the assessment of behavioral toxicity. Behavioral toxicity is operationally defined as reduced acquisition performance, as measured by a sequential learning task, following administration of a drug.

Working with great apes provides an opportunity to evaluate drug effects in nonhuman primate subjects that are closely related to man. However, the sheer physical size of these subjects places several constraints on the methods used. Compared with smaller animal species, which are less costly to acquire and maintain, a relatively small number of subjects can be utilized, thus the amount of data obtained from each subject must be maximized. As a result, drug effects must be evaluated with each subject serving as its own control, and experimental control of the target behavior must be satisfactorily maintained if drug effects are to be compared against baseline acquisition performance. Measuring repeated acquisition (learning) in individual subjects requires that the task used be designed in such a way that acquisition can be repeated literally hundreds of times in a highly controlled situation.

The particular sequential response task used in the present program was described in 1968 by Boren and Devine,[1] and was subsequently modified[2-5] and extended to psychopharmacological studies.[6]

This research was supported by Drug Enforcement Administration Contract J69-10. Basic support of the Yerkes Regional Primate Research Center was provided by PHS Grant RR 00165 of the Division of Research Resources, National Institutes of Health.

As modified for use with great ape subjects, this task is uniquely suited to measuring within-subject repeated acquisition in three major respects. First, each subject is required to learn a relatively complex response chain rather than a simple visual discrimination. Second, stimulus fading procedures are used to guide acquisition of the sequential response chain in a standardized manner. Initially, brightness cues are used to shape the animal's behavior. As the subject responds correctly, the light cue is gradually faded out and the length of the chain is extended. Third, and of particular importance, while the basic nature of the task is the same from session to session, the subject is required to learn a new lever sequence each day. Thus, the learning deficit or enhancement associated with the intake of various drugs can be assessed in individual subjects.

METHOD

Sequential Learning Task

A Lab-Care Co. cage (Model 5022), 1.6 m high, 1.0 m wide and 1.4 m long, was modified by replacing a section of one side with a 6 mm aluminum alloy plate (29 cm high × 46 cm long), which served as a mounting panel for six Lindsley response levers (Model 6310, Ralph Gerbrands Co.) mounted in a horizontal array on 7.5-cm centers. A stimulus light with a diameter of 6.2 cm was mounted 10 cm directly above each lever.

These lights served as visual cues signalling for the animal the correct lever. The saliency of these brightness cues was varied across eight levels of illumination, ranging from high contrast (the correct lever fully lighted with the other five off) to no contrast (all levers, including the correct one, at full brightness). Centered directly below the levers was a food receptacle into which M & M candy or peanut reinforcers were delivered from a dispenser. These reinforcers were dispensed each time the animal pulled the final lever in a correct sequence of levers. When an error was made, a 7-second timeout went into effect during which a buzzer was sounded and the house lights and all lever lights were extinguished. Testing began each day with maximum light cues followed by a gradual fading out of the discriminable brightness feature, thereby forcing the subject to learn the position of the correct levers. The length of the lever pulling sequence was also systematically increased from one lever to six levers. The fading procedure was first used with the shortest sequence length of one.

Each correct lever response was followed by a reduction in the brightness cue by one level while each error resulted in the light cue "backing up" to the level used on the previous trial. At the eighth level, all stimulus lights were identically illuminated and, consequently, no longer functioned as a cue. Therefore, a correct response at the eighth level indicated that the animal had learned the correct position of the lever(s). Thus, the brightness cue was systematically faded out through eight equal intensity changes, so that the stimulus lights provided no cue to the correct sequence of levers when acquisition of the behavioral chain was completed.

When the subject correctly completed sequence one, the sequence was increased to a two-lever chain. The subject was now required to pull two levers in the correct sequence to obtain reinforcement. Again, maximal brightness cues were used on the initial trials but were progressively faded out with each correct response. When the subject successfully completed the sequence of two levers at the eighth level of illumination, demonstrating that he had learned to discriminate the correct two-lever sequence by position, the sequence was lengthened to three levers and the process repeated.

Daily test sessions were terminated either when 50 minutes had elapsed or when the subject had successfully completed a sequence of six levers at the eighth light level, whichever occurred first. Since a new lever sequence was presented each day, a new sequence was learned each day. Thus, this task provided learning data for each day of testing. Therefore, learning (acquisition) on those days when a particular drug was administered could be compared with intervening control days when only placebo was given.

Multiple dependent measures can be derived from this task. Chain length completed, interresponse time and optimum divided by actual number of responses are included in this report. Additional measures, including number of reinforcements obtained, errors at each light level, and errors at each chain length, are presently being evaluated for possible further analysis.

Subjects Tested

A total of eight adult or young adult great apes have been tested on this task: two female and four male chimpanzees (*Pan troglodytes*) and two male orangutans (*Pongo pygmaeus*). At the present time, six of these animals (4 male, 2 female) are serving as subjects. Their estimated ages vary from 10–30 years (average = 18 years) and their current weights range from 30–85 kilograms (average = 53.3 kg).

Drugs and Procedures

Data on eight drugs in the general class of depressants or tranquilizers and ten compounds generally classified as stimulant or anorectic drugs (Table 1) are included in this report and will subsequently be referred to simply as "depressants" or "stimulants." Typically, three subjects are tested on low, medium, and high doses of each drug. A minimum of two control days (vehicle only) intervenes between drug days. Each ape is tested in at least three sessions on each dose of the drug. Determination of the low doses is based on the clinical literature and is usually slightly higher than the recommended clinical dose for humans. When information on clinical doses is unavailable, the low dose is estimated from similar drugs. The high drug doses are determined behaviorally and physiologically and are defined as the highest dose short of severe behavioral or physiological toxicity. That is, the dose is increased until the animal begins to show marked signs of physiological toxicity (e.g., vomiting, hyperactivity, sleep, etc.) or behavioral toxicity (e.g., failure to respond). The amount of drug administered is then lowered slightly and defined as a high dose. The medium dose is approximately equidistant between the low and high doses.

Table 1. Percent of control on high drug dose days

Name of drug[a]	Maximum Chain Length	Interresponse Time	Response Efficiency
Butabarbital (4)	87	100	80
Diazepam (3)	58	214	44
Glutethimide (2)	95	144	73
Halazepam (3)	96	119	62
Meprobamate (2)	97	154	82
Phenobarbital (2)	87	131	75
Scopolamine (2)	105	73	69
Secobarbital (3)	93	112	84
Benzphetamine (4)	40	630	141
Chlorphentermine (3)	76	237	156
Clortermine (3)	92	141	150
d-Amphetamine (3)	61	336	118
Diethylpropion (4)	46	267	125
Mazindol (3)	52	2184	93
Methamphetamine (3)	84	238	124
Methylphenidate (3)	39	93	95
Phendimetrazine (3)	67	196	124
Phentermine (3)	62	125	208

[a] The number of subjects tested with each drug is included in parentheses following the drug name.

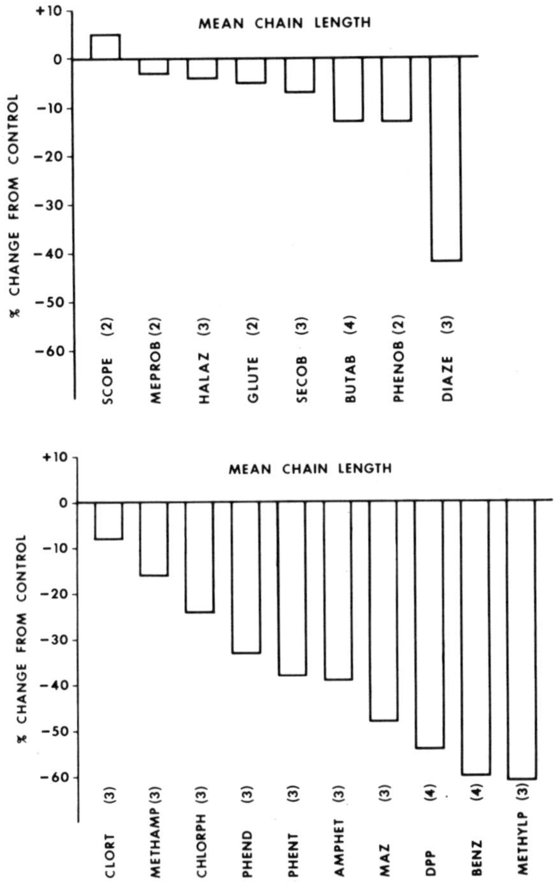

Figure 1. Average chain length achieved on high-dose drug days expressed as percent change from control. The number of subjects included in each *bar* is indicated within the parentheses next to the drug name (complete names in Table 1).

RESULTS

Chain Length

Percent change from control performance on the chain length measure following the high doses of drug is presented in Figure 1. There appears to be a marked difference between stimulant and depressant drugs on this measure. While animals receiving depressant drugs show relatively minor decreases from control levels (less than 15% in most cases), most stimulant drugs produced large decreases in maximum sequence length completed (over 35% in half the apes tested). The control days used in this and subsequent analyses are those days immediately preceding a drug administration day. Although a minimum of two control days are included between drug doses, additional control days are scheduled if the subject does not achieve criterion baseline performance on the second control day.

Interresponse Time

In Figure 2, the mean interresponse times (IRT) are depicted as percent changes from control levels. With few exceptions, administra-

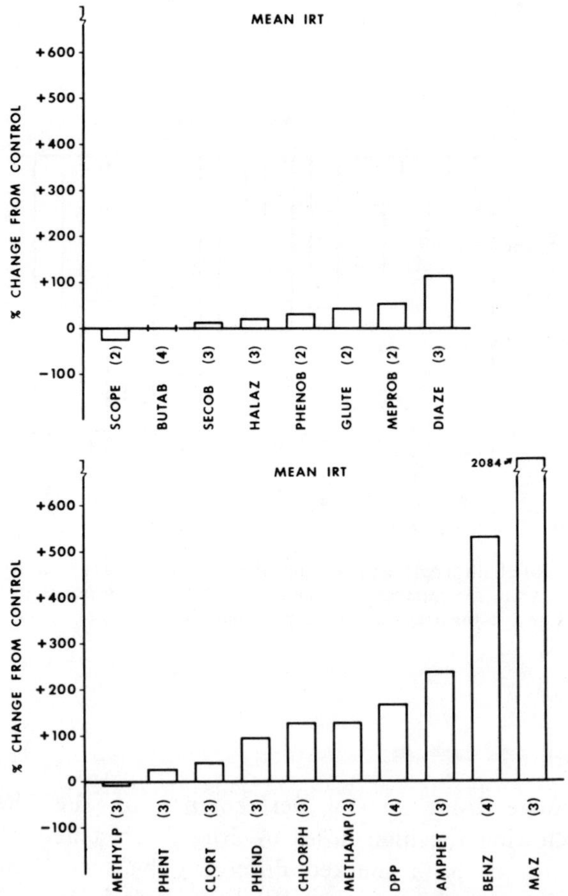

Figure 2. Average interresponse times obtained on high-dose drug days expressed as percent change from control. The number of subjects included in each *bar* is indicated within the parentheses next to the drug name (complete names in Table 1).

tion of these high doses of drug was associated with increases in mean IRT; however, this change is much more pronounced with stimulant drugs than with depressant compounds. Increases in this dependent measure probably reflect increased pausing by the subjects rather than actual changes in rate of responding. Visual observations of subjects during testing reveal that subjects tend to stop working on the lever task and move to another area of the testing cage more frequently if they have received a stimulant drug before testing. This is much less likely to occur if the animal has received a high dose of a depressant drug.

Response Efficiency

Figure 3 presents an additional dependent variable for the same drugs discussed above. This measure is obtained by calculating the optimum (minimum) number of responses required to complete the task at each of the chain lengths and comparing this to the actual number of responses required by the subject. The optimum number of responses required to complete a chain length of six levers is 168. This ratio is obtained for each control day and the average of these days is compared against the average performance following three high doses of any particular drug and expressed, as with the other measures, as a percent change from control.

In considering the results depicted in Figure 3, it may be noted that response efficiency is greater with the stimulant drugs than with the depressant drugs. Thus, even though the average chain length achieved is depressed for subjects receiving stimulant drugs before testing, and overall response rates are lower, as shown by the increase in mean IRT, those responses made by the subject when it responds tend to be correct. Following depressant drugs, however, neither chain length nor IRT is greatly affected, but efficiency of responding (optimum/actual responses) does decline.

DISCUSSION

The three dependent measures analyzed thus far suggest that this sequential learning task can yield information regarding the likelihood that a particular drug may produce behavioral toxicity, if administered at greater than therapeutic doses. Although the eight depressant drugs tested thus far produced relatively limited decrements from baseline performance with respect to two of the dependent measures, response efficiency is reduced. In this regard, it seems possible that these drugs are acting to attenuate the consequences of

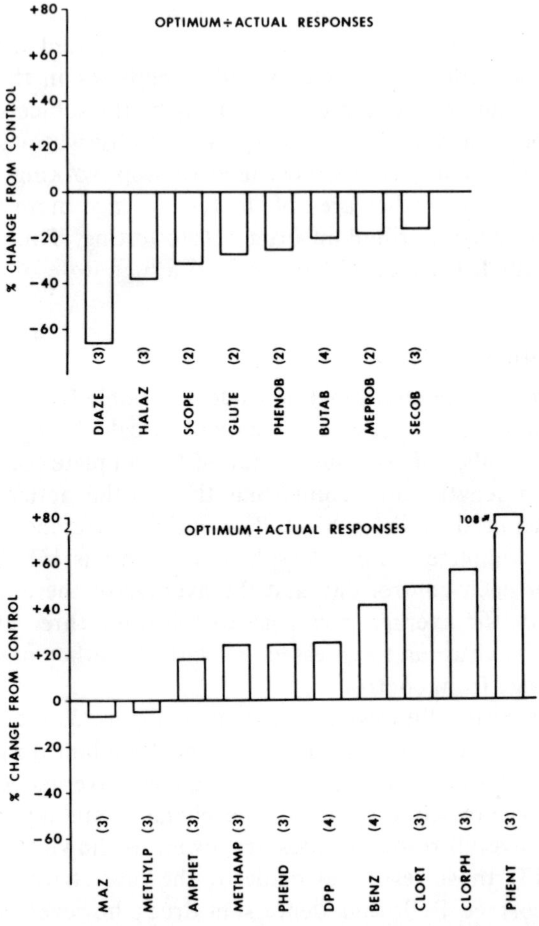

Figure 3. Average response efficiency achieved on high-dose drug days expressed as percent change from control. The number of subjects included in each *bar* is indicated within the parentheses next to the drug name (complete names in Table 1).

making errors. Specifically, when a subject pulls the incorrect lever, a 7-second timeout period is programmed where the house light is turned off and a buzzer sounds. This contingency can be viewed as punishment, which would ordinarily tend to reduce the probability of responding. In the case of depressant compounds, however, the drug state may be interacting with this punishment[7] and, therefore, the animals continue to respond even though they are making more errors and receiving more timeout periods (punishment). Because they persist in responding, however, they eventually complete the task. On the other hand, the interaction of stimulant drugs with punishment would be more likely to reduce responding than on control days and the subjects simply quit responding after a relatively few timeout periods. Thus, they complete the shorter chain lengths, which are presumably easier, but as they progress to the more difficult longer chains, they begin to make errors and, thus, stop responding. This could account for the somewhat paradoxical findings that deficits in the chain length and IRT measure are accompanied by increased response efficiency with eight of the ten stimulant drugs tested. More complete answers to these problems will require further analysis and listing.

In the past, drugs that were not effective orally and drugs that were judged by the subjects to be noxious tasting were difficult or impossible to evaluate since, until recently, the oral route of administration was used exclusively with these large subjects. Now, however, morphine is being successfully administered by intramuscular injection to two great ape subjects. Once this procedure has been extended to all six subjects, the possible range of drugs which can be tested using this task can be greatly extended.

LITERATURE CITED

1. Boren, J. J., and Devine, D. 1968. The repeated acquisition of behavioral chains. J. Exp. Anal. Behav. 11:651–660.
2. Boren, J. J. 1969. Stimulus fading variables affecting the maximum chain length a monkey can acquire. Paper presented at the Proceedings, 77th Annual Convention, A.P.A.
3. Boren, J. J. 1969. Some variables affecting the superstitious chaining of responses. J. Exp. Anal. Behav. 12:959–969.
4. Thompson, D. M. 1970. Repeated acquisition as a behavioral baseline. Psychonomic Science 12:156–157.
5. Thompson, D. M. 1971. Transition to a steady state of repeated acquisition. Psychonomic Science 24:236–238.
6. Thompson, D. M. 1973. Repeated acquisition as a behavioral baseline for studying drug effects. J. Pharmacol. Exp. Ther. 184:506–514.
7. McMillan, D. E. 1975. Determinants of drug effects on punished responding. Fed. Proc. 34:1870–1879.

Review of Research on Sedative Drug Dependence at the Addiction Research Center and University of Kentucky

Abraham Wikler

Before 1950, the German literature[1] contained numerous references to the occurrence of convulsions and of a delirious state resembling that of alcohol delirium tremens after withdrawal of barbiturates and other hypnotics in use at that time. In the United States, however, clinicians generally did not associate such phenomena with a sedative drug withdrawal syndrome, although there were scattered case reports to the contrary in the American literature.[2] At the Addiction Research Center, research on chronic barbiturate intoxication and withdrawal was stimulated by the observation that, among narcotic addicts admitted to the clinical division of the United States Public Health Service Hospital, a number had one or two generalized convulsions and/or psychosis shortly after admission. Members of the personnel at the Addiction Research Center were requested to see these patients as consultants and subsequent work-up revealed that all of them had taken large amounts of barbiturates (usually pentobarbital, secobarbital, and/or amobarbital) along with opioids prior to admission, and that such barbiturates had been either withdrawn abruptly or rapidly. From their histories, it appeared that there was a close relationship between previous seizures and barbiturate abuse, but this was not certain. At the time they were examined, no clear-cut abnormalities were found neurologically or in the electroencephalogram. It appeared, therefore, that the seizures and/or psychoses that occurred in these patients were due to barbiturate withdrawal, but as

Preparation of this review was supported, in part, by Research Grant DA 00044 from the National Institute of Drug Abuse with funds made available by the Special Action Office for Drug Abuse Prevention.

an underlying epileptic diathesis and/or prepsychotic personality state could not be ruled out, it was decided to investigate these questions experimentally.

STUDIES ON ADDICTION TO "SHORT-ACTING" BARBITURATES

The research at the Addiction Research Center[3-7] was carried out on addicts who volunteered for the studies after the purposes and risks, including the possible occurrence of seizures and/or delirium, had been explained to them. These subjects had been withdrawn from opioids several months before the investigation on barbiturate dependence was begun, or were taking both opioids and barbiturates on admission; in the latter case, chronic barbiturate intoxication was maintained at a known daily dose level, while opioids were withdrawn by the methadone substitution and withdrawal technique. Careful inquiry revealed no family histories of epilepsy, and except for an occasional subject who had had a seizure following sudden abstention from barbiturates, or had had a bout of alcoholic delirium tremens, none had had seizures or psychoses. In the drug-free subjects, control neurological examinations and electroencephalograms yielded no significant abnormal findings. The psychiatric diagnosis on all subjects was character disorder with various associated traits.

During the studies, the subjects (approximately 64 in all) were housed in a closed ward and were observed throughout the day and night by the investigators and trained male nursing personnel. Observations included written accounts of behavior and measurements of pulse and respiratory rates, blood pressure, body temperature, caloric intake, body weight, and hours of sleep. Neurological, electroencephalographic, and psychiatric examinations were made at appropriate intervals. Pentobarbital, secobarbital, or amobarbital was administered in multiple daily doses varying from 0.4 g to as much as 3.8 g (after partial tolerance had developed) for periods of 32–144 days; one subject received pentobarbital and another, secobarbital, 0.2 g at bedtime for 365 days.

During chronic intoxication on 0.4 g or more of these "short-acting" barbiturates, the subjects exhibited ataxia, dyssnergia, nystagmus, depression of the superficial abdominal and cremasteric reflexes, irritability, and varying degrees of impairment of the sensorium. Electroencephalograms were characterized by the appearance of low voltage, rhythmic fast (beta) and varying degrees of slowing of the alpha rhythm (Figure 1). On low daily doses of pentobarbital or secobarbital, e.g., 0.4 g/day, complete tolerance developed to the behavioral effects (Figures 2 and 3) and partial or complete tolerance developed to the electroencephalographic effects,[7] but at high daily doses, tolerance was only partial, though definite.[3,6]

Abrupt withdrawal of "short-acting" barbiturates at high daily dose levels (e.g., 0.8 to 2.2 g/day) was followed first by disappearance of signs of chronic intoxication and then, within 12–24 hr, by the rapid

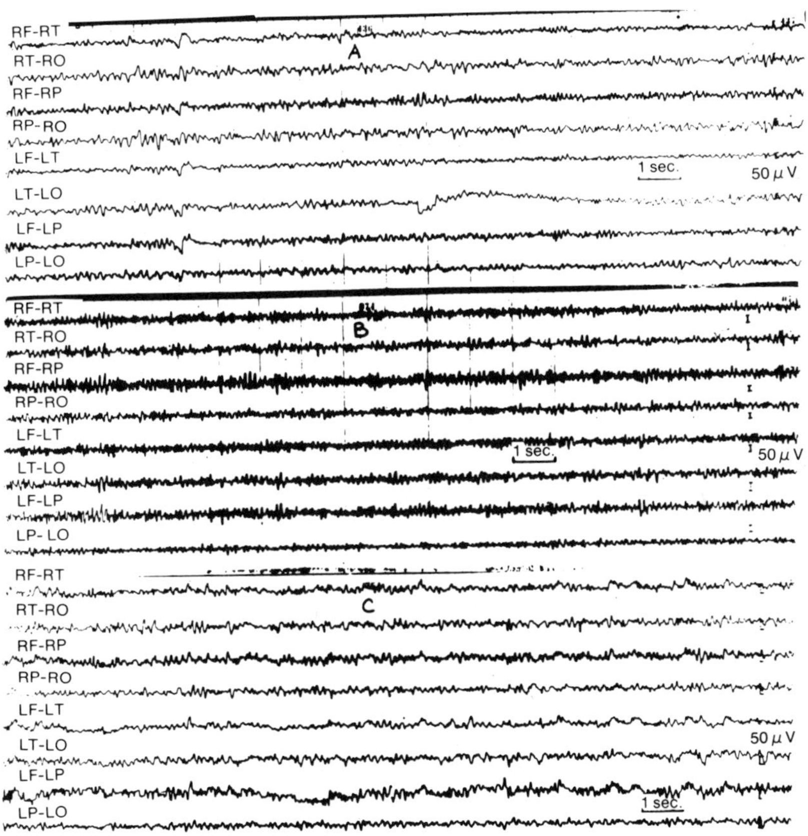

Figure 1. Electroencephalographic patterns during chronic barbiturate intoxication. Subject A, secobarbital 1.6 g/day after 19 days. Rhythmic and nonrhythmic 6–7 cps, random 4–5 cps and low voltage rhythmic 15 cps activity. Subject B, secobarbital 1.1 g/day after 55 days. Almost continuous 18 cps rhythmic activity. Subject C, secobarbital 0.6 g/day after 6 days. Pattern is intermediate between A and B. After recovery from experimental chronic barbiturate intoxication and withdrawal, all three records were normal. Bipolar tracings: F, frontal; T, temporal; P, parietal; O, occipital.

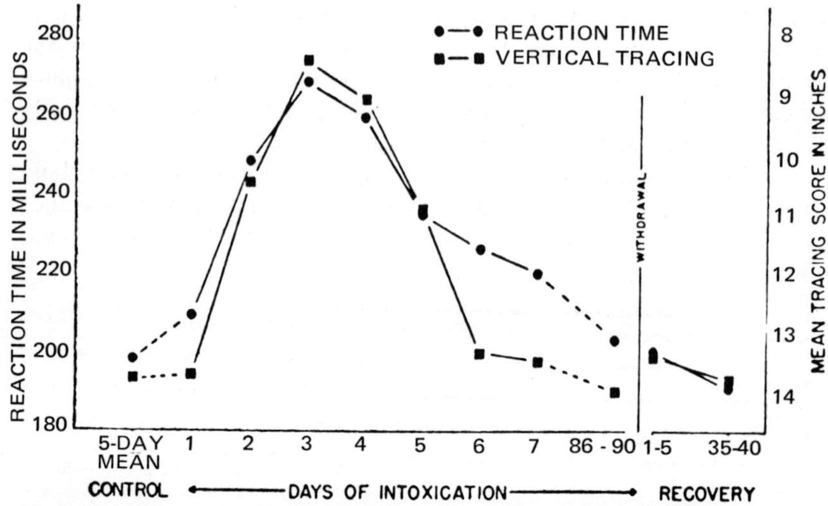

Figure 2. Tolerance to the effects of barbiturates on hours of sleep and degree of intoxication. Secobarbital: 10 SS, 0.4 g/day; pentobarbital: 8 SS, 0.4 g/day. Note tracing score on right ordinate is on inverted scale. Peak prolongation of reaction time and shortening of vertical tracing score is on days 3 and 4 of chronic intoxication, with tolerance developing subsequently. Reprinted with permission from Belleville, R. E., and Fraser, H. F. 1957. J. Pharmacol. Exper. Ther. 120:469–474. Copyright 1957, The Williams & Wilkins Co., Baltimore.

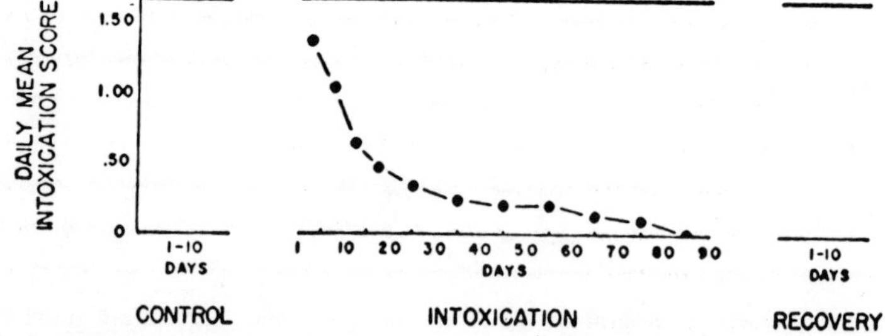

Figure 3. Tolerance to the effects of barbiturates on hours of sleep and degree of intoxication. Secobarbital: 10 SS, 0.4 g/day; pentobarbital: 8 SS, 0.4 g/day. *Indicates a significant difference from control ($p < 0.01$). Note tolerance to prolongation of hours of sleep develops by the 30th day. For the first 20 days of intoxication, daily mean intoxication scores during successive 5-day periods showed significant ($p < 0.01$) decreases in estimated degree of intoxication. Reprinted with permission from Belleville, R. E., and Fraser, H. F. 1957. J. Pharmacol. Exper. Ther. 120:469–474. Copyright 1957, The Williams & Wilkins Co., Baltimore.

evolution of an abstinence syndrome, the main features of which are shown in Table 1. As indicated, "minor" abstinence changes, including marked anxiety, restlessness, tremulousness (a coarse intention tremor), anorexia, nausea, vomiting, insomnia, diaphoresis, increase in cardiac and respiratory rates, postural hypotension, weakness, muscle twitches, and elevation of body temperature, became manifest within 24 hr and could persist for as long as two weeks. In some cases,

Table 1. The barbiturate abstinence syndrome (after abrupt withdrawal of secobarbital or pentobarbital following chronic intoxication at dose levels of 0.8 to 2.2 gm. per day orally, for 6 weeks or more)[a]

Clinical phenomenon	Incidence	Time of onset	Duration (Days)	Remarks
Apprehension	100%	1st day	3–14	Vague uneasiness, or fear of impending catastrophe.
Muscular weakness	100%	1st day	3–14	Evident on mildest exertion.
Tremors	100%	1st day	3–14	Coarse, rhythmic, nonpatterned, evident during voluntary movement, subside at rest.
Postural faintness	100%	1st day	3–14	Evident on standing up suddenly. Associated with marked fall in systolic and diastolic blood pressure, and pronounced tachycardia.
Anorexia	100%	1st day	3–14	Usually associated with repeated vomiting.
Twitches	100%	1st day	3–?	Myoclonic muscular contractions; or spasmodic jerking of one or more extremities. Sometimes bizarre patterned movements.
Seizures	80%	2nd–3rd day	8	Up to a total of 4 grand mal episodes, with loss of consciousness and post-convulsive stupor.
Psychoses	60%	3rd–8th day	3–14	Usually resemble "delirium tremens"; occasionally resemble schizophrenic or Korsakoff syndromes; or acute panic states may occur.

[a] Note: These data are based on a series of 19 cases of experimental addiction to barbiturates. Four developed seizures without subsequent psychosis; one exhibited delirium without antecedent seizures. Three escaped both seizures and delirium.

Reprinted with permission from Wikler, A., Amer. J. Psychiatr. 1968. 125:758–756.

these were the only abstinence phenomena and they subsided after 2–5 days without other sequelae.

However, in about 80% of the subjects, grand mal convulsions appeared, generally on the second or third day after barbiturate withdrawal but occasionally as late as the eighth day; these were not preceded by aurae, and in this group of subjects no one had more than four seizures (however, Wulff[8] reported that one subject had 11 seizures following barbiturate withdrawal). Prior to the onset of seizures, paroxysmal bursts of high voltage 4–6 sec waves appear in the electroencephalogram. Bursts of high amplitude 30–50/sec spikes have been recorded during the clonic phase of the convulsions and 1–6 sec "stupor" waves after the seizure has terminated.[3] The interseizure electroencephalograms display a variety of patterns. In subjects withdrawn from high daily dose levels of barbiturates (0.9 g/day or more), only 7% of the electroencephalograms recorded during the second and third abstinence days and 15% during the fourth to eighth abstinence days were within normal limits. The remaining records showed either diffusely slow abnormalities or, more often, paroxysmal bursts of bilaterally symmetrical, high voltage discharges, often consisting of 4/sec spike-and-wave complexes. Such slow and paroxysmal abnormalities persisted in the records of about 30% of the subjects up to the eighth day of abstinence, even in those that did not exhibit motor seizures, and in about 5% of the subjects during the "recovery" period, 2–4 weeks after barbiturate withdrawal.[6]

In about 60% of the subjects, a psychosis emerged between the third and eighth day of abstinence from high daily dose levels of barbiturates. During the first day or two, the clinical psychiatric syndrome was difficult to classify. In some cases it resembled a panic state, in others, schizophrenia, with retention of orientation; in still others, it was suggestive of the Korsakoff syndrome. However, by the second or third day, the syndrome was clearly delirioid, with disorientation, confusion, intense agitation, delusions, and visual and/or auditory hallucinations. This syndrome, indistinguishable from alcoholic delirium tremens, appeared in some subjects without prior seizures, and lasted 3–14 days. In one extremely agitated subject, with rising body temperature and marked tachycardia, it was deemed advisable to terminate the delirium. This was accomplished by administering 1.1 g of secobarbital sodium in divided doses parenterally until he slept; on the following day, he returned to his prewithdrawal daily oral dose of 1.3 g. Agitation and hallucinations subsided rapidly thereafter and eventually he was withdrawn very slowly over a 30-day period without untoward effects.[3]

As shown in Table 2, the intensity of the barbiturate abstinence syndrome is directly related to the total daily dose level from which the subjects were withdrawn. Thus, of 18 subjects withdrawn from 0.4 g of secobarbital or pentobarbital, only one had significant "minor" withdrawal symptoms and none had motor seizures or psychosis; however, paroxysmal discharges appeared in the electroencephalograms of five of these subjects.[7] The two subjects withdrawn from 0.2 g of pentobarbital or secobarbital for 365 days had no detectible abstinence phenomena. On the other hand, of 23 subjects withdrawn from 0.6–0.8 g of secobarbital, 14 had significant "minor" abstinence symptoms, three had seizures (Figure 4), and one had visual hallucinations without the other features of delirium. From these studies, it was concluded that for therapeutic purposes, 0.4 g/day of "short-acting" barbiturates was the maximal "safe" dose, not likely to produce clinically significant physical dependence.

Studies on the neurophysiologic and neurochemical bases of the barbiturate abstinence syndrome were carried out by Essig and his collaborators in dogs, using the long-acting barbiturate, sodium barbital (Veronal), given orally, for chronic intoxication. In intact control dogs, generalized seizures occurred reliably after abrupt withdrawal from sodium barbital, 118–178 mg/kg/day. Prior removal of the cerebellum had no effect on the occurrence of sodium barbital withdrawal seizures.[9] In intact dogs with potential epileptogenic foci produced by intracortial injection of aluminum hydroxide suspension some time before, both focal and generalized seizures occurred after withdrawal of sodium barbital, but these two kinds of seizures had different time courses and occurred independently.[10] After prior removal of the entire cerebral cortex, no motor seizures occurred after abrupt

Table 2. Summary of data on relationship of dosage of secobarbital or pentobarbital to intensity of physical dependence

Patients			Daily Dose of barbiturate, (g)	Days of Intoxication in hospital	No. of patients having symptoms and signs		
	No. receiving						
Total Number	Secobarbital	Pentobarbital			Convulsions	Delirium	Minor Symptoms of significant degree
18	16	2	0.9–2.2	32–144	14	12	18
5	5		0.8	42–57	1	0	5
18	18		0.6	35–57	2	0	9
18	10	8	0.4	90	0	0	1
2	1	1	0.2	365	0	0	0

Reprinted with permission from Fraser et al. 1958. JAMA 166:126–129.

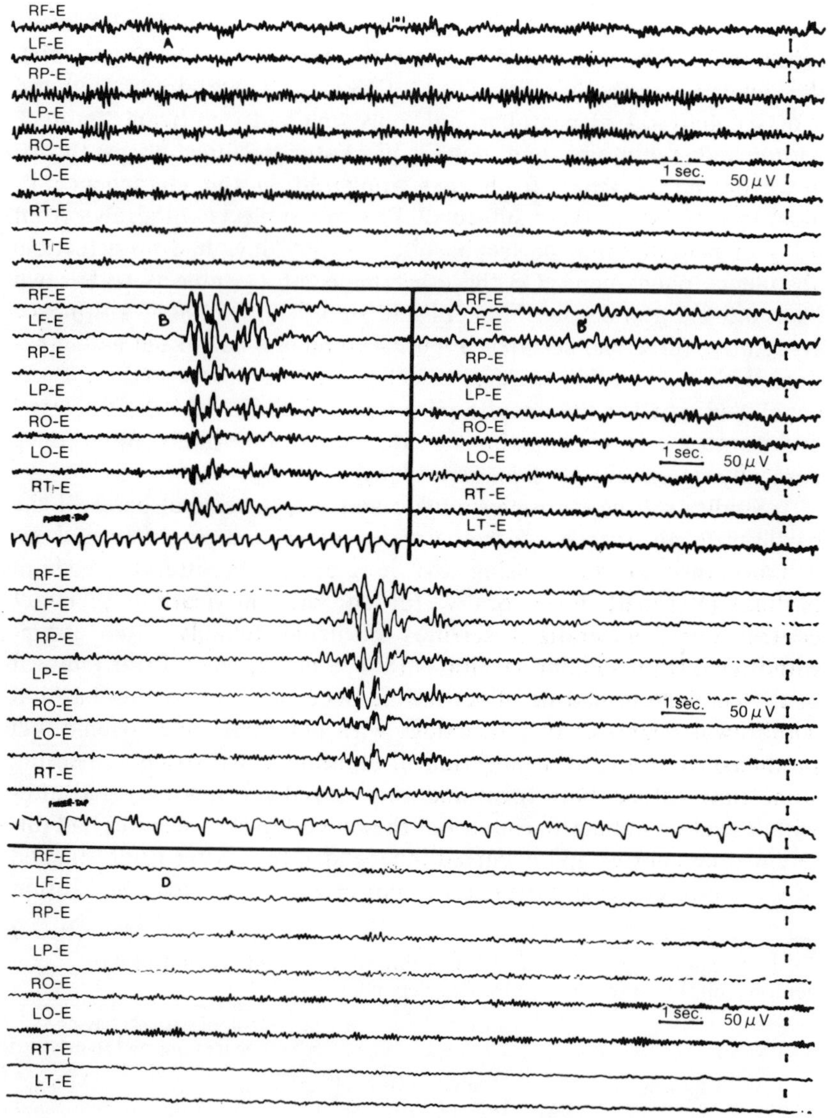

Figure 4. Electroencephalograms during chronic barbiturate intoxication, after abrupt withdrawal, and recovery in one subject. Monopolar recording. In B and C, lowest tracings are voluntary rhythmic finger taps, recorded by transduction. A, 17th day on secobarbital, 0.6 g/day. Dominant rhythmic activity is 7.5–9.5 cps with admixture of low voltage rhythmic fast (21 cps) activity (typical "barbiturate effect"). B, 26 hr after abrupt withdrawal (after 52 days on secobarbital, 0.6 g/day). Bilaterally synchronous spike and slow wave discharges, 54 of which occurred during 58 min of recording without interruption of finger tapping; however, one seizure occurred immediately after

withdrawal of sodium barbital (118–178 mg/kg/day), but one of the dogs displayed what seemed to be "sham rage" behavior. However, when the decorticated dogs were reintoxicated at a higher dose level, namely 190–248 mg/kg/day, tonic extension of the extremities (no clonus), generalized trembling and "sham rage" appeared after abrupt withdrawal of sodium barbital.[11] These studies suggested that the cerebral cortex as well as subcortical structures (but not the cerebellum) are involved in the genesis of the sodium barbital abstinence syndrome.

That chronic sodium barbital intoxication may produce a deficiency of the inhibitory neurotransmitter, gamma-amino-butyric acid (GABA) was suggested by the finding that in intact dogs, amino-oxyacetic acid (AOA), given in doses of 5–8 mg/kg every eight hours for up to seven days beginning 24 hours after abrupt withdrawal from sodium barbital, 150 mg/kg/day, reduced the incidence of withdrawal seizures by half, compared with intact dogs given physiological saline subcutaneously on the same schedule.[12] Inasmuch as AOA inhibits the transaminase that converts GABA into succinic semialdehyde, it might be expected that treatment with AOA would raise GABA levels in the nervous system. However, seizures did occur in the AOA-treated dogs, when the administration of AOA was discontinued. It may be, therefore, that either AOA did not elevate brain levels of GABA, or that the elevation of GABA levels by AOA was only temporary. Of clinical interest are the observations that in intact, otherwise untreated dogs, neither diphenylhydantoin[13] nor chlorpromazine[14] reduced the incidence of sodium barbital withdrawal seizures.

STUDIES ON ADDICTION TO NONBARBITURATE SEDATIVE DRUGS

Essig[15] demonstrated that following chronic around-the-clock intoxication of dogs with meprobamate, abrupt withdrawal of this nonbarbiturate sedative resulted in ultimately fatal status epilepticus in four of the five dogs used, while the remaining dog had withdrawal seizures but survived. Chronic intoxication with glutethimide (114–424 mg/kg

---

this recording. B′, immediately after seizure. Diffuse slowing, especially in frontals. Subject confused, does not recall seizure. C, 72 hours abstinent. Paroxysmal discharges, 20 of which were recorded during 42 min without interruption of finger tapping. D, 7 days abstinent. Electroencephalogram normal, dominant rhythmic activity is 10.5–11 cps. Fully recovered, no complaints. Reprinted with permission from Wikler et al. 1955. Electroenceph. Clin. Neurophysiol. 7:1–13.

over periods of 113–168 days) proved fatal to four out of five dogs used, but the remaining dog survived after having had four generalized seizures.[16] Reviewing the clinical literature, Essig[17] found evidence for the physical dependence-producing effects not only of meprobamate and glutethimide, but also of ethinamate, ethchlorynol, methyprylon, and chlordiazepoxide. In man, paroxysmal discharges in the electroencephalogram may occur after abrupt withdrawal of at least meprobamate in the absence of motor seizures (or delirium). An example of this is shown in Figure 5. This patient had used 3200 mg of meprobamate daily for about four months prior to abrupt withdrawal, which was not followed by any major abstinence phenomena.

STUDIES ON SUBSTITUTION OF ALCOHOL FOR BARBITURATES IN BARBITURATE-DEPENDENT PERSONS

Even more so than in the case of barbiturate dependence, the prevailing clinical opinion a quarter of a century ago was that "rum fits" and alcoholic delirium tremens were "toxic" effects of alcohol, and not alcohol abstinence phenomena. Because of the striking similarity of these phenomena to barbiturate withdrawal seizures and delirium, as demonstrated at the Addiction Research Center, an experimental study of chronic alcohol intoxication and the alcohol abstinence syndrome was undertaken at the addiction Research Center. These studies[18,19] proved conclusively that "rum fits" and delirium tremens were indeed alcohol abstinence phenomena, which differed from barbiturate abstinence phenomena mainly in time course: hallucinosis (without impairment of orientation or memory) could occur between drinks, when the blood alcohol level was falling rapidly; "minor" abstinence changes appeared sooner after the last drink and seizures appeared earlier, usually within the first two days of abstinence; the onset of delirium seemed also to occur somewhat earlier, by the third day of abstinence. Striking differences were found in the electroencephalogram. During chronic alcohol intoxication, frequencies were slowed progressively, with eventual development of partial tolerance; at no stage was there an increase in low voltage, fast rhythmic activity. On abrupt withdrawal of alcohol, the electroencephalographic pattern was usually that of low voltage, fast nonrhythmic activity, with paroxysmal discharges appearing only between the 15th and 18th hours of abstinence, when the blood alcohol concentration had fallen to zero.

Postulating that chronic alcohol and chronic barbiturate intoxi-

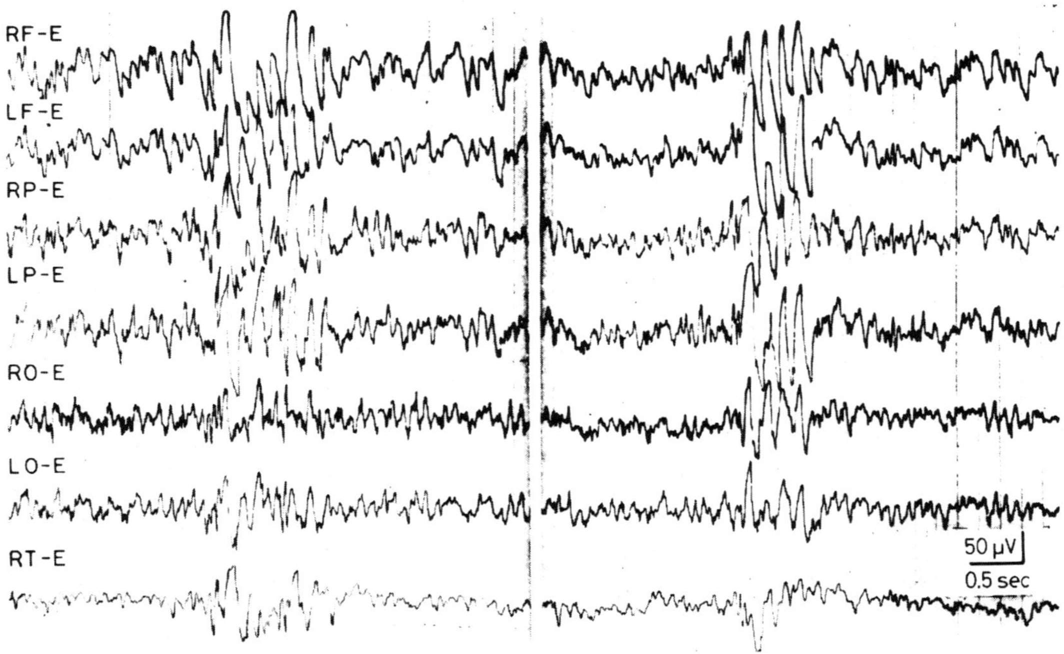

Figure 5. Two examples of spike and slow wave discharges from monopolar electroencephalogram recorded during 42nd hr after abrupt withdrawal of meprobamate in one patient who had used 3200 mg/day for approximately 4 months. Abstinence seizures did not occur. The left temporal tracing was obscured by artifact. Reprinted with permission from Wikler, A., and Essig, C. F. 1970. In: E. Niedermeyer (ed.), Epilepsy. Modern Problems of Pharmacopsychiatry, Vol. 4, pp. 170–184. S. Karger, Basel.

cation may be equivalent pathophysiologically and pharmacologically, a study was undertaken[20] to determine whether alcohol could be substituted for barbiturates in barbiturate-dependent persons, with prevention, or at least clear partial suppression, of the reliably predictable barbiturate abstinence phenomena.

Nine subjects who were taking large daily doses of barbiturates as well as, in some cases, opioids volunteered for the study, after the risks involved had been explained to them. Opioids were withdrawn by the methadone substitution and withdrawal technique, while the subjects were stabilized on pentobarbital sodium (1.67–2.3 g/day) or secobarbital (1.06–1.96 g/day) for periods of 22–44 days. On the first day of substitution, the morning dose of barbiturate was given at 6:00 a.m. and the first drink of alcohol (95% ethanol in three volumes of water or fruit juice) was given at 8:00 a.m. No further barbiturates were administered and drinks of alcohol were given at hourly intervals from 5:00 or 6:00 a.m. to midnight, and depending on the situation, additional drinks were given between 1:00 a.m. and 6:00 a.m. The amount of alcohol per dose was varied with the aim of maintaining a continuous state of intoxication, comparable in degree to that of chronic barbiturate intoxication. Drinking of alcohol was continued for 14 days, after which alcohol was abruptly and completely discontinued. During the period of alcohol substitution a vitamin preparation, given daily by i.m. injection, provided thiamin, 10 mg, riboflavin, 4 mg, and niacinamide, 200 mg. Average daily caloric intake from food varied from 1,738–2,706 calories (except in one subject, 785 calories), while alcohol provided 1,494–2,440 additional calories. Maintenance of a constant blood alcohol concentration proved to be difficult, as frequently the patient vomited after drinking a dose of alcohol. At the end of substitution, blood alcohol concentration varied from 32–352 mg/100 ml.

During alcohol substitution, one seizure followed by delirium of one or two days duration occurred in each of three subjects; at or shortly before the seizures, blood alcohol concentrations were 25 mg/100 ml, 42 mg/100 ml and 351 mg/100 ml in each of the three subjects. It appeared therefore that even a relatively high blood alcohol concentration did not protect one subject from the occurrence of a barbiturate withdrawal seizure. After abrupt withdrawal of alcohol, eight subjects exhibited generally mild "minor" alcohol abstinence phenomena; two subjects had one seizure each and delirium of two days duration, while one had one seizure without delirium. Thereafter, recovery proceeded rapidly.

Comparing these results with the frequency of withdrawal seizures and delirium following chronic intoxication with high daily doses of barbiturates (similar to those given in the course of the alcohol substitution study), it appears that substitution of alcohol reduces the number of barbiturate withdrawal seizures ($p < 0.004$ by the Mann-Whitney nonparametric test) and the frequency and duration of barbiturate withdrawal delirium. However, inasmuch as alcohol did not completely suppress major barbiturate abstinence phenomena, chronic barbiturate and chronic alcohol intoxications are only partially equivalent.

STUDIES ON THE INCIDENCE OF SEDATIVE DRUG DEPENDENCE AT THE UNIVERSITY OF KENTUCKY HOSPITAL PSYCHIATRIC WARD

Following the author's retirement from the U.S. Public Health Service, he joined the Department of Psychiatry at the University of Kentucky. On the University Hospital psychiatric ward, patients with admission diagnoses mainly a depression and anxiety, with or without associated character disorders, alcoholism, or disabling physical illness, frequently gave histories of taking variable quantities of sedative drugs (or such were found in their personal effects at time of admission) and, occasionally, patients developed seizures and/or delirium without their physicians' prior knowledge of sedative drug intake. To obtain an estimate of the incidence of sedative drug physical dependence among such patients, Bakewell and Wikler[21] carefully studied 132 consecutive admissions over a 14-month period with particular reference to their histories of sedative drug intake, their current medications (including those found in their personal effects), and the presence of signs of sedative drug intoxication or sedative drug abstinence phenomena on admission. If these gave any reason for suspecting sedative drug dependence, a pentobarbital cross-tolerance test was carried out, following the method described by Isbell[22] for treatment of barbiturate dependence.

The patient was given a "test" dose of 200 mg of pentobarbital orally or i.m., and observed one hour later (if, on admission, the patient showed signs of sedative drug intoxication, the test was postponed until such signs had vanished). If signs of intoxication were still detectable (ataxia, slurred speech, nystagmus, sleepiness), it was concluded that the patient was not tolerant or cross-tolerant to pentobarbital. If, on the other hand, no signs of pentobarbital intoxication were detectable, the patient was tentatively considered to be tolerant or cross-tolerant and physically dependent, and pentobarbital, 200 mg, was prescribed every six hours, with observation checks for pentobarbital intoxication or pentobarbital abstinence phenomena just before and one hour after each dose. If during the first 24 hours after the test dose the patient became progressively intoxicated, the dose was reduced to 100 mg of pentobarbital every six hours. If, on the other hand, no signs of intoxication appeared, or if abstinence phenomena were observed, the frequency of administration of 200 mg of pentobarbital was increased to every four hours. Thereafter, the dose and/or the frequency of pentobarbital was adjusted with the aim of maintaining a continuous state of mild pentobarbital intoxication throughout the 24 hours of the day. Generally, this could be accomplished within 48 hours after the test dose. The total daily dose of pentobarbital needed to maintain continuous mild intoxication was termed the "stabilization" dose. Inasmuch as Fraser et al.[5] had shown that 0.4 g/day or less of pentobarbital does not produce physical dependence to any significant degree, patients with stabilization doses of 0.4 g/day or less were not considered dependent or cross-dependent on pentobarbital and they were withdrawn rapidly. On the other hand, patients with stabilization doses of over 0.4 g/day of pentobarbital were considered to be both tolerant (or cross-tolerant) and dependent (or cross-dependent) on pentobarbital; in such cases, the stabilization dose of pentobarbital was maintained for 3–5 days, after which pentobarbital was withdrawn *slowly,* at a rate not exceeding 100 mg/day. If even "minor" abstinence signs appeared, the withdrawal procedure was suspended until these signs vanished; withdrawal was then resumed at a rate of 50 mg/day of pentobarbital. It was realized that, because of previous induction of hepatic microsomal nonspecific oxidative enzymes by a variety of sedative drugs or alcohol, a patient stabilized on daily doses of more than 0.4 g/day of pentobarbital might be tolerant or cross-tolerant, but not physically dependent or cross-dependent on pentobarbital; however, for clinical purposes, it was deemed better to be safe than sorry.

Of the 132 consecutive patients, 9 (6.8%) were found who were deemed to be dependent or cross-dependent on pentobarbital. Their daily pentobarbital stabilization doses, the sedative drugs that they had been taking before admission, and the estimated average daily intake of such drugs are given in Table 3. Of some interest is the finding that the sedative drug abused in five of the nine patients was glutethimide. Generally, this drug (as well as chlordiazepoxide and

Table 3. Case summaries

Patient no.	Sex	Age (years)	Drug of abuse: Agent	Drug of abuse: Est. av. daily intake (Mg)	Daily pentobarbital stabilization dose level (Oral, Mg)
1	M	36	Glutethimide	2,500	800
2	F	59	Glutethimide	5,000	1,200
3	F	44	Glutethimide	2,000	900
4	M	60	Glutethimide	4,000	1,200
5	F	49	Glutethimide	1,000	800
			Meprobamate	4,000	
6	F	60	Glutethimide	?	800
			Chlordiazepoxide	100?	
7	F	53	Amphetamine-amobarbital (elixir)	?	800
			Pentobarbital (elixir)	?	
			Aprobarbital (elixir)	?	
8	M	61	Secobarbital	?	1,000
			Pentobarbital	?	
			Butabarbital	?	
			Phenobarbital	?	
			Propantheline and phenobarbital	?	
			Diazepam	?	
9	M	29	Paraldehyde	?	800

Reprinted with permission from Bakewell, W. E., Jr., and Wikler, A. 1966. JAMA 196:710–713.

diazepam) had been prescribed by physicians, but the patients increased the dose and frequency of administration at their own discretion, utilizing refills to obtain the additional quantities of the drug. Also interesting is the fact that *only* 6.8% of 132 psychiatric patients was found to be dependent or cross-dependent on sedative drugs; 93.2% were not dependent or cross-dependent. This raises some questions about the validity of the popular opinion that only persons with "emotional" or "characterological" disorders are likely to abuse sedative drugs.

SUMMARY

Experimental studies in man at the Addiction Research Center demonstrated that during chronic barbiturate intoxication partial tolerance develops to the behavioral and (to a lesser extent) electroencephalographic effects of pentobarbital, secobarbital, or amobarbital. Abrupt withdrawal of barbiturates from chronic intoxication levels of more than 0.4 g/day is followed by "minor" abstinence phenomena (anxiety, tremulousness, muscle twitches, weakness, postural hypotension, anorexia, and insomnia), which first appear within 12–24 hours after the last dose. Withdrawal is generally followed on the second or third day of abstinence by generalized seizures and/or delirium that begins on the third to the eighth day of abstinence. The frequency of occurrence of withdrawal seizures and/or delirium was directly related to the chronic intoxication daily dose level, over a range of 0.6–2.3 g/day. Paroxysmal discharges appeared in the electroencephalogram after abrupt withdrawal of barbiturates even when no abstinence seizures occurred.

Substitution of ethanol for "short-acting" barbiturates in barbiturate dependent subjects *partially* suppresses barbiturate abstinence seizures and delirium.

In dogs, decortication but not decerebellation elevates the daily dose of barbital required for the occurrence of seizures after abrupt withdrawal, and modifies their characteristics, the seizure consisting of tonic extension (no clonus) and "sham rage." Amino-oxyacetic acid suppressed barbital withdrawal seizures, but seizures occurred after withdrawal of amino-oxyacetic acid. Neither diphenylhydantoin nor chlorpromazine suppressed barbital withdrawal seizures.

Among 132 consecutive patients admitted to the University of Kentucky Hospital psychiatric ward, with primary diagnoses other than drug dependence, 9 (6.8%) were found to be tolerant or cross-tolerant and presumably dependent or cross-dependent on pentobarbital by the pentobarbital "stabilization test" (daily "stabilization dose," 0.8–1.2 g/day). It is remarkable that 93.2% of such patients with psychiatric disorders were not found to be dependent or cross-dependent on pentobarbital.

LITERATURE CITED

1. Pohlisch, K., and Panse, F. 1934. Schlafmittelmissbrauch. Georg Thieme, Leipzig.
2. Kalinowsky, L. 1942. Arch. Neurol. Psychiat. 48:949.

3. Isbell, H., Altschul, S., Kornetsky, C. H., Eisenman, A. J., Flanary, H. G., and Fraser, H. F. 1950. Arch. Neurol. Psychiat. 64:1.
4. Fraser, H. F., Isbell, H., Eisenman, A. J., Wikler, A., and Pescor, F. T. 1954. Arch. Int. Med. 94:34.
5. Fraser, H. F., Wikler, A., Essig, C. F., and Isbell, H. 1958. Amer. Med. Ass. 166:126.
6. Wikler, A., Fraser, H. F., Isbell, H., and Pescor, F. T. 1955. Electroenceph. Clin. Neurophysiol. 7:1.
7. Essig, C. F., and Fraser, H. F. 1958. Electroenceph. Clin. Neurophysiol. 10:649.
8. Wulff, M. H. 1959. Electroenceph. Clin. Neurophysiol. 14 (Suppl.):173.
9. Essig, C. F. 1964. Int. J. Neuropharmacol. 3:453.
10. Essig, C. F. 1962. Psychopharmacologia 3:432.
11. Essig, C. F. 1962. Arch. Neurol. 7:471.
12. Essig, C. F. 1963. Int. J. Neuropharmacol. 2:199.
13. Essig, C. F., and Carter, W. W. 1962. Neurology 12:481.
14. Essig, C. F., and Fraser, H. F. 1966. Clin. Pharmacol. Ther. 7:466.
15. Essig, C. F. 1958. Arch. Neurol. Psychiat. 80:414.
16. Essig, C. F. 1963. Amer. J. Psychiat. 119:993.
17. Essig, C. F. 1964. Clin. Pharmacol. Ther. 5:334.
18. Isbell, H., Fraser, H. F., Wikler, A., Belleville, R. E., and Eisenman, A. J. 1955. Quart. J. Stud. Alcohol 16:1.
19. Wikler, A., Pescor, F. T., Fraser, H. F., and Isbell, H. 1956. Amer. J. Psychiatr. 113:106.
20. Fraser, H. F., Wikler, A., Isbell, H., and Johnson, N. K. 1957. Quart. J. Stud. Alcohol 18:541.
21. Bakewell, W. E., Jr., and Wikler, A. 1966. JAMA 196:710.
22. Isbell, H. 1950. Med. Clin. North America 34:425.

Drug-Maintained Performance Procedures and the Assessment of Drug-Abuse Liability

Joseph V. Brady

and

Roland R. Griffiths

The experimental analysis of drug-maintained performances over the past decade has provided evidence of a good correspondence between compounds self-administered by laboratory animals and those abused by man.[1-3] More recently, research attention has been directed toward the assessment of relative abuse liability or the rank ordering of such compounds with respect to the range of drugs self-administered by laboratory animals.[4-7] Behavioral assessment procedures for evaluating such comparative abuse liability have been based generally upon research involving the performance-maintenance potential (e.g., reinforcing properties) of different environmental stimuli (e.g., food, drugs, etc.). Differential performance-maintenance potency has been assumed to reflect the "strength" (Hodos, 1961 (Ref. 20)) or "efficacy"[8] of stimuli as response-contingent reinforcers, though interpretive caution is required in extrapolating such hypothetical intervening processes to the comparative assessment of drug abuse liability. Behavioral measurement procedures for evaluating the differential reinforcing effects of stimuli, however, do seem to provide useful information about the relative reinforcing strength of various doses of a single drug, as well as the rank ordering of different drugs for their abuse potential.

A number of studies involving the analysis of intravenous drug reinforcement in laboratory animals have examined a range of

This research was supported by DEA Contract J-69-15 and NIDA Grant DA 01147.

chemical substances utilizing continuous reinforcement schedules.[9-13] The rates of responding maintained by such continuous drug reinforcement schedules have proven difficult to use as a measure of relative abuse liability because response rate under these conditions is often inversely related to the dose of a given compound. Where the schedule of reinforcement does not involve such a close relationship between response rate increases and elevations in drug intake, however, the rate of responding may reflect differential reinforcement magnitude independently of reinforcement frequency.[14] Under conditions involving the use of two concurrently available equally valued reinforcement schedules producing different drug reinforcers, response rates have been reported to reliably reflect relative reinforcement efficacy.[15,16] In addition, closely related discrete-trial choice or preference procedures for assessing the relative reinforcing properties of stimulus events have recently been shown to effectively discriminate between different doses and types of drugs.[6,8,17-19]

Perhaps the earliest and most extensively developed behavioral assessment procedure for evaluating relative drug abuse liability has involved the application of progressive ratio performances and response cost measures of reinforcement strength. This methodological approach to the evaluation of abuse liability generally requires two steps focusing on: 1) establishing a substitution baseline on which drug reinforcement is delivered contingent upon emission of a specified operant performance, and 2) systematically increasing the number of responses required for each drug reinforcement until responding falls below some criterion level. The response requirement at which this criterion is met is referred to as the breaking point, and a number of studies have reported orderly increasing relationships between breaking point and such variables as degree of food deprivation,[20] concentration and volume of liquid reinforcer,[21] and the intensity and train duration of electrical intracranial stimulation.[22,23] In addition, two recent reports have described drug comparisons using this method in which cocaine was found to maintain consistently higher breaking points than several other compounds, including methylphenidate, SPA, methylamphetamine, and amphetamine.[5,7] Although the results of those studies showing that breaking point varies as a function of several "motivational" conditions are suggestive that progressive ratio procedures may provide a meaningful comparative measure of the relative strength or efficacy of a reinforcing stimulus, the studies on drugs in this regard are limited to the extent that only a narrow range of doses have thus far been examined.

The studies to be described in the present report focus on two interrelated measures, derived from the two-part sequence involved in the application of a progressive ratio procedure to the comparative assessment of drug abuse liability with laboratory primates. Male baboons (*Papio anubis*) weighing 12–25 kg served as subjects in these experiments. Details of the special restraint and housing system, cannulation technique, and multiple drug infusion system have been previously described in detail.[4] Briefly, a special chair was designed,[24] which restrained the baboon by means of moveable arm cuffs and a waist plate. This system effectively minimized physical stress while at the same time affording the positive protection of indwelling catheters essential for chronic studies. Each animal, fitted to his own cart, was individually housed within a 0.8 × 0.8 × 1.2 m sound-resistant experimental chamber. The baboon faced an "intelligence" panel containing necessary stimulus displays and associated behavioral control devices as illustrated in Figure 1. The animals were maintained within this space, subject to the continuous conditions of a given experiment, although once each day the chamber was opened for maintainence of the equipment and close inspection of the baboon. Water was freely available via a drinking tube and food pellets were continuously available to the subject by means of a modest fixed-ratio response requirement on the food lever.

After initial behavioral training of approximately two months on

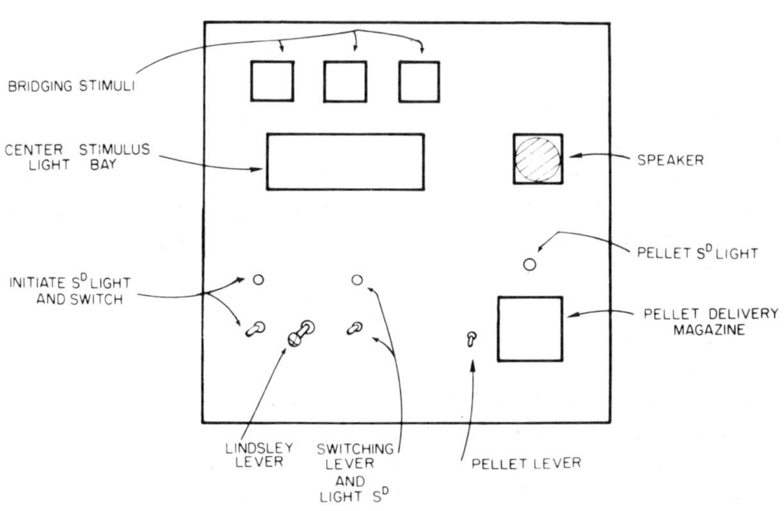

Figure 1. Intelligence panel within experimental chamber.

the progressive-ratio paradigm (described below) with food reinforcement, each subject was surgically prepared with an intravenous catheter using the general procedure reported by Deneau, Yanagita, and Seevers.[2] The catheter infusion system and procedures for preparation and administration of the drugs involved in these studies have been previously described in detail.[6,7]

The initial question addressed in the application of this methodology focused on a determination of drug reinforcement properties as measured by the maintenance of a self-infusion performance. Availability of a single drug infusion occurred at a minimum interval of 3 hours since the last infusion, thus limiting the maximum number of possible infusions to 8 each day. Infusion availability was indicated by a 5-second tone and illumination of a jewel light directly over the lever located slightly to the left of center at the bottom of the subjects' intelligence panel (see Figure 1). The lever was a standard leaf switch that required a downward force of approximately 150 g for closure. When the jewel light was illuminated, each response on the lever produced a brief feedback tone (approximately 0.3 sec). Upon completion of a fixed-ratio requirement of 160 responses (FR 160), the jewel light over the lever was extinguished and a 5 × 5 cm stimulus light was illuminated in the upper left hand corner of the intelligence panel for a 1-hour period. In addition, the drug infusion began at this time.

Self-infusion performance was first established with cocaine at a dose of 0.4 mg/kg per infusion. After five consecutive days of cocaine availability, during which six or more infusions were taken each day, a specified dose of the test drug or saline was substituted for the cocaine. At least seven days access to each dose of drug or saline was permitted. Cocaine was then reinstated, and when the criterion of five consecutive days of six or more infusions per day had been met, another dose or drug was again substituted. The order of exposure to drugs, saline, and different doses was mixed; all subjects were given twelve days of access to saline several times during the examination of different drugs at different doses. This basic approach thus provided a standardized procedure for evaluating the reinforcing properties of drugs, and a number of compounds have been examined in this way including a recent series of phenylethylamine amphetamine derivatives marketed as clinical anorectics.

Figure 2, for example, illustrates results obtained with the substitution in one baboon. The figure shows that when saline or a low dose (0.1 mg/kg) of diethylpropion was substituted for cocaine, the self-

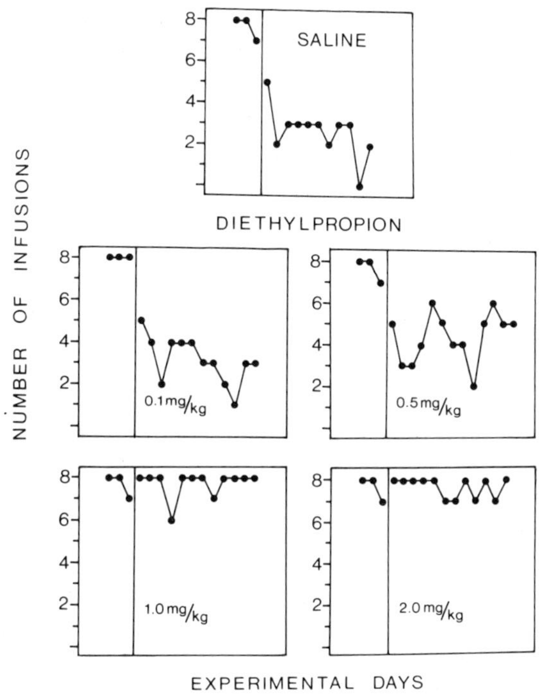

Figure 2. Daily pattern of self-infusion maintained by various doses of diethylpropion, HCl, and saline in the same subject. The initial three-day period of each determination shows the self-infusion performance maintained by cocaine (HCl, 0.4 mg/kg) before substitution of saline or the indicated dose of diethylpropion. Drug doses are expressed as the salt. The infusion duration was approximately 100 seconds.

infusion performance decreased during the twelve-day substitution period until the subject received only two or three infusions per day. At a dose of 0.5 mg/kg diethylpropion, self-infusion performance was maintained at an average rate of about five infusions per day, which was higher than saline but lower than the preceding cocaine control periods. Finally, at the highest doses tested, 1.0 and 2.0 mg/kg, the figure shows that relatively stable rates of self-infusion were maintained at overall rates comparable to cocaine control periods (seven or eight infusions per day).

In the course of evaluating the reinforcing properties of the anorectic stimulants, it has been possible to measure the average number of food pellets consumed per day as a function of the average self-infused daily drug dose. In general, the results show that increasing doses of all such drugs were associated with decreases in food pellet consumption. Furthermore, the dose-effect relationships derived from the two measures of reinforcing efficacy and anorectic potency provide the basis for calculating a "toxicity ratio," which is somewhat akin to the more conventional Therapeutic Index. In this case, however, the ratio numerator is provided by a measure of the lowest drug dose that suppresses food intake, and the denominator is derived from a measure of the lowest drug dose that maintains stable self-administration. Extrapolating from this relationship, it is obvious that the ideal anorectic would suppress food intake without having any reinforcing properties, and the most undesirable compounds in this regard would have only weak anorectic effects combined with powerful reinforcing effects. In fact, the range of anorectic stimulants that we have thus far studied can be shown to yield very orderly and systematic ratio data that provide a potentially useful measure of the relationship between the apparently therapeutic and toxic properties of the compounds in this category.

As useful as the substitution procedure may be for providing information about whether or not a drug is a reinforcer, as well as some pertinent facts about dose-effect relationships, it is of but limited value in determining relative reinforcing strength compared to other self-administered drugs. Indeed, there are few if any reliable methods for which extensive data has been developed in this regard, as the introductory paragraphs of this chapter have indicated. At least one such procedure, however, the progressive ratio or response cost method, appears to hold some promise for a productive yield in this complex domain of relative abuse liability assessment, although as indicated, the extent to which dose-effect relationships with a range of compounds have been investigated to date is unfortunately limited. The remainder of the present chapter is devoted to the data we have thus far developed in extending the application of this procedure to a comparative assessment of abuse liability with a number of stimulant and depressant drugs.

An outline of the behavioral sequence involved in the initial progressive ratio procedure used in our laboratory is illustrated in Figure 3. As with the previously described substitution procedure, the availability of a trial occurred at an interval of three hours since the completion of the preceding trial. The availability of a trial was indicated by an 8-second auditory tone stimulus, followed by the illumination of a jewel light directly over the "initiate" lever located at the far left of the subject's intelligence panel. The initiate lever was a standard leaf switch that required a downward force of approximately 150 g

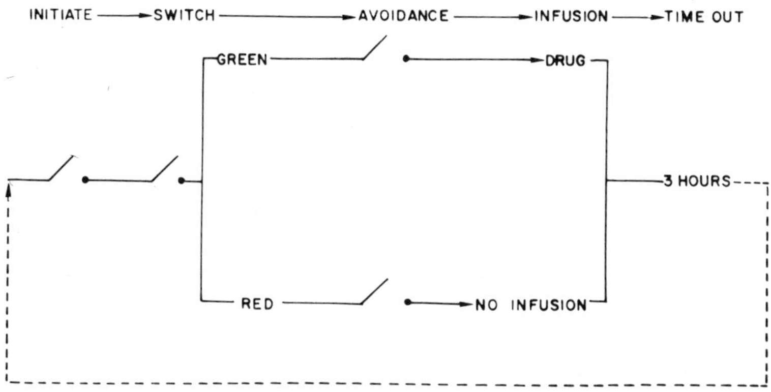

Figure 3. Diagrammatic representation of progressive-ratio behavioral sequence.

for closure. A fixed-ratio response requirement (FR X) on the initiate lever was necessary to proceed with the trial. Upon completion of this initiate ratio, the jewel light over the initiate lever was extinguished while a second jewel light was illuminated over the "switching" lever (standard leaf switch) located slightly to the left of center at the bottom of the intelligence panel. Simultaneously the subject was presented with a 5-second tone and one of two colors (red or green) in the 5 × 15 cm stimulus light bay on the upper center of the intelligence panel; the color initially presented was alternated on each trial.

At this point in the behavioral sequence, the subject had the opportunity to "lock in" the color presented or change the color. Responding on the switching lever changed the color in the stimulus bay on every fifth response (FR 5 schedule). However, the first response on the Lindsley lever (located between the initiate and switching levers) "locked in" the prevailing color in the light bay and set up a shock avoidance requirement on the same lever. Under this schedule, every 2 minutes a 3-second illumination of a white light in the stimulus light bay was followed by an electric shock (4 ma, 0.25 sec) through a tail electrode, unless the animal made 15 responses within the 2 minutes. The avoidance requirement was identical for both red and green colors and was included to provide a possible measure of some of the nonspecific behavioral effects of the drugs. When the avoidance requirement was fulfilled, the center stimulus bay light was extinguished while a smaller 5 × 5 cm bridging stimulus light of the same color was illuminated in the upper section of the

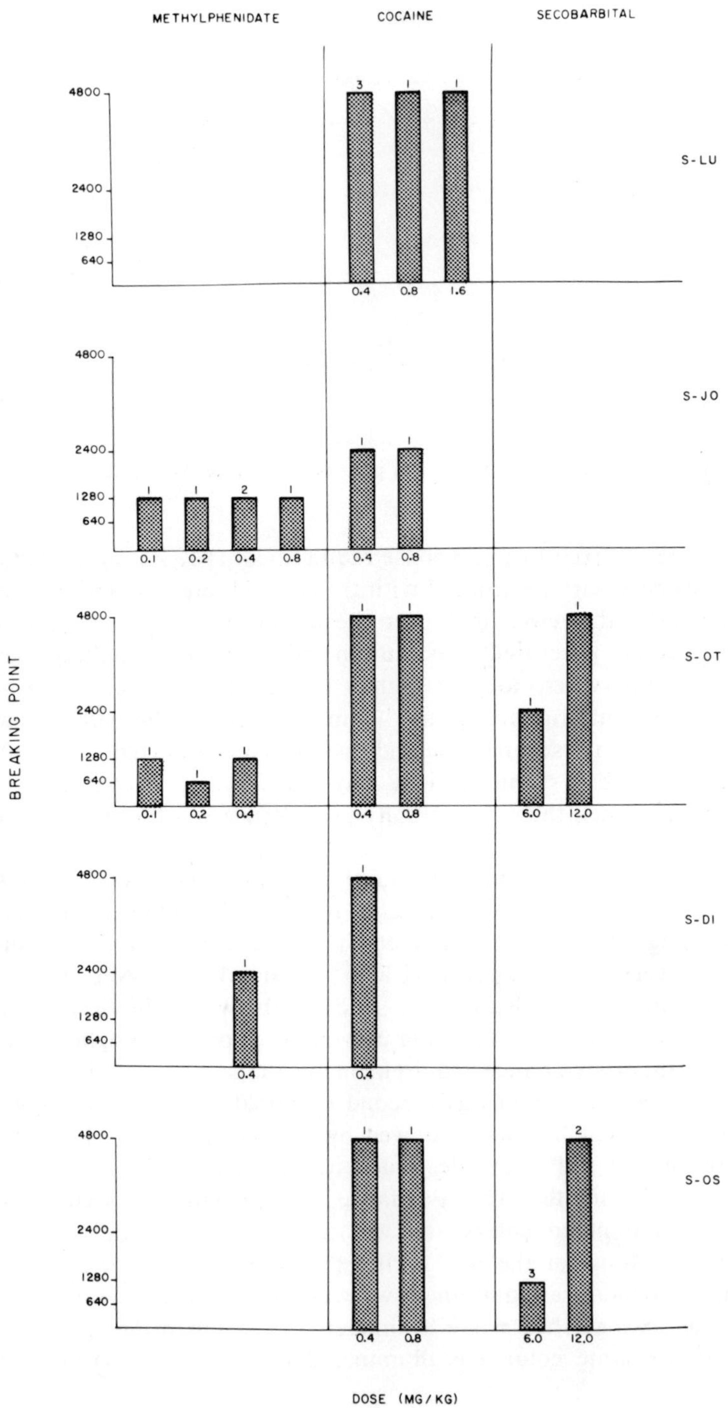

METHYLPHENIDATE
COCAINE
SECOBARBITAL
BREAKING POINT
4800
2400
1280
640
S-LU
S-JO
S-OT
S-DI
S-OS
0.1
0.2
0.4
0.8
1.6
6.0
12.0
DOSE (MG/KG)

intelligence panel for a 1-hour period. The drug infusion also began at this time, provided that the trial has been completed in the drug-associated color (green). Completion of the trial in red resulted in no infusion.

On the basis of subsequent experience, a substantially simplified behavioral sequence was developed for use in some of the later progressive ratio studies described below. The simplified procedure involved omitting the switching and avoidance components of the behavioral sequence. The intelligence panel was identical except for the absence of the switching and avoidance levers and their corresponding stimulus lights. Trials were identical in all respects except that the 5-second tone was presented at the onset of trial availability and that completion of the response requirement on the initiate lever resulted in the immediate infusion of drug and illumination of the bridging light (upper left) on each trial.

A breaking point experiment involved first introducing a drug on the progressive-ratio procedure with a low ratio requirement on the intiate lever (usually FR160), and obtaining a baseline performance of a high and stable frequency of trial completion, and a consistent selection of the drug alternative. Once this performance was established, the ratio requirement on the initiate lever was systematically increased every seven days until the rate of completing trials fell below a criterion level (two or less trials per day for three consecutive days, or four of the seven days at the fixed-ratio value). A breaking point was defined as the ratio value at which criterion performance disruption occurred. The sequence of ratio values used was: 160, 320, 640, 1280, 2400, 4800, and 9600. Following disruption of performance, the ratio requirement on the initiate lever was lowered, and the original performance recovered before the replication of the experiment or substitution of another dose or drug.

The results of our initial series of breaking point comparisons with a limited range of stimulant and depressant compounds is summarized in Figure 4. Above each bar is indicated the number of determinations at that condition, while the absence of a bar indicates the subject was not exposed to that condition. Twelve breaking point determinations were obtained with cocaine in a total of five subjects. Within-subject comparisons show that dose manipulations had no

Figure 4. Breaking point values for doses of methylphenidate, cocaine, and secobarbital in five subjects. Each *bar* represents breaking point obtained at indicated dose of drug. Numeral above *bar* indicates the number of determinations at that dose. In all cases, multiple determinations resulted in identical breaking point values. Absence of *bar* indicates subject was not exposed to that condition.

effect on absolute breaking point. Of the four subjects exposed to multiple doses of cocaine, all showed identical breaking points at doses of 0.4 and 0.8 mg/kg cocaine. Furthermore, the one subject exposed as well to a higher dose of cocaine (1.6 mg/kg) showed the same breaking points at all three doses.

Illustrative daily data for one subject (S-LU) are presented in Figure 5, which shows the results of five successive breaking point determinations with cocaine at doses ranging from 0.4 to 1.6 mg/kg. The first two determinations and the last determination are at a constant dose of 0.4 mg/kg and demonstrate within-subject replication. In the first determination, although the breaking point criterion was met at FR 4800, the ratio was increased to 9600 for five days. Following recovery of performance at an FR 160, a replication of the breaking point determination at this dose revealed clear disruption of performance at FR 4800 (the ratio value of 320 was inadvertently omitted from this determination). Subsequent determinations at doses of 0.8, 1.6, and 0.4 mg/kg of cocaine all produced a breaking point of 4800 responses.

Samples of ratio initiate performance on cocaine reinforced trials of S-LU are presented in Figure 6. As described previously, trial availability was indicated by the sounding of a tone and illumination of the initiate panel light. Under low ratio values, subjects typically showed little or no pausing before responding at a high stable rate until the ratio was completed. Under high ratio values, subjects typically showed considerable pausing with intermittent response bursting before responding at a high, relatively stable rate until completion of the ratio.

Figure 4 summarizes nine breaking point determinants with methylphenidate in a total of three subjects. As with cocaine, within-subject comparison suggests that dose manipulation with methylphenidate had no effect on absolute breaking point. For one subject (S-JO), five separate determinations over an 8-fold dose range (0.1–0.8 mg/kg) all produced identical breaking points. The second subject (S-OT) showed breaking points at 1280, 640, and 1280 at doses of 0.1, 0.2, and 0.4 mg/kg, respectively.

Illustrative daily data for S-JO presented in Figure 7 show the results of five breaking point determinations with methylphenidate, with doses ranging from 0.1 to 0.8 mg/kg. Examination of the figure with respect to number of trials completed per day shows a clear disruption of trial completion at 1280 responses at each dose, with some weakening of performance at 320 and 640 responses.

Following the fourth determination with this subject, cocaine was substituted for methylphenidate and two breaking points of 2400 were obtained. Subsequently, the subject was returned to 0.4 mg/kg methylphenidate and replication of the breaking point determination at this dose indicated again a criterion disruption of performance at 1280.

The within-trial response pattern of initiate performance with methylphenidate was similar to that described with cocaine. Under low fixed-ratio values there was little or no pausing, while under higher ratios there was considerable pausing with some response bursting before responding at a high, relatively stable rate until completion of the ratio.

Figure 4 summarizes seven breaking point determinations with secobarbital in two subjects. Within-subject comparison shows that for both subjects increasing the dose of secobarbital from 6.0 to 12.0 mg/kg resulted in higher breaking point values.

Illustrative daily data for S-OS, presented in Figure 8 show the results of five breaking point determinations with secobarbital. At a dose of 6.0 mg/kg a high number of trials were completed at low ratio values. The figure shows that clear disruption of a trial completion occurred and was immediately replicated at a ratio value of 1280. The performance baseline was then recovered and the dose increased to 12.0 mg/kg. Although the trial completion showed some variability at ratio values of 1280 and 2400 at this dose, the criterion for disruption was first obtained at 4800. As shown, additional replication at doses of 6.0 and 12.0 mg/kg confirmed the breaking point values of 1280 and 4800 responses, respectively. The within-trial response pattern of initiate performance with secobarbital was similar to that described for cocaine and methylphenidate.

Since all three drugs were examined in behaviorally active dose ranges (i.e., at doses that were self-administered) and in some cases at identical absolute doses within the same subjects, some between-drug comparisons are possible. One interesting comparison is that between methylphenidate and cocaine. Examination of Figure 4 shows that three subjects were exposed to the same absolute dose of both drugs (0.4 mg/kg). In each case, cocaine produced a higher breaking point than methylphenidate. Furthermore, at the range of doses studied, within-subject comparison reveals that all of the cocaine breaking points (five determinations total) were higher than all of the breaking points obtained with methylphenidate (nine determinations total).

Another interesting comparison is the dose-response difference in

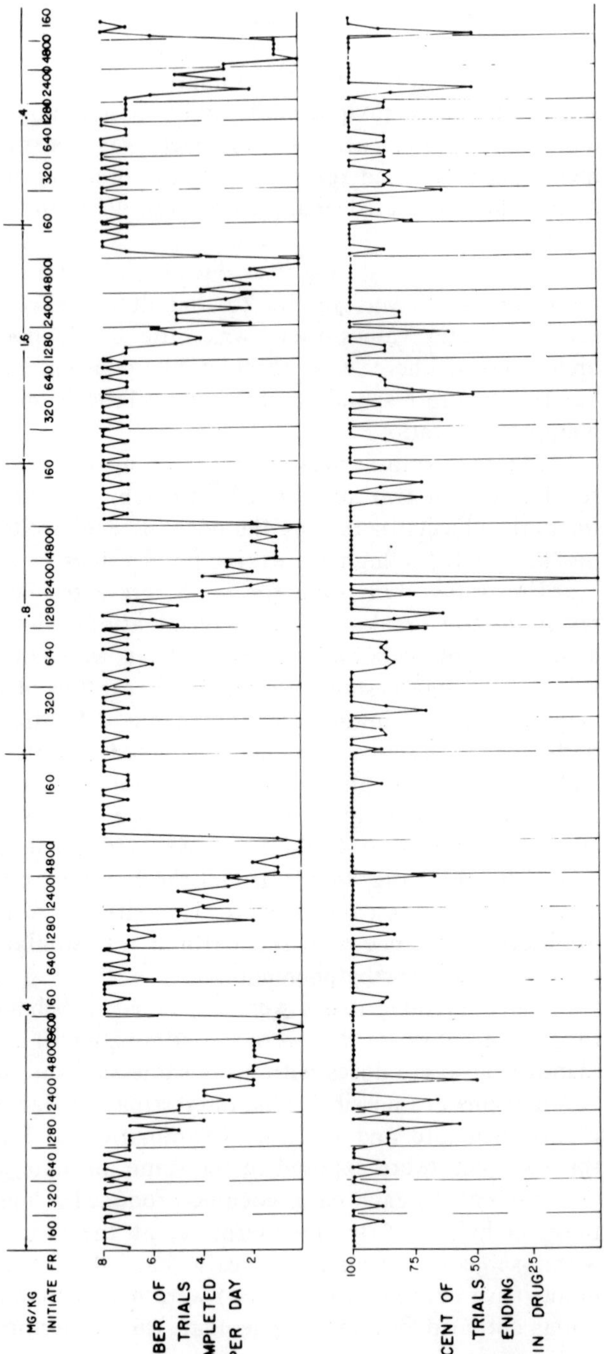
S-LU
MG/KG
INITIATE FR
NUMBER OF TRIALS COMPLETED PER DAY
PERCENT OF TRIALS ENDING IN DRUG

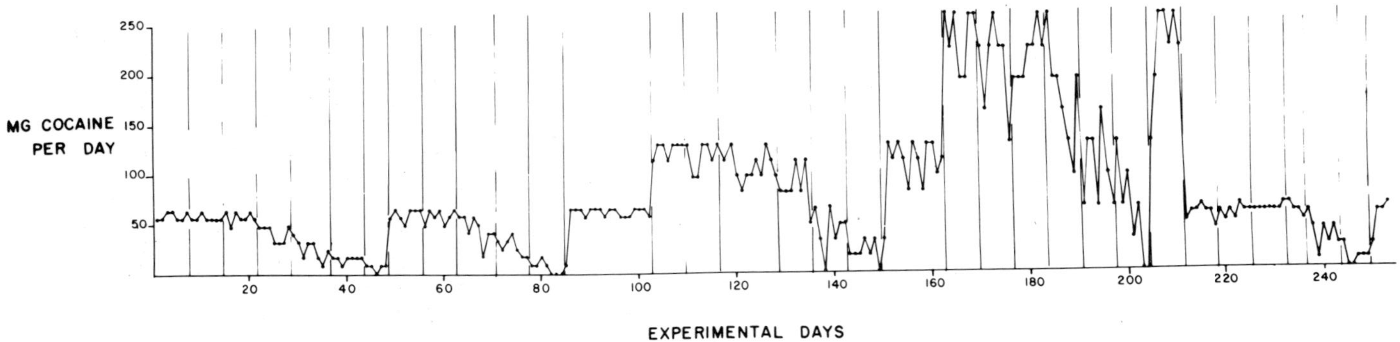

Figure 5. Five successive breaking point determinations with cocaine at doses of 0.4, 0.4, 0.8, 1.6, and 0.4 mg/kg, respectively, in S-LU.

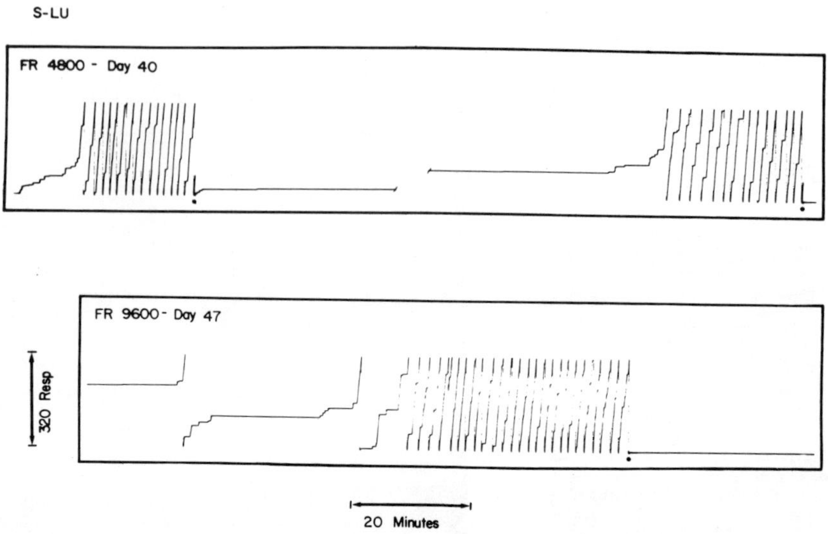

Figure 6. Representative cumulative records of initiate performance with cocaine (0.4 mg/kg) in S-LU. Recorder was turned off during three-hour timeout period during which responding had no consequence. Dots indicate completion of preceding trial and availability of next trial.

secobarbital versus methylphenidate and cocaine. At the range of doses studied, the manipulation of doses of the stimulant compounds (methylphenidate and cocaine) had little or no effect on breaking points; whereas increasing doses of secobarbital produced increased breaking point values. Of the six occasions (involving a total of 19 determinations) in which multiple doses of a stimulant compound were examined within the same subject, there was only one instance in which identical breaking points were not obtained. In that instance, S-OT showed breaking point values of 1280, 640, and 1280 at doses of 0.1, 0.2, and 0.4 mg/kg of methylphenidate, respectively. Given that the intermediate dose produced the lowest breaking point value (an unlikely dose-response effect) and that the effect was not obtained in S-JO, who showed identical breaking points over a wide range of methylphenidate doses, it seems likely that this difference may have been eliminated upon further replication. In any case, in five out of six occasions on which subjects were exposed to multiple doses of stimulant drugs, identical breaking points were obtained at all doses studied and for all replications (a total of 19 separate determinations). These observations involved a 4-fold dose range for cocaine and an 8-fold range for methylphenidate. In contrast, the two subjects exposed to two doses of secobarbital (7 determinations total) both showed increases in breaking points when the dose was increased from 6.0 to 12.0 mg/kg. Furthermore, both of these subjects had demonstrated dose independence with respect to stimulant drugs.

Subsequently, additional procedural modifications involving not only elimination of the switching and avoidance components, but also a fore-shortening of the seven-day ratio sequence and alteration of the breaking point criterion, were instituted with a view to increasing the efficiency of the method and permitting more complete dose-effect analyses. Under these circumstances, it has been possible to undertake breaking point comparisons between a number of compounds including cocaine, diethylpropion, chlorphentermine, and fenfluramine based upon more extensive dose-response determinations. Doses examined have ranged from those that did not maintain stable self-infusion, through those that maintained stable breaking points, up to doses so high that criterion self-infusion levels could not be maintained. The results obtained reflect orderly and systematic dose-effect relationships between various compounds thus far examined, with cocaine generally maintaining the highest breaking points, followed in order by diethylpropion, chlorphentermine, and fenfluramine. Moreover, there were doses of cocaine that maintained higher average breaking points than all tested doses of the other three drugs, and there were doses of diethylpropion that maintained higher breaking points than all doses of either chlorphentermine or fenfluramine. Finally, there were doses of chlorphentermine that maintained higher breaking points than all doses of fenfluramine.

Clearly, these results suggest that the progressive ratio procedure has the potential for providing useful information pertinent to the assessment of relative drug abuse liability. It is essential that until additional data is developed, the current breaking point differences between compounds be interpreted with caution, because in some instances maximum breaking point data involves considerable overlap. The present findings involve an examination of the indicated compounds over a substantial dose range, thus reducing the possibility that the observed differences are merely artifacts of the tested doses. Moreover, the correspondence between the rank ordering that emerges from such an analysis and the reported experiences with abuse problems at the human level is encouragingly good.

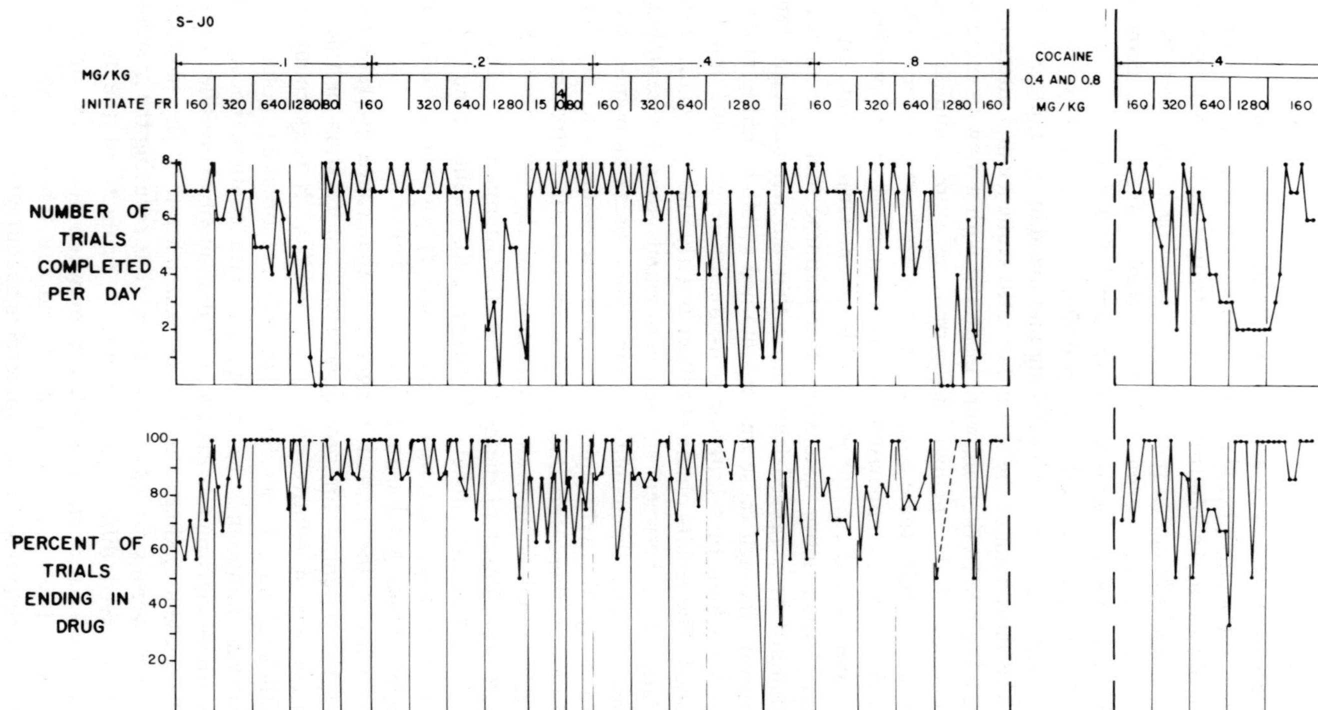
S-JO
MG/KG
INITIATE FR
.1
.2
.4
.8
160
320
640
1280
80
15
4
COCAINE
0.4 AND 0.8
MG/KG
NUMBER OF TRIALS COMPLETED PER DAY
8
6
4
2
PERCENT OF TRIALS ENDING IN DRUG
100
80
60
40
20

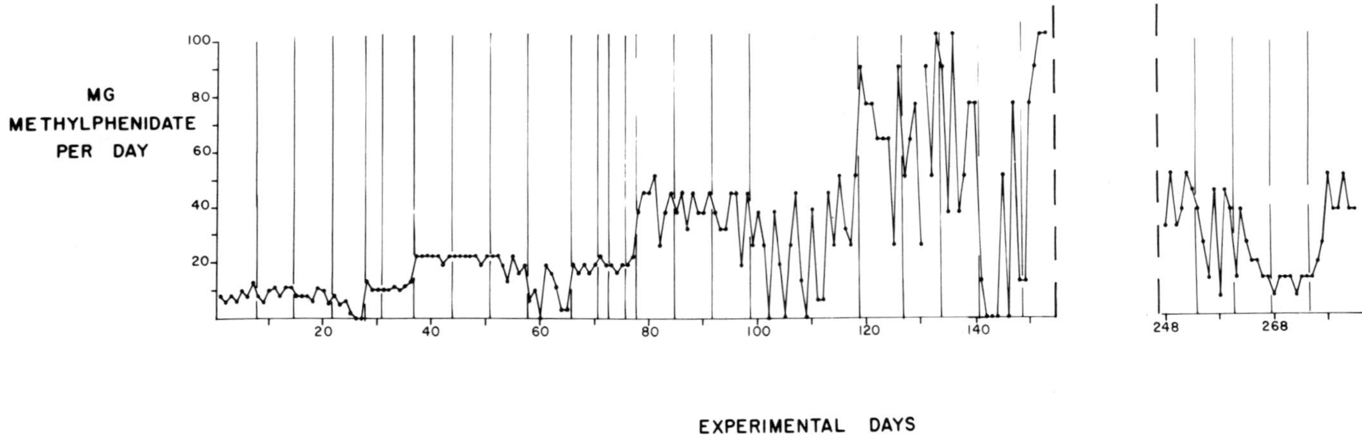

Figure 7. Five breaking point determinations with methylphenidate at doses of 0.1, 0.2, 0.4, 0.8 and 0.4 mg/kg, respectively, in S-JO. On experimental days 154–247 breaking point determinations were made with cocaine at indicated doses.

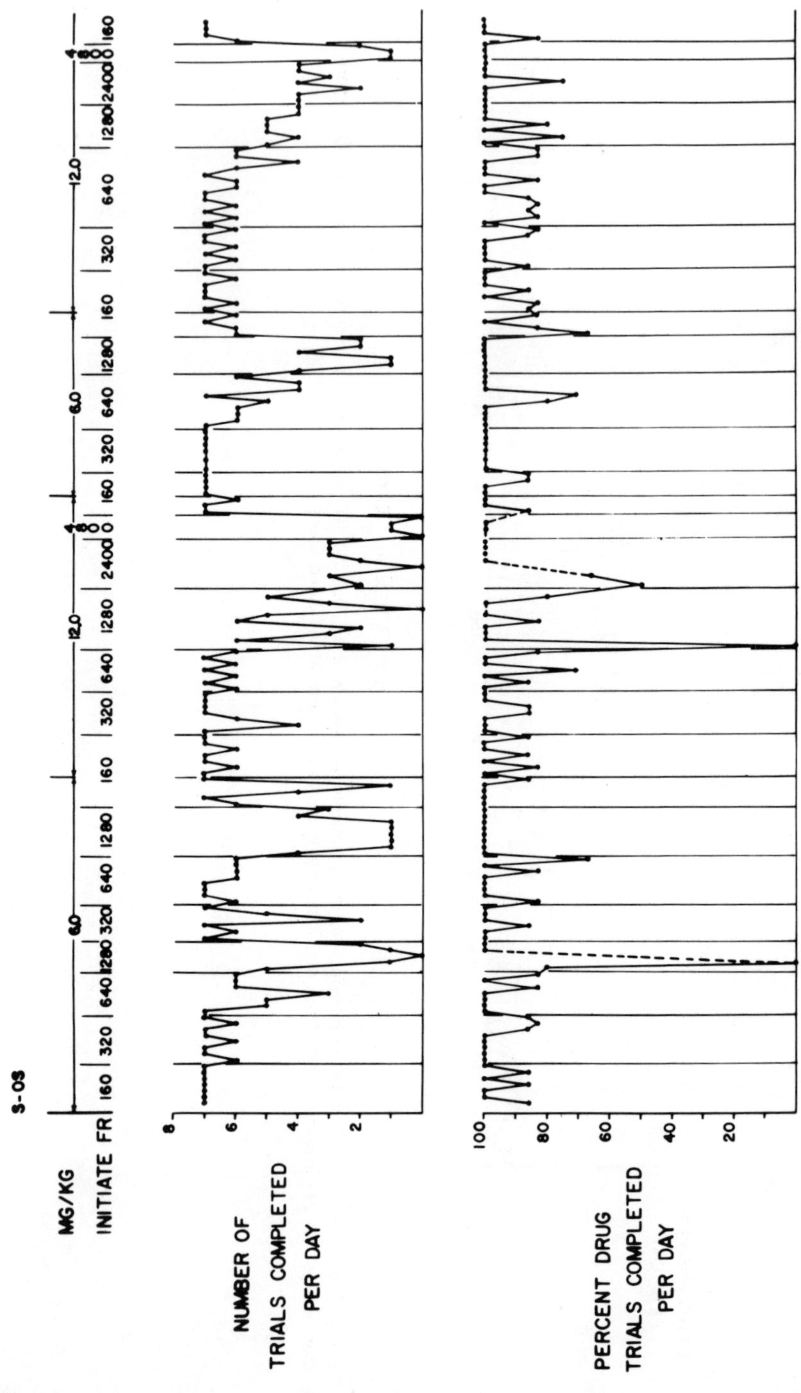
S-03
MG/KG
INITIATE FR
NUMBER OF TRIALS COMPLETED PER DAY
PERCENT DRUG TRIALS COMPLETED PER DAY

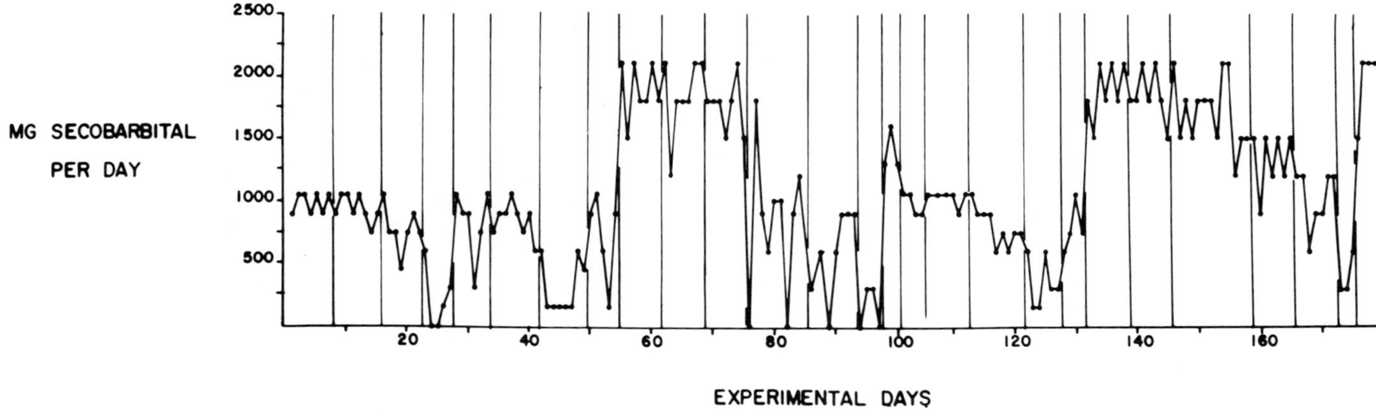

Figure 8. Five successive breaking point determinations with secobarbital at doses of 6.0, 6.0, 12.0, 6.0, and 12.0 mg/kg, respectively, in S-OS.

LITERATURE CITED

1. Schuster, C. R., and Thompson, T. 1969. Ann. Rev. Pharmacol. 9:483–502.
2. Deneau, G. A., Yanagita, T., and Seevers, M. H. 1969. Psychopharmacologia 16:30.
3. Woods, J. H., and Tessel, R. E. 1974. Science 185:1067–1069.
4. Findley, J. D., Robinson, W. W., and Peregrino, J. 1972. Psychopharmacologia 26:93–114.
5. Yanagita, T. 1973. Bull. Narc. 1:25–57.
6. Brady, J. V., Griffiths, R. R., and Winger, G. 1975. Hypnotics: Methods of Development and Evaluation, pp. 221–235. Spectrum Publications Inc., New York.
7. Griffiths, R. R., Findley, J. D., Brady, J. V., Gutcher, K., and Robinson, W. W. 1975. Psychopharmacologia 43:81–83.
8. Johanson, C., and Schuster, C. R. 1975. J. Pharmacol. Exp. Ther. 193:676–688.
9. Pickens, R., and Harris, W. 1968. Psychopharmacologia 12:158–163.
10. Pickens, R., and Thompson, T. 1968. J. Pharmacol. Exp. Ther. 161:122–129.
11. Woods, J. H., and Schuster, C. R. 1968. Int. J. Addic. 3:231–237.
12. Wilson, M. C., Hitomi, M., and Schuster, C. R. 1971. Psychopharmacologia 22:271–281.
13. Goldberg, S. R., Hoffmeister, F., Schlicting, U. V., and Wuttke, W. 1971. J. Pharmacol. Exp. Ther. 179:277–283.
14. Balster, R. L., and Schuster, C. R. 1973. J. Exp. Anal. Behav. 20:119–129.
15. Iglauer, C., and Woods, J. H. 1974. J. Exp. Anal. Behav. 22:179–196.
16. Llewellyn, M. E., Iglauer, C., and Woods, J. H. 1976. J. Exp. Anal. Behav. 25:81–91.
17. Brady, J. V., and Griffiths, R. R. 1976. In: Cocaine and Other Stimulants. Contemporary Issues in Stimulant Research. E. H. Ellinwood and M. M. Kilbey (eds.), p. 599–613. Plenum Press, New York.
18. Johanson, C. E. 1976. Control of Drug Taking by Schedules of Reinforcement. Pharmacol. Rev. 27:343–355.
19. Griffiths, R. R., Wurster, R. M., and Brady, J. V. 1976. Control of Drug Taking by Schedules of Reinforcement. Pharmacol. Rev. 27:357–365.
20. Hodos, W. 1961. Science 134:943–944.
21. Hodos, W., and Kalman, J. 1963. J. Exp. Anal. Behav. 6:387–392.
22. Keesey, R. E., and Goldstein, M. D. 1968. J. Exp. Anal. Behav. 11:293.
23. Hodos, W. 1965. J. Comp. Physiol. Psychol. 59:215.
24. Findley, J. D., Robinson, W. W., and Gilliam, W. A. 1971. J. Exp. Anal. Behav. 15:69–71.

Assessment of Reinforcing Properties of Stimulant and Depressant Drugs in the Rhesus Monkey as a Tool for the Prediction of Psychic Dependence-Producing Capability in Man

Friedrich Hoffmeister

The World Health Organization Expert Committee on dependence-producing drugs defined the state of psychic dependence in man "as a condition in which a drug produces a feeling of satisfaction and psychic drive that requires periodic or continuous administration of the drug to produce pleasure or to avoid discomfort."[1]

The notion underlying this statement is that there are distinct psychopharmacological properties of drugs that will produce in an organism the conditions described. In other words, there are certain substances that have biochemical properties that change the functions of the central nervous system in such a way that an organism will become forced, by their ingestion, to become psychologically dependent.

On the other hand, it is well known that the abuse liability of a drug depends on, or at least varies with, nonpharmacological variables such as the psychopathological status of an individual, environmental contingencies, and even fashions.

Since the variety of these nonpharmacological variables can never be *fully* mimicked in animal experiments, psychopharmacology is bound to assess the behavioral pharmacological properties contributing to drug abuse of human beings under a number of controlled and, to a certain extent, necessarily artificial conditions.

Parts of these experiments have been submitted to J. Pharmacol. Exp. Ther. for publication.

As a consequence, reports of animal experiments referring to abuse liability of drugs have to confine themselves to psychopharmacological statements and thereby leave more or less alone the special influence nonpharmacological variables will have.

For this reason many scientists in describing their results have confined themselves to the behavioral-pharmacological terminology, e.g., to report on reinforcing properties of drugs assessed under given experimental conditions.[2]

Standardization of experimental conditions generally involves simplification of the experimental procedure. This might limit their predictive value for abuse liability in man, since interindividual differences of drug actions are excluded. Therefore, it seems to be appropriate not to rely on results achieved only with one given experimental set up.

The general rule in psychopharmacology, that the assessment of a profile of actions usually correlated much better with the effects of a drug in man than do the results achieved with a sophisticated single method, should be followed in the application of methods to assess drug self-administration behavior.

The question whether "method a" gives better predictive values than "method b" seems to be of secondary importance.

A second pharmacological rule that should be followed in the use of animal experimental techniques as tools for the prediction of human abuse liability is that as many drugs, the abuse liability of which is known, as possible should be compared by a broad number of techniques and the resulting profile of actions correlated with the data known from the same drugs in man.

Finally, drug interactions that clearly contribute to the abuse liability in man are an important field in animal experiments, since such interactions sometimes might explain otherwise inexplicable drug-taking behavior in man.

Thus, the problem of assessment of abuse liability of drugs in animal experiments is basically not different from other problems in pharmacology.

For example, the predictive value of animal experiments for antianginal or antischizophrenic properties of a compound in man is as difficult to judge as the predictive value of the animal experimental methods presently available for the abuse liability.

Following the notion of assessing a behavioral pharmacological profile of drugs as a tool for the prediction of abuse liability in man, I now give a short survey of results achieved with relatively simple self-administration techniques in the rhesus monkey.

RESULTS

Continuous self-administration tests allow animals to self-administer a drug without time or dose limitation 24 hours a day for several weeks. This procedure permits assessment of reinforcing effects, the pattern of drug taking, and the manifestation of pharmacological effects of a drug at self-medicated dose levels.

This important procedure, originally invented by Deneau, Yanagita, and Seevers,[3] yields a variety of information about the reinforcing effects under the conditions described above.[4,5] Conclusions drawn from its results might, however, be misleading because physical and psychic dependence-producing effects contribute to the extent of self-administration, since during the course of such experiments the motivation of an animal to self-administer a drug might change.

If, for example, an animal is offered morphine (see Figure 1), a drug with physical dependence-producing properties,[6] it becomes evident that at least two different properties of the compound might be involved in the maintenance of self-administration. At the beginning of the experiment, responding for the drug infusions is initiated and maintained by the psychopharmacological properties, e.g., the positive reinforcing properties of the compound. The appearance of withdrawal symptoms following saline replacement demonstrates that the monkey has become physically dependent during the course of the experiment. Thus the question remains open about what extent responding for morphine is maintained by the positive reinforcing psy-

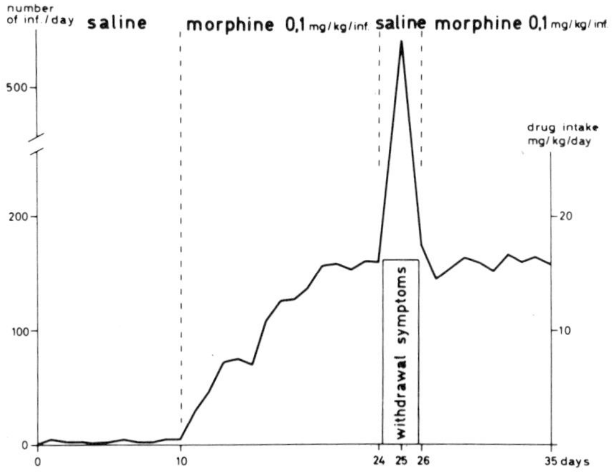

Figure 1. Self-administration of morphine (0.1 mg/kg infusion) by one rhesus monkey. No limitation in time or amount of drug availability.

chopharmacological properties of the substance, or by the negative reinforcing properties of the ongoing withdrawal symptoms.

To overcome the difficulties in interpreting such results among several other procedures, the cross self-administration technique has been introduced. This technique has the advantage that well-trained

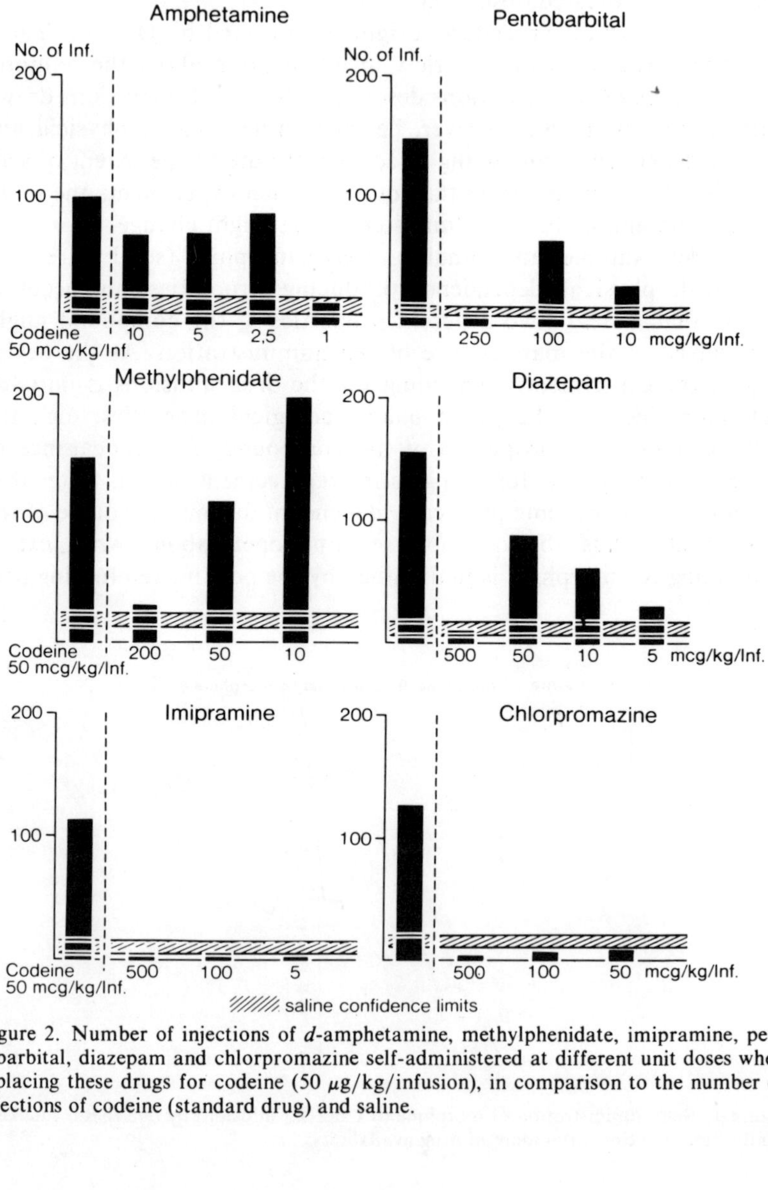

Figure 2. Number of injections of *d*-amphetamine, methylphenidate, imipramine, pentobarbital, diazepam and chlorpromazine self-administered at different unit doses when replacing these drugs for codeine (50 μg/kg/infusion), in comparison to the number of injections of codeine (standard drug) and saline.

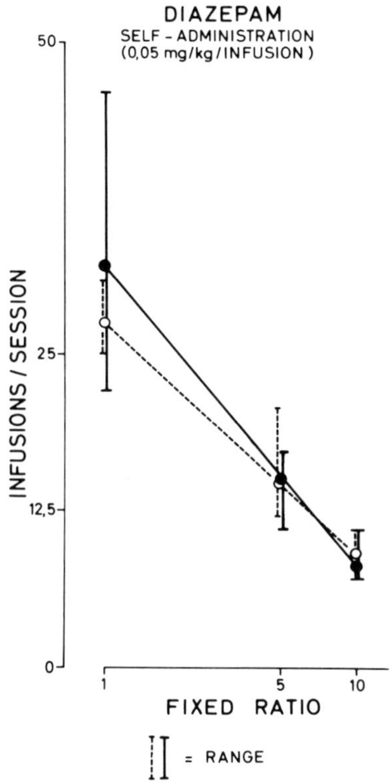

Figure 3. Effects of varying FR response requirement on the number of self-administered diazepam infusion. *Abscissa*, FR value; *ordinate*, infusions per session. Each circle represents the mean of two observations in each of the two monkeys. *Vertical lines* are standard areas. FR value was varied in ascending order (●——●) or in descending order (○----○).

animals can be exposed to different drugs and dosages over the course of relatively few test sessions. The rate of self-administration is stabilized and maintained by response-produced infusions of a standard drug (see Figure 2); other test drugs are then substituted for several consecutive sessions to determine the extent to which the substituted drug is self-administered. Using this technique it is possible to show that different doses of *d*-amphetamine or methylphenidate are self-administered above saline range, whereas imipramine, a drug with basically stimulant properties, is not self-administered.[6]

The depressants pentobarbital and diazepam are also self-administered, whereas the depressant drug chlorpromazine is not (see Figures 3 and 4).[6]

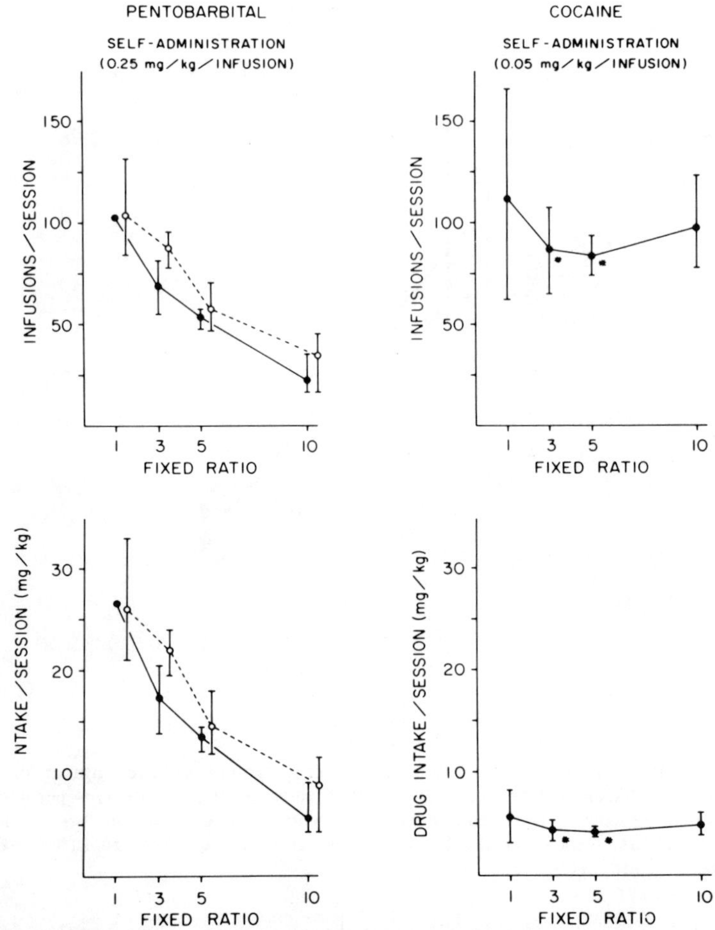

Figure 4. Effects of varying the FR response requirement on the number of self-administered infusions and drug intake per session. *Abscissa,* FR value; *ordinate,* infusions per session (top) and drug intake per session (bottom). Each *circle* represents the means of two observations in each of the three monkeys. *Vertical lines* are standard errors. FR value was varied in ascending order (●——●) or in descending order (○----○).

Self-administration of pentobarbital and diazepam is, however, significantly influenced by increasing the number of lever presses required for drug infusion.

In contrast, self-administration of the psychostimulant cocaine is less susceptible to changes of the ratio[7] (Hoffmeister, unpublished results).

Thus, even these few examples show that cross self-administration methods give mainly "yes" or "no" answers; the main disadvantage of these methods, however, is the lack of quantitativity with regard to the relative reinforcement strength of drugs.

Because there are drugs that are not assessed as positive reinforcers in this technique, investigations on possible negative reinforcing properties are certainly of value.

For example, chlorpromazine and perphenazine (Figure 5) have been shown to be not reinforcing in continuous self-administration tests or cross self-administration tests.[8,3] Since the class to which these drugs belong is known to have an extremely potent rate of depressing effects, the question remains open whether or not the lack of self-administration is due to their rate of depression or due to the lack of positive reinforcing properties.

As Figure 6 shows, the stimuli associated with the infusions of perphenazine would engender and maintain avoidance responding in the same dose range in which the drug depresses avoidance responding maintained by stimuli associated with noxious electric shock.

The same applies for the major tranquilizer chlorpromazine

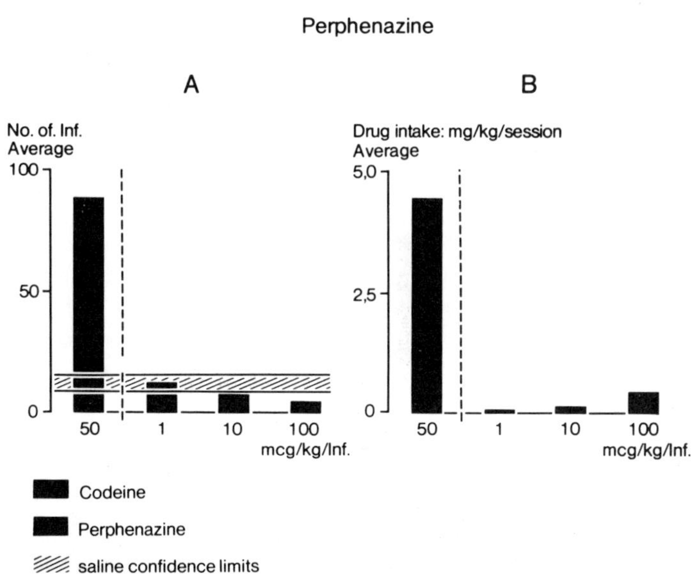

Figure 5. Number of injections of perphenazine self-administered at different unit doses when substituting the drug for codeine, in comparison to the number of injections of codeine (standard drug) and saline.

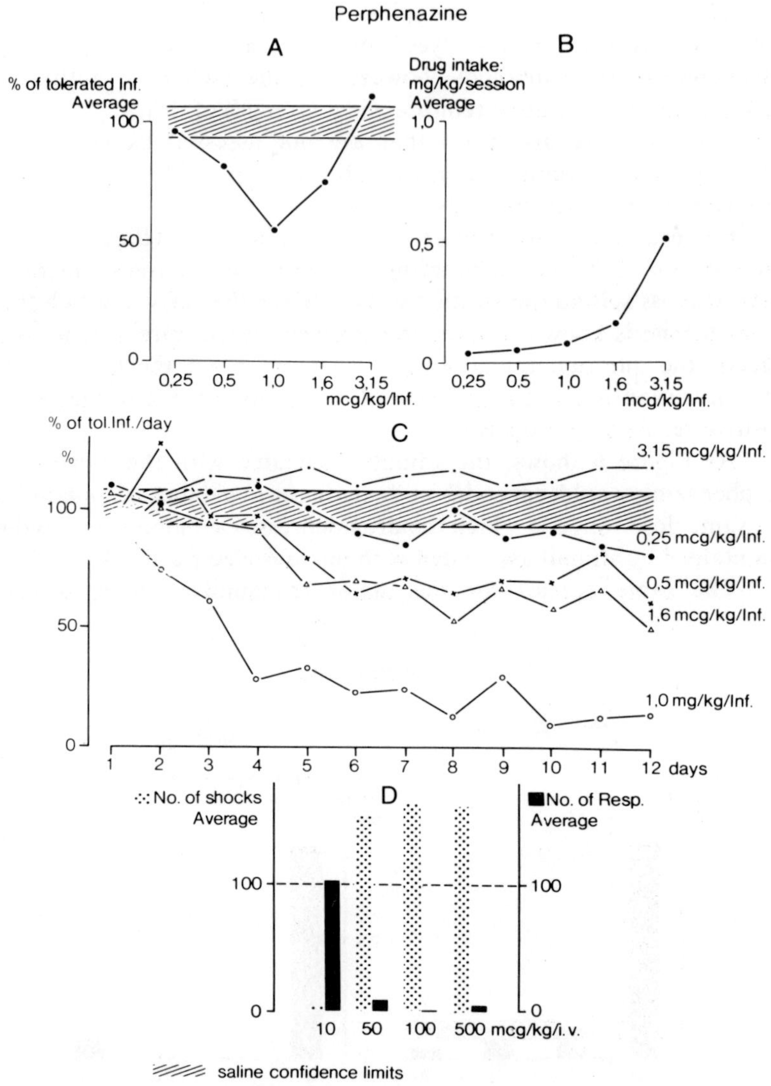

Figure 6. Effects of varying perphenazine infusion doses on the percentage of infusions tolerated, the drug intake during a 12th day replacement period. *A:* Average percentage of tolerated infusions during the 12-day replacement period. *B:* Average drug intake (mg/kg/session). *C:* Effect on mean number of infusions tolerated per 2-hour session plotted as percentage of the saline infusions tolerated per 2-hour session (ordinate) by the same subjects during the extinction periods. *D:* Effect of perphenazine on mean number of responses and shocks per session under a schedule of termination of a stimulus associated with electric shock.

(Figures 7 and 8), whereas stimuli associated with infusions of pentobarbital (Figure 9) are ineffective in this respect.[9]

Scheduled infusions of the antidepressant imipramine (Figure 10) also do not engender and maintain avoidance responding, although this compound, like chlorpromazine, depresses the rate of responding to avoid a noxious electric stimulus.[10]

Figure 11 summarizes qualitatively the results achieved in these three simple methods. As can be seen, it is possible to differentiate various types of mood-elevating substances, for example *d*-amphetamine and the antidepressants, as well as different kinds of central depressants such as barbiturate-like compounds and major tranquilizers.

This might be considered to be a poor result, and there might be pharmacologists who will claim to be able to differentiate in the same

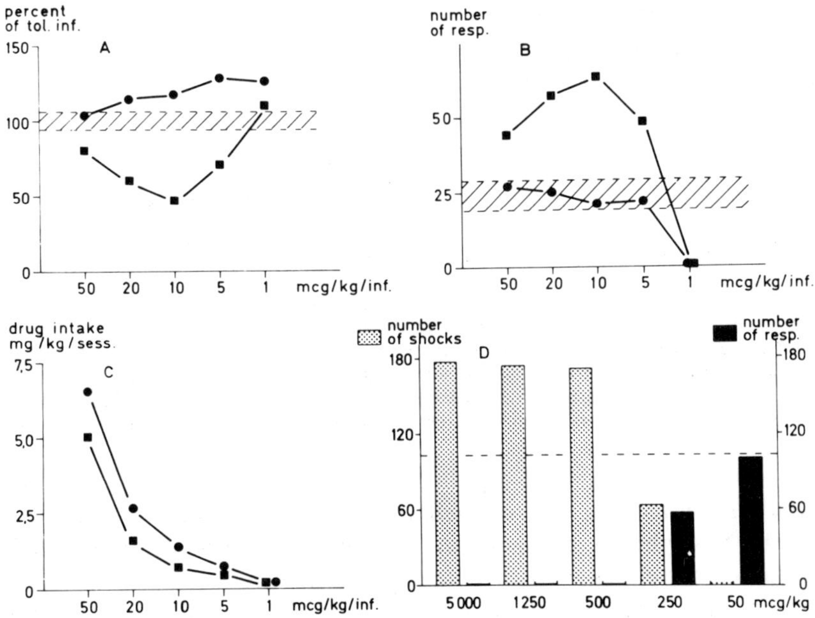

Figure 7. *A* to *C*: Effects of varying infused doses of chlorpromazine on the percentage of infusions tolerated (*A*), number of responses (*B*), and drug intake (*C*) during the first and second half of the six-session drug period. *D*: Effects of chlorpromazine on mean number of responses and electric shocks per session under the schedule of termination of a stimulus associated with electric shock. *Circles* indicate means of the first half of drug period; *horizontal dashed lines* indicate confidence limits of saline infusions tolerated and number of responses with saline infusions.

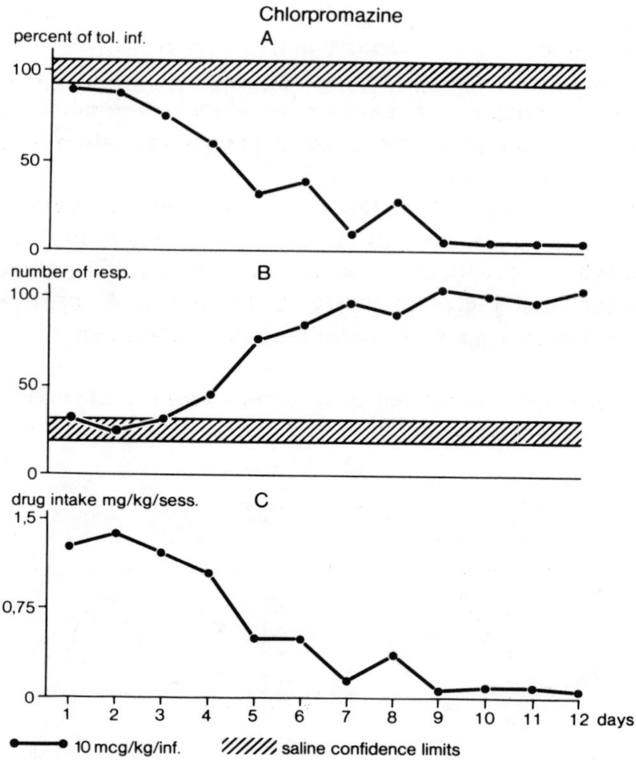

Figure 8. Effect of 10 μg/kg/infusion of chlorpromazine on the percentage of infusions tolerated, number of responses and drug intake at the individual days of a 12-day replacement period. *A:* Effect on mean number of infusions tolerated per two-hour session plotted as percentage of the saline infusions tolerated per two-hour session (*ordinate*) by the same subjects during the extinction periods. *B:* Effect on mean number of responses per two-hour session. *C:* Effect on mean drug intake per session.

way just by looking at cross-behavior of a mouse injected with these drugs. Nevertheless, the fact that the influence of these drugs on cross-behavior correlates with their reinforcing effects is pure chance, and reinforcing effects and the effects on cross-behavior of different drugs belonging to these groups are certainly different.

On the other hand, the results clearly correlate qualitatively with the abuse liability of the compounds investigated. Thus, they should have some predictive value when applied to new psychotropic drugs.

Moreover, this predictive value of self-administration methods will certainly improve as soon as quantitative methods of assessing relative efficacy of drugs, such as drug choice procedures, second-order schedule procedures, or progressive ratio test and others, will be applied to such an extent that correlations with human drug-taking behavior will become possible.

The importance of drug interactions has been stressed by several authors,[11] especially in the field of narcotic analgesics and narcotic antagonists. This field of research is certainly important in the field of nonnarcotics.

Combinations of pentobarbital with *d*-amphetamine are self-administered to a greater extent in cross self-administration procedures than either drug alone (Figure 12).[12]

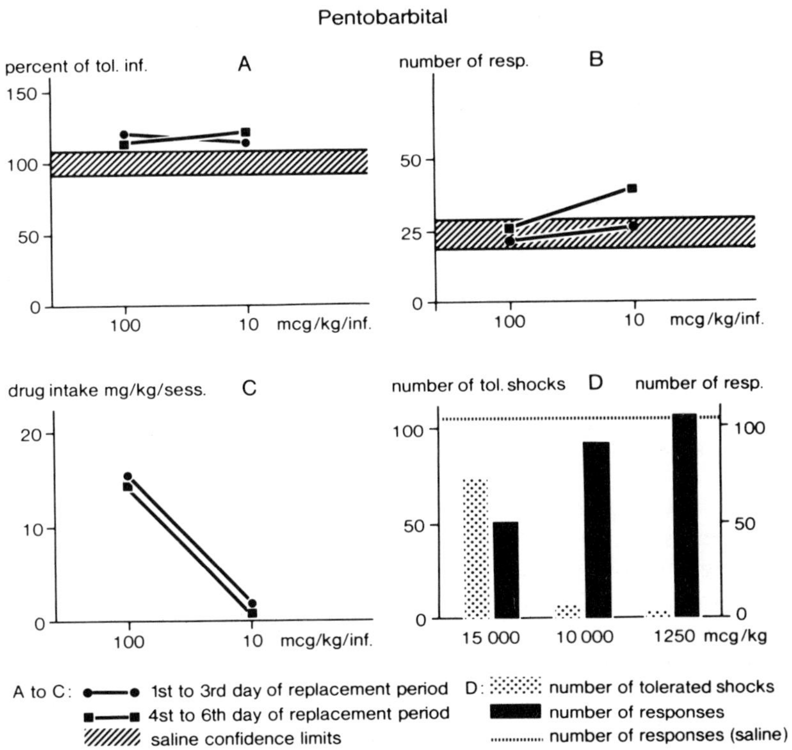

Figure 9. *A* to *C:* Effects of varying the infused doses of pentobarbital on the percentage of infusions tolerated (*A*), number of responses (*B*), and drug intake (*C*) during the first and second half of a six-session drug period. *D:* Effects of pentobarbital on mean number of responses and electric shocks per session under a schedule of termination of a stimulus associated with electric shock. *Circles* indicate means of first half of drug period; *squares* indicate means of second half of drug period.

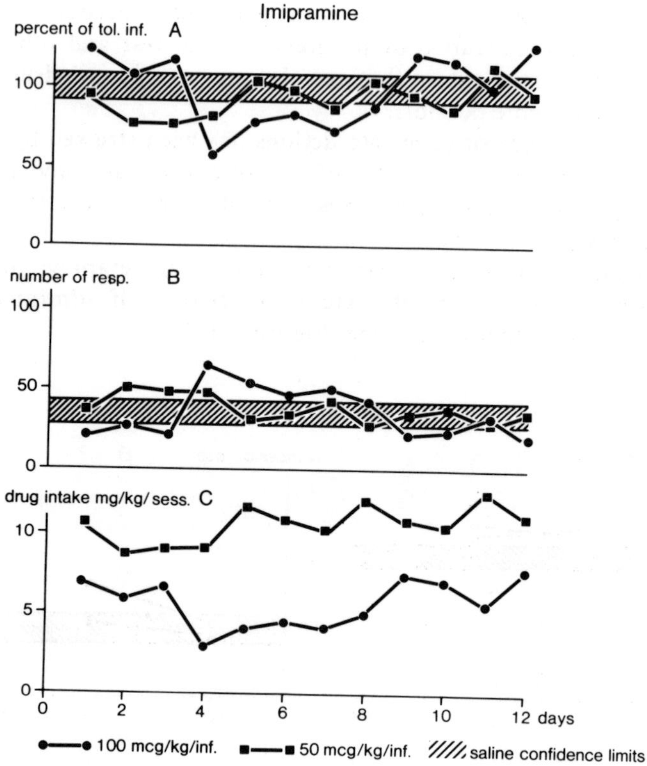

Figure 10. *A* to *C:* Effects of imipramine (50 and 100 μg/kg/infusion) on the percentage of infusions tolerated (*A*), number of responses (*B*), and drug intake (*C*) at the individual days of a 12-day replacement period.

Acetylsalicylic acid is devoid of either positive or negative reinforcing properties and consequently is not self-administered by rhesus monkeys. Codeine is self-administered when offered under a schedule of continuous self-administration (Figure 13). The doses of the self-administered substance are well tolerated by the animals.

If, however, codeine is offered in combination with acetylsalicylic acid, monkeys self-administer toxic or even lethal doses of the combination (Figure 14).

These few results show that drug interaction studies are a field of major importance in the assessment of abuse liability of the effects that abuse will have on an organism.

To summarize; at our present state of knowledge there are methods that permit assessment of reinforcing effects of psychotropic drugs. Insofar as the pharmacological property of a reinforcer is correlated with abuse liability, these methods have a considerable predictive value for the abuse liability of drugs in man.

Substance	Positive reinforcing Properties				Negative reinforcing Properties	
	Continuous Self-administration		Cross Self-administration		Drug Avoidance	
	Maintenance of Initiation behavior	Initiation of behavior	Maintenance of behavior	Extinction of behavior	Initiation of avoidance behavior	Complete extinction of avoidance behavior
Cocaine	+ + +	+ + +	+ + +	+ + +	∅	+
Amphetamine	+ + +	+ + +	+ + +	+ + +	∅	+
Methylphenidate	+ +	+ +	+ +	+ +	∅	+
Imipramine	∅	∅	∅	∅	∅	∅
Amitryptyline	∅	∅	∅	∅	∅	∅
Pentobarbital	+ +	+ +*	+ +*	+ +	∅	+
Diazepam	+ +	+	+*	+*	∅	∅ - (+)
Haloperidol	∅	∅	∅	∅	+	∅ - (+)**
Chlorpromazine	∅	∅	∅	∅	+ (+)	∅ - +**
Perphenazine	∅	∅	∅	∅	+ + +	∅ - +**
Acetylsalicylic Acid	∅	∅	∅	∅	∅	∅

** Dependent on dose
* Dependent on schedule

Figure 11. Positive and negative reinforcing properties of central stimulant and depressant drugs in continuous self-administration, cross self-administration and drug 014
avoidance experiments (schematic).

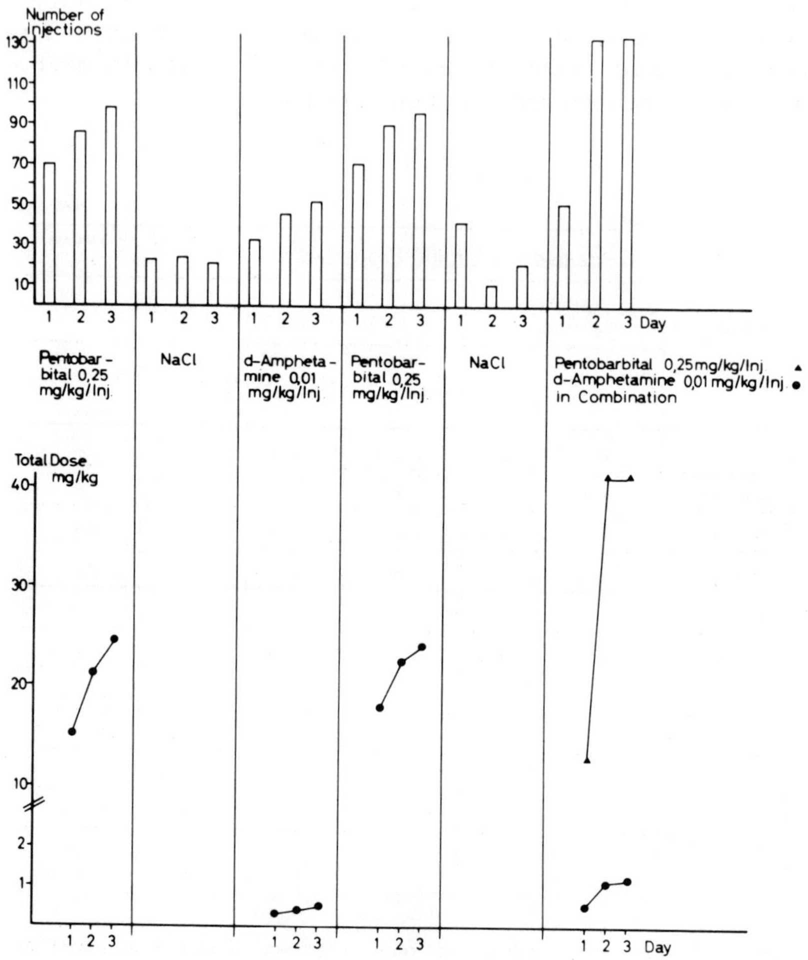

Figure 12. Self-administration of a combination of pentobarbital and *d*-amphetamine as compared with the self-administration of either drug alone.

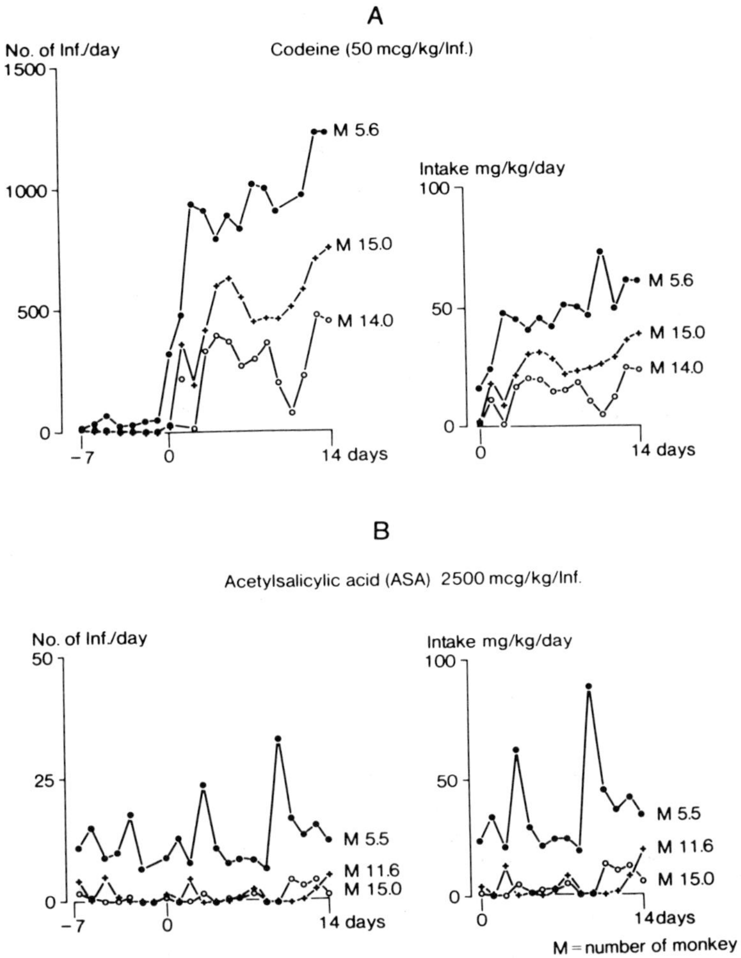

Figure 13. *A, left side:* Self-administration of 50 μg/kg/infusion of codeine of three monkeys over a period of 14 days; *right side:* Daily codeine intake in mg/kg of the same monkeys. *B, left side:* Self-administration of 2500 μg/kg/infusion of ASA over a period of 14 days by three monkeys; *right side:* Daily ASA intake in mg/kg of the same monkeys.

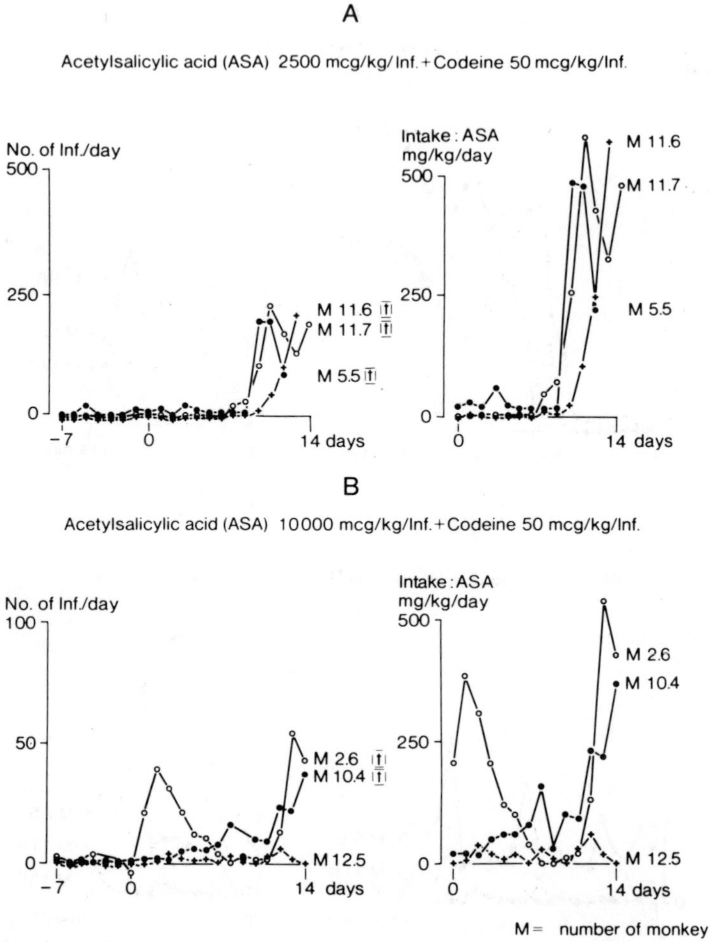

Figure 14. *A, left side:* Self-administration of a combination of 50 μg/kg/infusion of codeine plus 2500 μg/kg/infusion of ASA of three monkeys over a period of 14 days; *right side:* Daily ASA intake in mg/kg of the same monkeys. *B, left side:* Self-administration of a combination of 50 μg/kg/infusion of codeine plus 10,000 μg/kg/infusion of ASA over a period of 14 days of three monkeys; *right side:* Daily ASA intake in mg/kg of the same monkeys. † = death of monkey.

LITERATURE CITED

1. World Health Organization. 1976. World Health Org. Techn. Rep. Ser. 526.
2. Woods, J. H., and Schuster, C. R. 1970. Regulation of drug self-administration. In: R. T. Harris, W. M. McIsaac and C. R. Schuster (eds.), Advances in mental science II, Drug dependence, pp. 158–169.
3. Deneau, G. A., Yanagita, T., and Seevers, M. H. 1969. Self-administration of psychoactive substances by the monkey. Psychopharmacologia 16:30–48.
4. Weeks, J. R. 1962. Experimental morphine addiction: Method for automatic intravenous injection in unrestrained rats. Science 138:143–144.
5. Thompson, T., and Schuster, C. R. 1964. Morphine self-administration, food-reinforced, and avoidance behaviors in rhesus monkeys. Psychopharmacologia 5:87–94.
6. Hoffmeister, F. 1974. Positive and negative reinforcing properties of psychotropic drugs in rhesus monkeys. Neuropsycho-pharmacology. Exc. Med. Int. Congre. Ser. 359:245–252.
7. Goldberg, S. R., Hoffmeister, F., Schlichting, U., and Wuttke, W. 1971. A comparison of pentobarbital and cocaine self-administration in rhesus monkeys: Effects of dose and fixed-ratio parameter. J. Pharmacol. Exp. Ther. 179:277–283.
8. Hoffmeister, F., and Goldberg, S. R. 1973. A comparison of chlorpromazine, imipramine, morphine and *d*-amphetamine self-administration in cocaine-dependent rhesus monkeys. J. Pharmacol. Exp. Ther. 187:8–14.
9. Hoffmeister, F. 1975. Negative reinforcing properties of some psychotropic drugs in drug-naive rhesus monkeys. J. Pharmacol. Exp. Ther. 192:468–477.
10. Hoffmeister, F., and Wuttke, W. 1976. Psychotropic drugs as negative reinforcers. Pharmacological Reviews. (In press.)
11. Woods, J. H., Downs, D. A., and Villarreal, J. E. 1973. Changes in operant behavior during deprivation- and antagonist-induced withdrawal states. In: L. Goldberg and F. Hoffmeister (eds.), Psychic dependence, pp. 114–121. Springer Verlag, New York.
12. Schlichting, U., Goldberg, S. R., Wuttke, W., and Hoffmeister, F. 1970. *d*-Amphetamine self-administration by rhesus monkeys with different self-administration histories. Exc. Med. Int. Congr. Ser. 220:62–69.

Procedures for the Preclinical Assessment of Abuse Potential of Psychotropic Drugs in Animals

Chris E. Johanson

and

Charles R. Schuster

The use of animals for the prediction of the abuse liability of new compounds began with the screening of analgesics for physical dependence of the opiate type.[1,2] In this simple procedure, rhesus monkeys were initially made physically dependent on morphine by subcutaneous injections given four times daily. When a new compound was tested, it was merely substituted for morphine and observations for signs of withdrawal were made. The same preparation could be used to determine whether or not the compound was an opiate antagonist as well. The elegance of this screening procedure was due to its simplicity and efficiency. Many compounds over a wide range of doses could quickly be assessed for abuse liability at a relatively low cost. This rapid and economical procedure undoubtedly helped to make pharmaceutical houses willing to submit their compounds for testing and led to the FDA adopting this test as mandatory for analgesic testing. Subsequently, procedures that directly determine the dependence-producing properties of drugs have been included in the testing of new analgesic compounds to improve the specificity of the screening program. These procedures have proven so useful over the years that the general concept of using animals for the preclinical assessment of analgesics is well accepted. Indeed, a large segment of the interests of the Committee on Problems of Drug Dependence has been devoted to the continuance of this type of screening.

In 1932, the amphetamines were introduced into the medical pharmacopaeia as decongestants and, in addition, as a replacement for ephedrine in the treatment of bronchial asthma. Although they were relatively ineffective in this latter regard, their impressive central nervous system stimulant effects soon became obvious, and led eventually to their use in the treatment of obesity, hyperkinesis, and narcolepsy. Only over the last 10–15 years have clinicians recognized the abuse liability of the amphetamines and related compounds.[3-5] Because of this potential abuse, there have been increasing efforts on the part of the pharmaceutical industry to develop new psychomotor stimulant drugs with lower abuse potential than those currently available. This search is analogous to the attempts to find an analgesic compound that does not produce physical dependence. The methodology used with analgesics, however, was not applicable, since the chronic administration of psychomotor stimulant drugs does not result in physical dependence.[6] However, there is little question that with the psychomotor stimulants a state of psychological dependence characterized by the repeated use of this class of drugs is developed in certain individuals. One approach that may be useful in assessing the capacity of a drug to produce psychological dependence is offered by procedures involving repeated intravenous self-administration of drugs by infra-human organisms. The development of such procedures may provide the methodology for the preclinical screening of anorectic agents similar to that available for analgesics.

Research over the last decade has demonstrated that animals repeatedly make responses that are followed by intravenous injections of psychomotor stimulant drugs.[7] This property is shared by a number of drugs of that class, including cocaine, the amphetamines, methylphenidate, phenmetrazine, and pipradrol, to mention a few. With few exceptions, every stimulant tested with infra-human animals has been shown to maintain responding under a wide variety of environmental circumstances. Therefore, it appears that one of the pharmacological properties shared by all psychomotor stimulant drugs is their ability to act as positive reinforcers in that each will initiate and maintain an increased frequency of the behavior it follows.[8]

The illicit use of a drug by humans is undoubtedly related to its reinforcing properties. If the drug reinforcement mechanism is common to both animals and man, it is possible to develop an animal model of human drug abuse. Evidence for the validity of this animal model is rapidly accumulating. Animals self-administer the same drugs that humans use for nonmedical purposes; these include not only the psychomotor stimulants but opiates, barbiturates, and alcohol as well.[7,9] In addition, the pattern of intake of these drugs in experimental animals is very similar to the pattern of their illicit use by man. Stimulants, for instance, are taken in cycles with days of high intake alternating with days of low intake.[10,11] This pattern is reminiscent of that reported for humans.[5] Finally, the physiological and behavioral consequences of the repeated self-administration of drugs is similar in animals and man.[12,13] This information strongly suggests that an animal model of intravenous drug self-administration can be useful in studying factors that influence the nonmedical use of drugs in man.

As mentioned previously, pharmaceutical companies are eagerly trying to develop new psychomotor stimulant drugs of lower abuse potential. If such drugs are developed, the production of psychomotor stimulant drugs with high abuse potential could be sharply curtailed, thus reducing the quantities available for rediversion into the illicit market. If animal studies are valid predictors, it should be possible to evaluate new stimulant compounds for their dependence potential during their preclinical testing. Although it is true that some drugs appear to lack positive reinforcing properties (e.g., chlorpromazine, fenfluramine), it is unlikely that the psychomotor stimulants can be replaced in all of their applications with drugs completely devoid of positive reinforcing properties. A more realistic goal is to find drugs with significantly less dependence potential than those currently available. The problem then is to develop procedures to determine first whether or not a drug is capable of serving as a positive reinforcer, and if so, to be able to measure its relative reinforcing efficacy. In operant terms, this is comparable to assessing the strength of a positive reinforcer.[8]

This chapter describes procedures used in our laboratory at The University of Chicago to assess the abuse potential of psychomotor stimulant drugs and other compounds (Figure 1). Every drug is initially tested using the substitution procedure, which is very similar to the physical dependence substitution procedure used for analgesic testing. This procedure is designed to quickly evaluate a wide range of

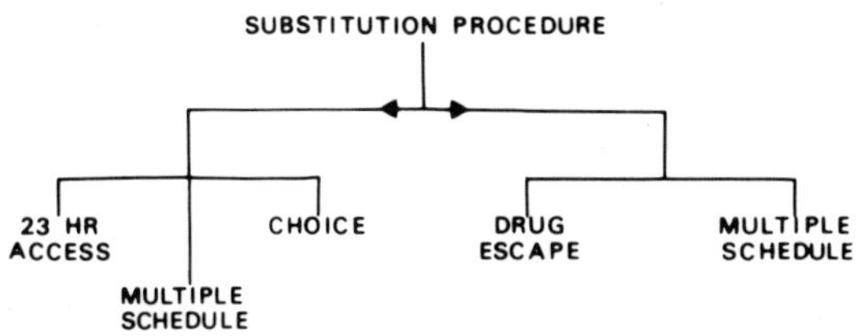

Figure 1. Outline of procedures used at The University of Chicago for the preclinical assessment of the abuse potential of drugs using rhesus monkeys.

doses of a given compound but is inadequate for assessing relative reinforcing properties. If the results of this test indicate that the drug is, at some dose, a positive reinforcer, it will be tested in a procedure (choice) designed to more clearly rank it in terms of reinforcing efficacy. In addition, two other tests, the unlimited access and multiple schedule procedures, are used to assess the behavioral effects produced by the drug.

The unlimited access procedure is used to determine whether a drug is a positive reinforcer in untrained animals. Measuring drug intake, intake pattern, and food intake, provides multiple measures for characterizing a drug relative to other drugs. In addition, gross behavioral observations can be useful in determining drug side-effects. The multiple schedule is also useful in determining the behavioral consequences of a drug. Since this procedure produces stable responding over indefinite periods, complete dose-response curves can be generated in the same organism. Comparison of the dose-response function generated by this procedure to that generated by the substitution procedure, can give an indication of the drug's toxicity relative to its reinforcing properties.

If the results of the substitution test indicate that the drug is not a positive reinforcer but may actually have aversive properties, it is tested using a drug-escape procedure, not only to assess toxicity but also to determine whether or not the results of the substitution test could have been due to the use of doses that were not pharmacologically active.

In order to describe these procedures, illustration from our own work will be used. Over the last 3 years, we have been conducting research principally on two drugs, diethylpropion and perphenazine. Diethylpropion, a psychomotor stimulant, is an example of a drug giving positive results on the substitution test, and perphenazine, a phenothizine, is an example of a drug giving negative results. In order to more fully evaluate the reinforcing efficacy of these drugs, several additional studies, as outlined above, were done.

TESTING OF DIETHYLPROPION

Substitution

By and large, the majority of the studies that demonstrate that psychomotor stimulants, opiates, barbiturates, and alcohol can function as positive reinforcers have utilized some modification of the substitution procedure.[7] Animals equipped with intravenous catheters are initially trained to respond for drugs such as cocaine or pentobarbital (baseline drug) usually on a fixed-ratio (FR) schedule of injection. After responding becomes stable, a test compound is substituted. Responding may be maintained by the test compound or decline to minimal levels (Figure 2). By alternating the baseline drug and different doses of the test compound, a dose-response function can be quickly obtained. Using a variation of this procedure, diethylpropion has been tested in our laboratory.[14,15] Rhesus monkeys were initially trained to press a lever on a fixed-ratio 10 schedule to receive 0.2 mg/kg cocaine during a 3-hour daily session. After responding became stable, saline or different doses of diethylpropion were substituted for the cocaine solution for 6 consecutive sessions. The doses of diethylpropion tested and the order of testing are given in Table 1. Prior to the substitution of the next dose of diethylpropion, the animals were returned to the baseline conditions of 0.2 mg/kg/inj cocaine for three sessions.

Figure 3 shows number of injections obtained on the FR 10 schedule at various doses of diethylpropion for each animal. The means and ranges were calculated from data obtained from the last three sessions at each dose. The overall mean and standard error of 0.2 mg/kg/inj cocaine and saline injections are also shown. In general, the dose-response curves for animals A041 and A065 had an inverted U shape, but for A069 responding was inversely related to

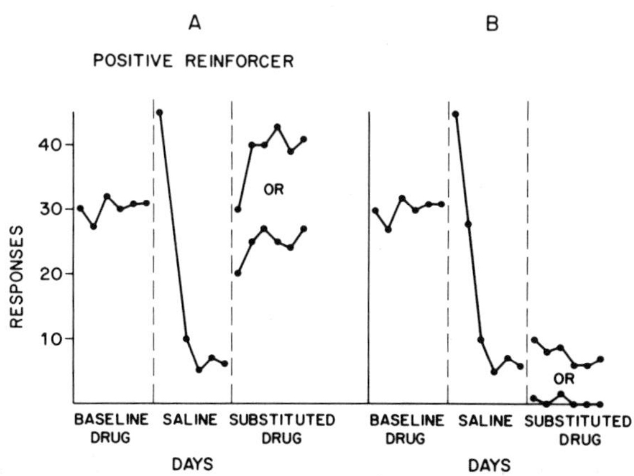

Figure 2. Possible outcomes of the substitution procedure. (Reprinted from Schuster, C. R., and Johanson, C. E. 1974. The use of models for the study of drug abuse. *In* R. J. Gibbons, Y. Israel, H. Kalant, R. E. Popham, W. Schmidt, and R. G. Sinart (eds.), Research Advances in Alcohol and Drug Problems, Vol. 1., pp. 1–31. John Wiley and Sons, Inc.)

Table 1. Order of diethylpropion testing dose (mg/kg/inj)

Animal	0.01	0.05	0.2	0.5	1.0	1.5	3.0
A041	3	6	4	2	7	1	5
A065	5	2	4	1	3	6	7
A069	4	3	1	2	5	6	7

Modified from Ref. 15.

dose. For all three animals responding was maintained above saline levels by doses ranging from 0.05 mg/kg to 1.0 mg/kg. At higher doses of diethylpropion responding did not exceed that generated by saline injections. This data demonstrates that, like other psychomotor stimulant drugs, diethylpropion can act as a positive reinforcer. In addition, the shape of the dose-response curve in the present study is

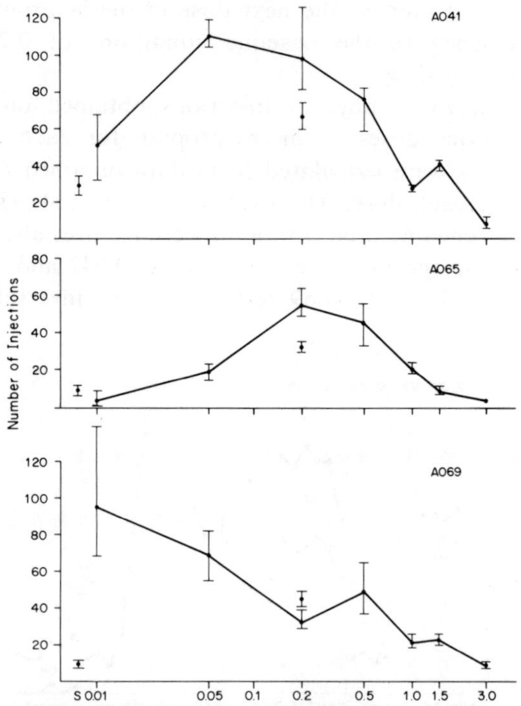

Figure 3. Dose-response functions showing the mean number of injections self-administered at different doses of diethylpropion for three animals in the substitution procedure. These means are derived from data obtained on the last three sessions at each dose. Means for saline and 0.2 mg/kg cocaine are also shown. *Brackets* indicate range. (Reprinted from Ref. 15.)

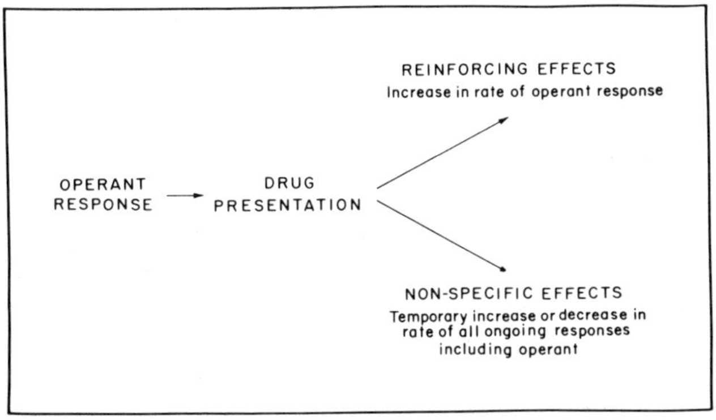

Figure 4. Diagram of two types of effects that drug delivery contingent on an operant response can exert.

similar to those generated with other stimulants.[16,17] Responding increased as dose was increased at the lower end of the range and then decreased as dose was further increased; the total daily dose received remained relatively constant compared to the magnitude of the increase in dose. Inspection of Figure 3 shows that the mean number of injections of 0.2 mg/kg cocaine was about the same as the number of injections obtained when testing 0.5 mg/kg diethylpropion. Cocaine, therefore, is more potent than diethylpropion by a factor of 2.5. Although this estimate of relative potencies is based upon only one dose of cocaine, it is generally accurate because additional observations in our laboratory indicate that the dose-response functions for cocaine and diethylpropion are parallel.

Although the substitution procedure is useful in determining whether or not a drug possesses positive reinforcing properties, it is inadequate for assessing these properties relative to other drugs. As has been explained elsewhere,[15] responding maintained by a drug is influenced not only by its reinforcing actions but as well by its other pharmacological properties. As shown in Figure 4, a drug that is a positive reinforcer will increase responding leading to its delivery. This effect is dependent on the contingency relationship. The drug, however, also has direct effects on responding regardless of the event maintaining it. These direct effects may either increase or decrease responding depending on the environmental situation. Most important, the direct effects are not dependent on the contingency relationship between responding and drug delivery. In the substitution procedure, rate of responding is determined by both the reinforcing properties and direct effects of a drug. Therefore, it is impossible to compare different drugs on reinforcing properties alone.

Choice

In the following studies, a procedure was designed to obviate the problem described above, in order to assess more clearly the relative reinforcing efficacy of psychomotor stimulant drugs. As demonstrated in this book, there are a variety of procedures that may be useful for this purpose. Unlike many of these other tests, however, the choice paradigm involves concurrent alternatives. Diethylpropion can be used to illustrate this point. Diethylpropion is a psychomotor stimulant that is similar in its profile of pharmacological actions to cocaine and the amphetamines.[18] Despite this similarity and its availability on the market for over 15 years, there is little evidence for nonmedical use, except when more preferred stimulant drugs are unavailable.[19] The animal substitution procedure seems to be analogous to that situation. It is also important to determine, however, whether or not this drug is ever preferred to other stimulants available concurrently. A procedure in which animals are given a choice between two stimulants can begin to assess this aspect of abuse liability.

Figure 5 shows a diagram, in Findley notation,[20] of the choice procedure used in the studies to be described. As in the substitution procedure, monkeys were equipped with an intravenous catheter and trained to press a lever to receive a drug injection. However, in this study, the catheters were double lumen so that two drugs could be delivered without intermixing.

Each daily session (see Figure 5) consisted to two sampling periods followed by several choice trials. During the first sampling period, a red or green stimulus light (S_1) was illuminated above the left lever while the stimulus light about the right lever remained dark. Five responses on the left lever resulted in the injection of 1 ml of drug A. Responses on the right lever were recorded but had no other pro-

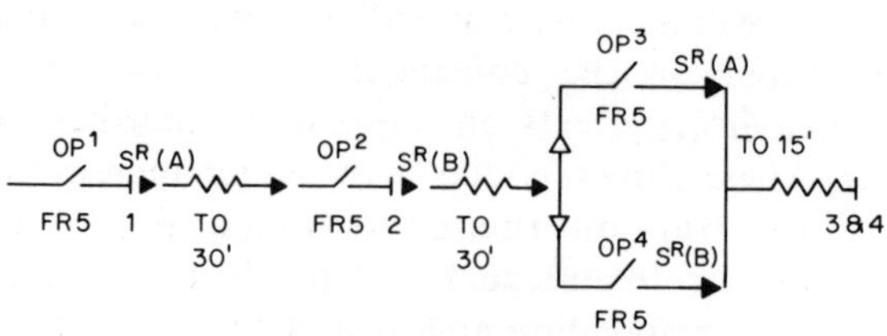

Figure 5. Diagram of the choice procedure in Findley notation.

grammed consequences. The position of S_1 switched to the right lever box and thereafter alternated with each injection of drug A. Five injections were permitted during the first sampling period. After the fifth injection, a 30-minute timeout occurred during which only the white ceiling light was illuminated, and responding was recorded but had no additional programmed consequences. After the timeout, the second sampling period began in which five opportunities were given for self-injection of drug B. The stimulus (S_2) associated with availability of drug B was different in color from S_1. If S_1 was red, S_2 was green, and vice versa. In all other respects, however, the procedures used during this second sampling period were identical to those used during the first sampling period. After the fifth injection of drug B, another 30-minute timeout was initated.

The remainder of the session consisted of choice trials during which S_1 and S_2 were simultaneously presented, one over each lever. Five responses on the lever illuminated by S_1 resulted in the injection of 1 ml of drug A, whereas five responses on the lever illuminated by S_2 resulted in the injection of 1 ml of drug B. The first response on one lever terminated the stimulus over the other lever and made responses on that lever inconsequential for the remainder of the trial.

This procedure was repeated on all choice trials with the restriction that S_1 and S_2 randomly appeared above each lever on 50% of the trials. A session lasted until all choice trials were completed or until 24 hours had passed.

Since this procedure has not been used extensively, it is necessary to review some previous work to support its validity. Initially, in order to determine whether this procedure could even distinguish between a positive reinforcer and saline, choices were given between various doses of cocaine (0.05–1.5 mg/kg/inj), methylphenidate (0.075–0.7 mg/kg/inj), or diethylpropion (0.5 and 1.0 mg/kg/inj) and saline.[14,15,21] In all instances, animals chose the drug rather than saline. In the next series of studies, higher doses of a drug (cocaine, methylphenidate, or diethylpropion) were compared to lower doses of the same drug.[14,15,21] In most instances, the animals chose the higher dose. Figure 6 shows the results of comparisons between 0.1 mg/kg cocaine and both lower and higher doses of cocaine in three animals. As can be seen, this dose was preferred to lower doses but higher doses were preferred to it. Given limited intake (i.e., a limit of 20 trials per session), it is logical that higher doses, below the level of toxicity, would be chosen.

In the next study, cocaine and methylphenidate were compared to

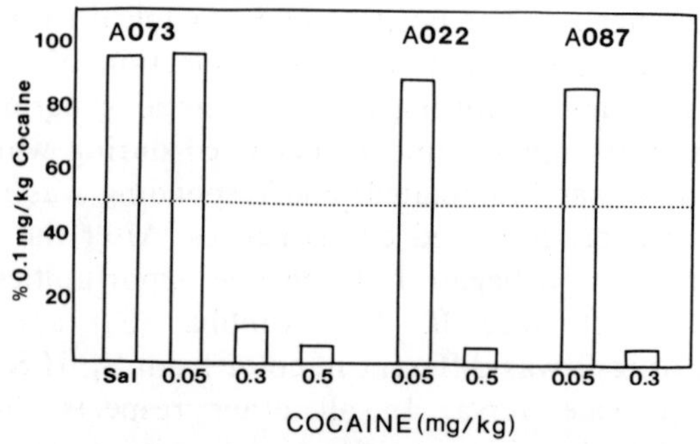

Figure 6. Mean percent of trials 0.1 mg/kg cocaine was chosen over alternatives by three animals. The alternative is indicated on the *abscissa*. The *dotted line* indicates 50%. Means are based on last three sessions of each comparison.

each other across a wide range of doses. Generally, higher doses were chosen over lower doses regardless of the drug.[21] Figure 7 shows the results from one animal of comparisons between 0.1 or 0.5 mg/kg cocaine and several doses of methylphenidate. At the two lower doses (0.075 mg/kg methylphenidate and 0.1 mg/kg cocaine) neither solution was preferred. Higher doses of methylphenidate, however, were preferred. The higher dose of cocaine was preferred to both 0.075 and 0.2 mg/kg methylphenidate, but when both drugs were equal to dose (0.5 mg/kg), neither was preferred. The higher dose of 0.7 mg/kg methylphenidate was chosen over cocaine. It seems then that these two drugs were equal in terms of both potency and efficiency.

The situation was different when cocaine and diethylpropion were compared. In virtually all cases where preferences were shown, cocaine was preferred. Figure 8 shows the results from two of the four

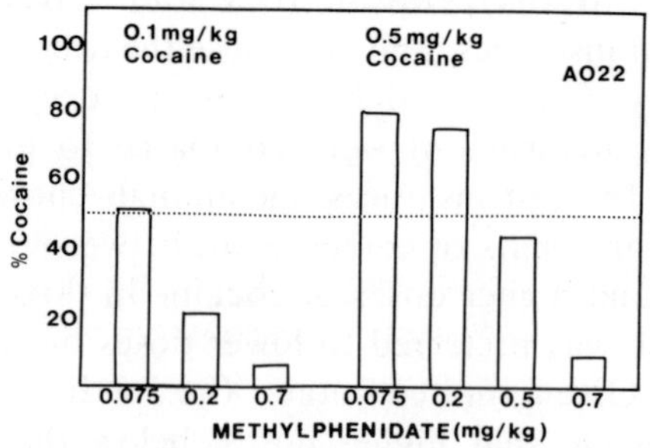

Figure 7. Mean percent of trials cocaine was chosen over methylphenidate by A022. The dose of cocaine was 0.1 mg/kg or 0.5 mg/kg. The doses of methylphenidate are shown on the *abscissa*. The *dotted line* indicates 50%. Means are based on last three sessions of each comparison.

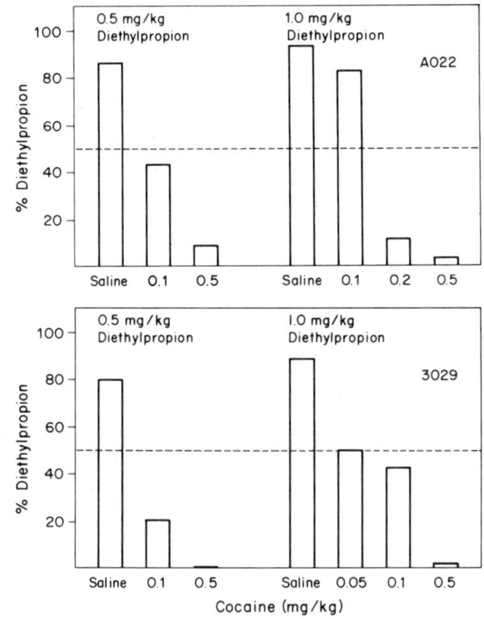

Figure 8. Mean percent of trials diethylpropion was chosen over cocaine by two animals. The dose of diethylpropion was either 0.5 or 1.0 mg/kg. The doses of cocaine are shown on the *abscissa*. The *dotted line* indicates 50%. Means are based on last three sessions of each comparison.

animals tested. In only one comparison was diethylpropion preferred to cocaine, and this occurred when a dose ten times that of cocaine was used. This difference in potency is greater than that seen in the substitution procedure (2.5:1). These data also suggest that diethylpropion is not only less potent but also less efficacious than cocaine, since no animal other than A022 ever demonstrated a preference for diethylpropion, even when there was a 20-fold difference in dose. This finding corresponds well with reports of the relative incidence of the abuse of diethylpropion and demonstrates the possible usefulness of the choice procedure in predicting the abuse liability of psychomotor stimulant drugs.

Unlimited Access

In order to fully characterize the abuse potential of any drug, it can also be useful to assess its toxicity or the behavioral consequences of its ingestion, under conditions where no time limitations are placed on the animal's access to drug.[22] A simple procedure is to allow naive animals unlimited access to the drug. In both the substitution and choice procedure, animals were initially trained to lever-press using cocaine. Such an experimental history may alter the animal's propensity to self-inject other compounds. The unlimited access procedure is primarily useful, however, in assessing the behavioral consequences of chronic drug intake. By assessing intake over a relatively long period of access, the development of tolerance can be seen. In addition, the pattern of intake can be compared to that generated by drugs from the major classes of abused drugs. Measures of the effects of the drug on food intake and gross observations of behavior can be useful in evaluating the toxicity of the compound. Finally, observations following a period of drug availability can indicate whether or not the drug has produced physical dependence.

Deneau, Yanagita, and Seevers,[10] using rhesus monkeys, found that animals initiated and maintained responding for cocaine and *d*-amphetamine. Self-administration was cyclic, with randomly alternating days of high and low intake, and, in addition, the behavioral effects were characteristic of high dose amphetamine intoxication in monkeys[12] and man.[5] We conducted a similar study to confirm and extend the observations of Deneau et al.[10,11] Naive monkeys equipped with intravenous catheters could self-administer a drug at any time during the day by pressing the lever one time (FR 1). The drug available was either 0.2 mg/kg cocaine, 0.05 mg/kg *l*-amphetamine, 0.025 mg/kg *d*-methamphetamine, 0.05 mg/kg *d*-amphetamine, or 0.5 mg/kg diethylpropion. These doses are within a range that maintains response rates above saline operant levels in the substitution procedure.[14,16,17] The animals were given access to these drugs for 28–30 days until they died or were moribund.

Animals initiated responding, usually within the first 24-hour period for all 5 drugs. Animals given access to cocaine, *d*-methamphetamine, and *d*-amphetamine all died in less than 15 days. One of the two animals given access to *l*-amphetamine and 3 of the 5 animals given access to diethylpropion survived the 30-day period. Even the two diethylpropion animals who died survived longer than those who died given access to the other four drugs. Figure 9 shows the results for 2 animals given access to cocaine and Figure 10 shows the results for the 3 animals who survived access to diethylpropion. The latter figure demonstrates the cyclic pattern of intake similar to that reported by Deneua et al.[10] The other four drugs showed a similar pattern. For most animals, food intake was initially suppressed and became highly variable for the remainder of the experiment. Inspection of the data failed to reveal any systematic relationship between food and drug intake. The results of this study show that

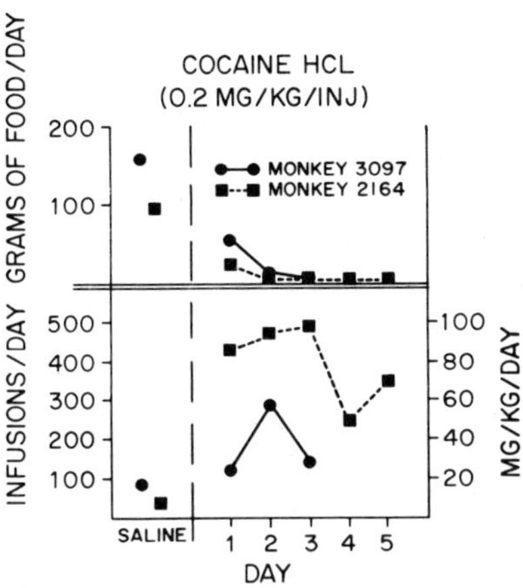

Figure 9. Number of infusions and drug intake (bottom panel) and food intake (top panel) on each day of access to 0.2 mg/kg/inf cocaine hydrochloride for monkeys 3097 and 2164. Mean number of saline infusions and mean food intake for the three days prior to drug access are shown to the left of both panels. (Reprinted from Ref. 11.)

diethylpropion shares many of the properties of other stimulants. Naive animals initiate responding leading to its injection. Food intake is suppressed and, in addition, animals show typical psychomotor stimulant effects. However, despite these similarities, these studies suggest that diethylpropion, even at extremely high doses, is less toxic than the amphetamines and cocaine.

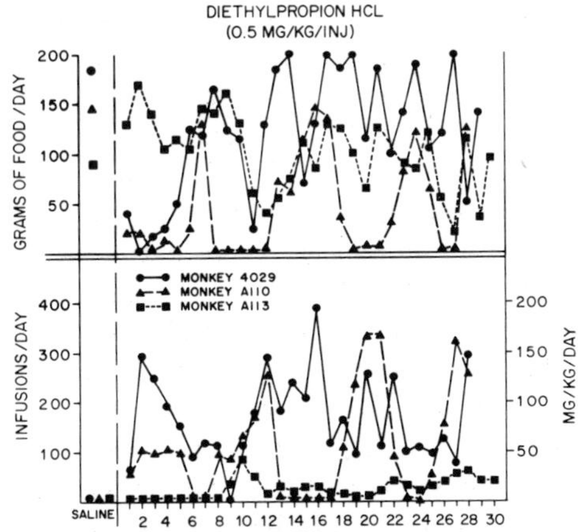

Figure 10. Number of infusions and drug intake (bottom panel) and food intake (top panel) on each day of access to 0.5 mg/kg/inf diethylpropion hydrochloride for monkeys 4029, A110, and A113. Mean number of saline infusions and mean food intake for the three days prior to drug access are shown to the left of both panels. (Reprinted from Ref. 11.)

Multiple Schedule

A second procedure used to assess and compare the behavioral effects of diethylpropion to other psychomotor stimulant drugs involves a multiple schedule of reinforcement. Responding is maintained by food delivery or shock stimulus termination and the drug is given non-contingently. One of the advantages of this procedure is that it is possible to maintain stable rates of responding over extremely long periods of time. Therefore, using the same animals, entire dose-response functions can be generated with several drugs to facilitate comparisons. This allows a comparison of the relative potencies of psychomotor stimulant drugs, both in terms of their reinforcing effects and their effects on behavior generated by the multiple schedule. However, since the drugs are not self-administered in this procedure, but are given acutely by the experimenter, the effects are not necessarily those which would be seen when the drug is taken repeatedly at doses determined by the animal.

Rhesus monkeys, seated in a restraining chair, are trained to respond on a three-ply multiple schedule during a 3-hour daily session. The first component, which is 3 minutes in duration, is a fixed-ratio (FR) schedule (20 or 30) maintained by food. In the second component, 9 minutes in duration, responding is also maintained by food but the schedule is a DRL 45 seconds (differential reinforcement of a low rate). In this schedule, responses result in food delivery if spaced by at least 45 seconds. Responses occurring before that time has elapsed reset the 45 second clock and are not reinforced. The final component, which is 3 minutes in duration, is also a fixed-ratio 20 or 30 schedule maintained by shock stimulus termination. If the animal fails to complete the ratio in 15 seconds, a 10 ma shock is delivered, whereas the completion of the ratio results in a 15-second safe period. All components are separated by timeout periods, during which responding has no consequences. The entire sequence, including timeouts; is 30 minutes in length and is repeated six times. In addition, each component is associated with a different color discriminative stimulus above the lever. After responding is stable for 2 days, drug injections are given intravenously after 1 hour of the session. Figure 11 shows cumulative response records to two animals during control sessions and after various doses of cocaine for the last 2 hours of each session. It should be noted that the control performances and the sensitivity to cocaine are considerably different for the two animals; if two drugs are to be compared, therefore, it is important to use the same animal. Figure 12 shows the dose-response function for cocaine

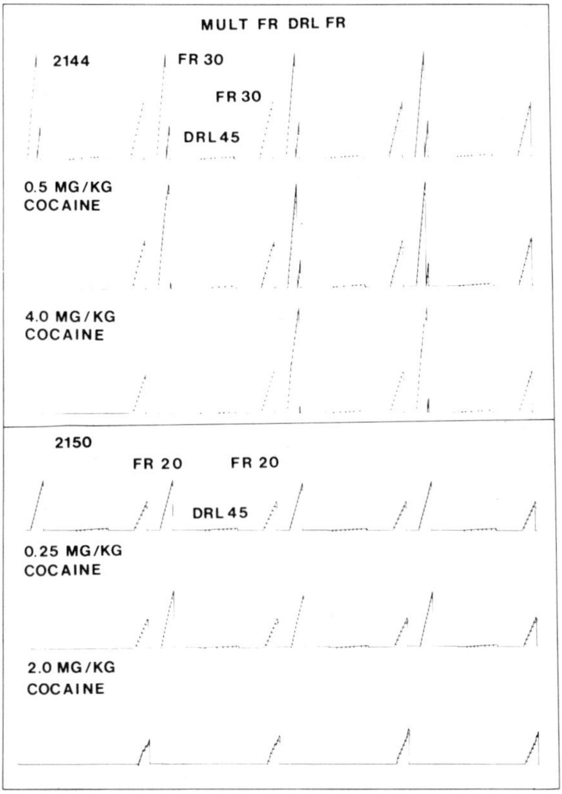

Figure 11. Cumulative response records for animals 2144 (top) and 2150 (bottom) responding on a MULT FR DRL FR schedule. Responding during the first two components is maintained by food delivery and responding during the third component is maintained by shock stimulus termination. Records are shown during baseline conditions and during sessions where cocaine has been given intravenously.

for animal 2144. Rates of responding maintained by food on both the FR and DRL schedules decreased but this was not dose-related (Figure 12: top and bottom panels). The decrease in rate of responding is also reflected in the decreased number of reinforcers earned on the DRL schedule (Figure 12: middle panel). The failure of cocaine to increase low rates of responding such as that maintained by DRL schedules is surprising, since psychomotor stimulants often increase low rates of responding.[23] Rate of responding maintained by shock avoidance, on the other hand, despite the fact that it was almost identical to the rate of responding for food on the FR schedule, was not decreased but, in fact, increased (Figure 12: top panel). No

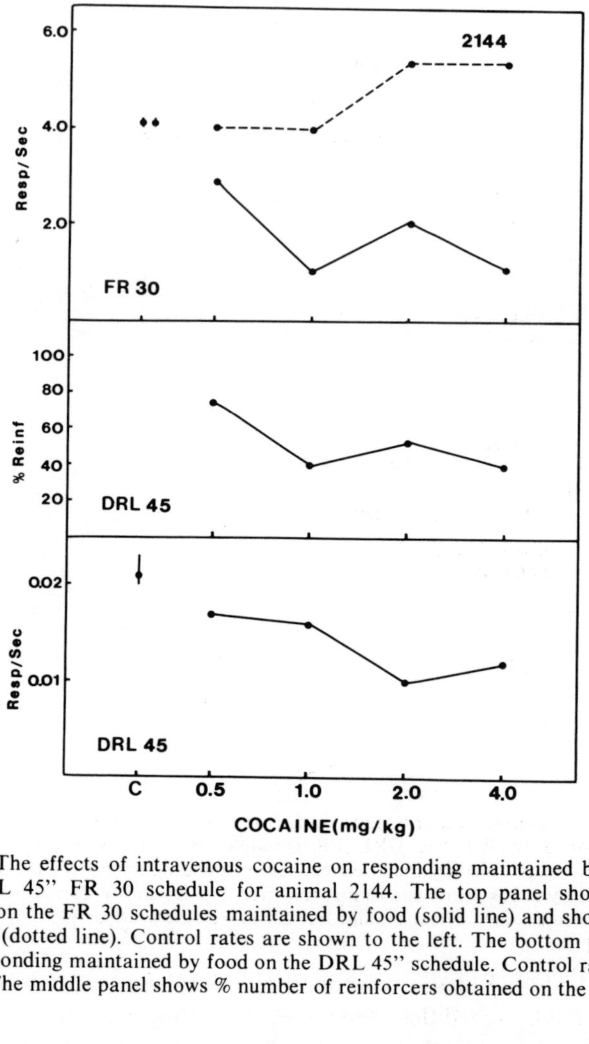

Figure 12. The effects of intravenous cocaine on responding maintained by a MULT FR 30 DRL 45" FR 30 schedule for animal 2144. The top panel shows rates of responding on the FR 30 schedules maintained by food (solid line) and shock stimulus termination (dotted line). Control rates are shown to the left. The bottom panel shows rates of responding maintained by food on the DRL 45" schedule. Control rate is shown to the left. The middle panel shows % number of reinforcers obtained on the DRL 45".

attempts were made to increase the cocaine dose because 4.0 mg/kg precipitated convulsions in this animal on many occasions. When this occurred, sessions were terminated and diazepam (10 mg/kg) was used to control the convulsions.

Figure 13 shows the dose-response function for diethylpropion for the same animal. It is important to note that control rates of responding maintained by all three schedules were strikingly similar to control rates for cocaine shown in Figure 12. Rates of responding maintained by food on the FR 30 schedule were decreased at 2.0 mg/kg and showed a maximal decrease at 12 mg/kg (Figure 13: top panel). DRL performance as measured by number of reinforcers earned was disrupted at 1.0 mg/kg (Figure 13: middle panel), but as with cocaine, rate of responding maintained by shock avoidance was unaffected even at 12 mg/kg (Figure 13: top panel). A dose of 16 mg/kg resulted in convulsions that were terminated by diazepam. Unlike cocaine, response rate on the DRL schedule increased so that the IRT distribution shifted to the left. These increases, however, were unrelated to dose (Figure 13: bottom panel). Although several measures could be

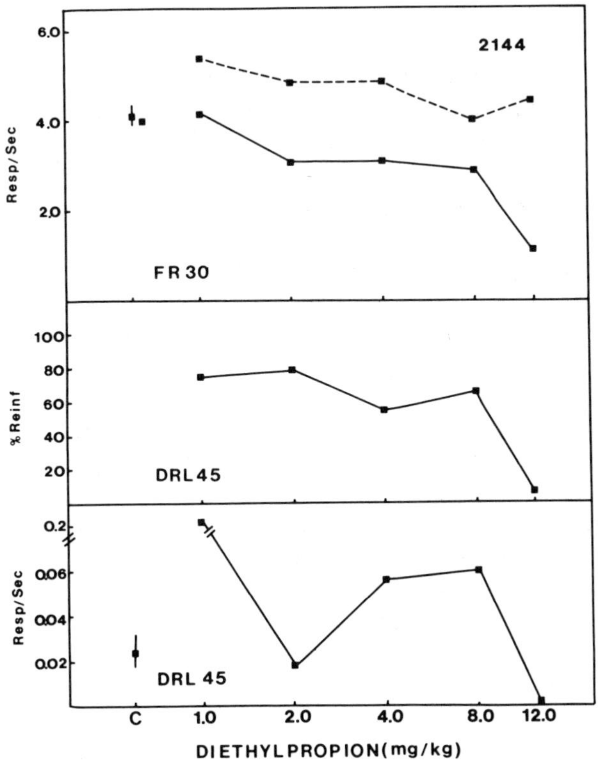

Figure 13. The effects of intravenous diethylpropion on responding maintained by a MULT FR 30 DRL 45" FR 30 schedule for animal 2144. The top panel shows rates of responding on the FR 30 schedules maintained by food (solid line) and shock stimulus termination (dotted line). Control rates are shown to the left. The bottom panel shows rates of responding maintained by food on the DRL 45" schedule. Control rate is shown to the left. The middle panel shows percent number of reinforcers obtained on the DRL 45".

used to compare the relative potencies of cocaine and diethylpropion (lowest effective dose for 3 schedules, maximum tolerated dose, ED 50, etc.), on the average there seems to be a 4-fold difference, with cocaine being more potent. This is similar to the potency differences found in the substitution procedure (2-1/2:1) but is very different from that seen in the choice study. Therefore, it is possible that the results of the substitution test largely reflect diethylpropion's direct effects but not its reinforcing effects.

TESTING OF PERPHENAZINE

Substitution

Diethylpropion is an example of a test drug giving positive results in the substitution procedure. Perphenazine, on the other hand, produced very different results during this initial testing.[24] The substitution procedure used was similar to that described for diethylpropion with two exceptions. Both 0.2 mg/kg cocaine and 0.5 mg/kg pentobarbital were used as baseline drugs because it has been shown that past history can affect pattern of intake.[25] In addition, sessions for two of the six animals were separated by at least three days and no sessions were conducted on the other days. Sessions were separated by three days to control for cumulative drug effects. Five doses of perphenazine were tested in three of the monkeys: 0.0001, 0.001, 0.01, 0.1 and 1.0 mg/kg/infusion. The highest dose was omitted for a fourth monkey. For the two monkeys with sessions separated by three days, only 0.01 mg/kg perphenazine was tested.

Figure 14 shows the mean number of infusions of perphenazine self-administration as a function of dose per infusion. These means were calculated from the last three sessions at each dose of perphenazine. The mean and range of saline infusions are indicated to the right of each curve. On the last three days of substitution, animals A043 and 4029, whose sessions were separated by 3 days, self-administered a mean of 11 and 4 infusions of 0.01 mg/kg perphenazine, respectively. For each animal, no dose of perphenazine maintained more responding than that maintained by saline. Table 2 indicates mean perphenazine intake for each dose tested. While intake increased as a function of dose, the number of infusions taken was small and they occurred in the first few minutes of the session.

Clearly, perphenazine is not a positive reinforcer, since rates of responding were consistently below those maintained by saline. Since

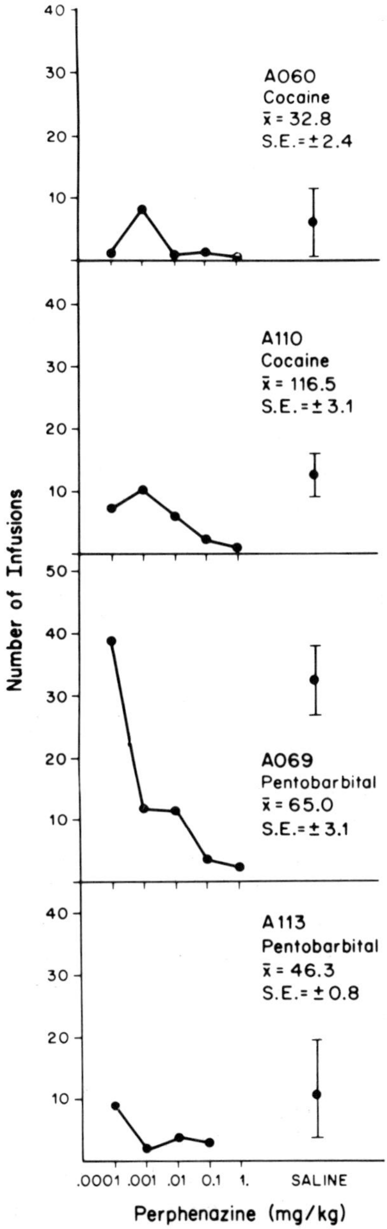

Figure 14. Dose-response functions showing the mean number of infusions self-administered at different doses of perphenazine for 4 animals in the substitution procedure. These means are derived from data obtained on the last three sessions at each dose. Means for saline and baseline drugs are also shown. (Modified from Ref. 24.)

Table 2. Mean perphenazine intake (mg/kg) for each animal as a function of dose, calculated from the last three days of substitution

	Dose (mg/kg/inf)				
Animal	0.0001	0.001	0.01	0.1	1.0
A043	NT[b]	NT[b]	0.11	NT[b]	NT[b]
A060	0.0001	0.008	0.01	0.1	0
A069[a]	0.0039	0.012	0.11	0.3	2.0
A110	0.0007	0.01	0.06	0.2	1.0
A113[a]	0.0009	0.002	0.04	0.3	NT[b]
4029	NT[b]	NT[b]	0.04	NT[b]	NT[b]

Reprinted from Ref. 24.

[a] Baseline drug of pentobarbital.

[b] NT: Dose not tested.

similar results have been found in studies using chlorpromazine, these data suggest that this is a property of the entire class of phenothiazines.[10,26,27] However, it is not possible using this procedure to determine whether perphenazine has no effect on responding producing it (i.e., is neutral) or whether it has negative reinforcing properties.

Multiple Schedule

One explanation of the substitution data may be that the doses of perphenazine tested were either pharmacologically inactive (i.e., were too low) or suppressed responding to such a degree that the reinforcing effects were masked (i.e., were too high). The effects of these doses on schedule-controlled behavior are therefore important additional data. The multiple schedule of reinforcement maintained by food delivery and shock stimulus termination, as previously described, was used to assess the effects of noncontingent intravenous injections of perphenazine. As before, injections were given 1 hour after the beginning of the 3-hour daily session. Figure 15 shows the results from one animal on all three schedules. Rates of responding showed a similar dose-dependent decrease on both fixed-ratio schedules (Figure 15: top panel). Doses ranging from 0.0001 to 0.01 mg/kg had minimal effects; a dose of 0.05 mg/kg decreased responding and 0.1 mg/kg almost totally suppressed responding. The dose function was similar for the number of reinforcers earned on the DRL schedule (Figure 15: middle panel). The effects of perphenazine on rate of DRL responding was erratic, largely because of the extreme variability in control rates. This variability is attributable to response bursting. Nevertheless, the highest dose, 0.1 mg/kg, did suppress responding. These results demonstrate that the doses used in the substitution procedure were neither too low nor too high. For instance, five injections of 0.01 mg/kg (giving a total dose of 0.05 mg/kg) clearly would have produced discernible pharmacological actions. In addition, however, at least 500 injections of 0.0001 mg/kg could have been self-administered before

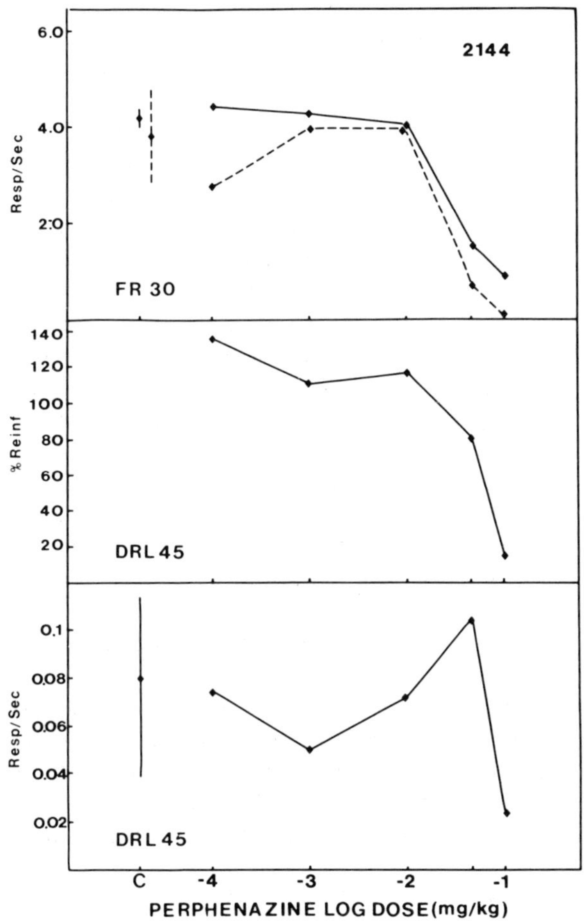

Figure 15. The effects of intravenous perphenazine on responding maintained by a MULT FR 30 DRL 45" FR 30 schedule for animal 2144. The top panel shows rates of responding on the FR 30 schedules maintained by food (solid line) and shock stimulus termination (dotted line). Control rates are shown to the left. The bottom panel shows rates of responding maintained by food on the DRL 45" schedule. Control rate is shown to the left. The middle panel shows percent number of reinforcers obtained on the DRL 45".

responding would in any way be suppressed and the reinforcing actions masked.

Escape

Although it can be concluded that perphenazine is not a positive reinforcer across a range of pharmacologically active doses, these procedures are not able to differentiate between compounds that are aversive and ones that are neutral. If a compound is aversive, animals should respond to avoid or terminate (i.e., escape) an injection. In the last few years it has been shown that morphine-dependent rhesus monkeys will escape or avoid injections of morphine antagonists.[28-31] The aversiveness of the antagonists is probably related to their ability to produce withdrawal symptoms, although it has also been shown that monkeys who are not dependent on opiates can be trained under schedules of negative reinforcement to escape and avoid antagonists.[30]

In a study by Kandel and Schuster (in preparation), rhesus monkeys physically dependent on morphine were trained to escape injections of nalorphine. After being withdrawn from morphine, these same animals were given an opportunity to escape perphenazine.

Figure 16 shows a schematic representation of the procedure. At the beginning of the session, a white house light and blue lever light were illuminated. At the same time, a continuous intravenous infusion of the drug was begun. Completion of a FR 5 requirement on the lever resulted in a 1- or 3-minute timeout period. During this time, no drug was infused. In addition, the blue lever light and white house light were terminated, and a blue house light was illuminated. Sessions were terminated after two hours or when a fixed amount of drug had been given.

Figure 17 shows the results from two animals. Response rates and latencies are shown for the first hour as well as the total session. Response rates increased and latencies decreased as the dose of perphenazine increased from 0.00025 to 0.001 mg/kg/10-sec infusion. As the dose was increased further, response rates tended to decrease and

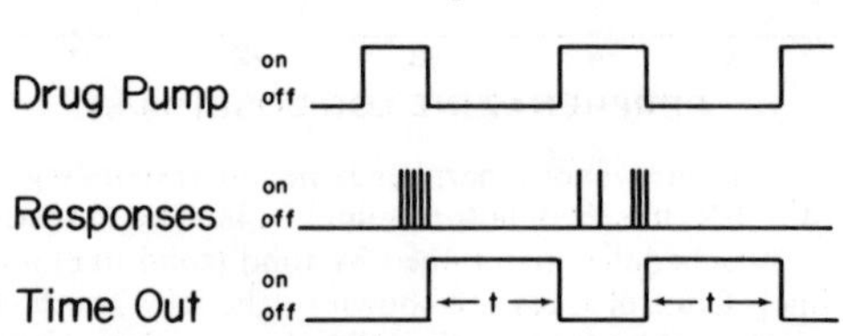

Figure 16. Diagram of drug escape procedure. (Reprinted from Kandel, D. A., and Schuster, C. R. 1977. An investigation of nalorphene and perphenazine as negative reinforcers in an escape procedure. Pharmacol. Biochem. Behav. 6:61–71.)

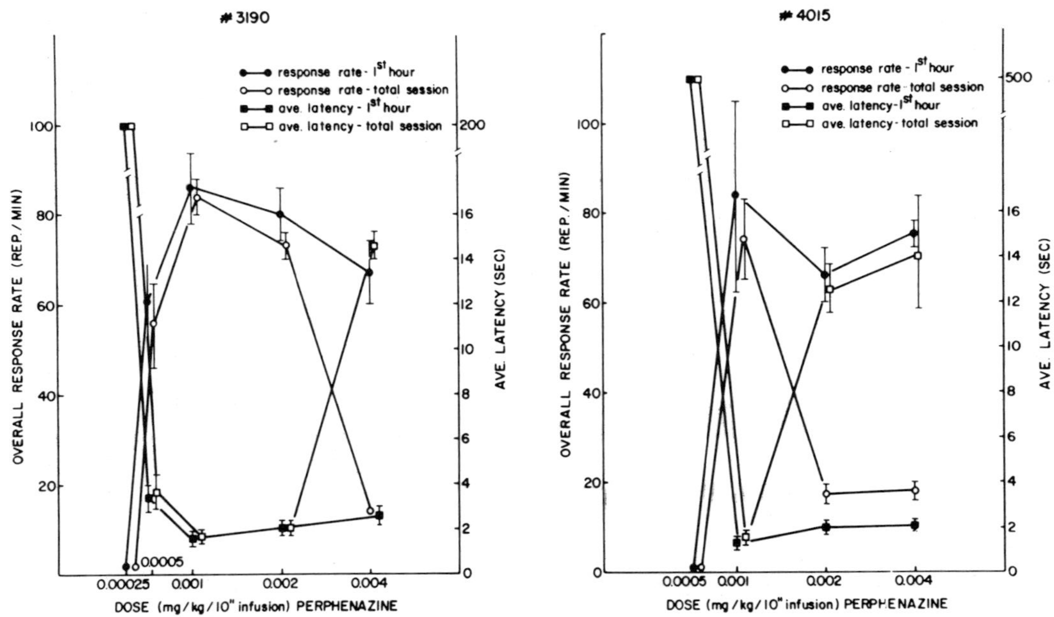

doses of perphenazine. (Reprinted from Kandel, D. A., and Schuster, C. R. 1977. An investigation of nalorphene and perphenazine as negative reinforcers in an escape procedure. Pharmacol. Biochem. Behav. 6:61–71.)

latencies tended to increase. This trend was more pronounced for rates and latencies derived from the entire session. It seems then that perphenazine does possess aversive properties, because rhesus monkeys will respond to escape its infusion. Animals are able to perform this task despite the general rate-decreasing effects of perphenazine. At high doses, however, despite the high rate of responding during the first hour of the session, enough drug is infused so that during the second hour of the session, response rates are decreased and latencies are increased.

CONCLUSIONS

The results described in this report show clearly that perphenazine is not a positive reinforcer, but indeed, has aversive properties. Test procedures allowing this type of conclusion are important for two reasons: 1) it demonstrates the specificity of the self-administration procedures, and 2) it outlines procedures useful in determining properties of drugs relevant to therapeutic use as well as abuse considerations. If a drug is aversive, i.e., will be escaped, it may be difficult to ensure that patients will consistently follow the physicians' orders to take the drug despite its demonstrated efficacy. In fact, this is exactly what often occurs with the phenothiazines. The results of the investigation of the abuse potential of diethylpropion illustrate that it is possible to discriminate between drugs in terms of their reinforcing efficacy. There is little question that diethylpropion is a positive reinforcer capable of maintaining responding under a variety of conditions. This was shown in all three self-administration procedures: substitution, unlimited access, and choice. The latter procedure, however, seemed to indicate that, relative to cocaine and methylphenidate, diethylpropion was not as powerful a reinforcer. If reinforcing properties are related to abuse potential, diethylpropion may have less abuse liability than those other compounds. There is, in fact, some clinical evidence to support this conclusion. In addition, the results of the unlimited access procedure seem to show that diethylpropion is less toxic than other stimulants although it shares many of the same properties.

The results presented in this report suggest that the behavioral procedures employed show promise in their ability to quantitatively predict the abuse potential of drugs. There are several factors that must be considered, however, in evaluating the utility of these procedures. First, the complete testing of any compound is time-consuming. The procedures outlined for the testing of diethylpropion required 1–2 years to be carried out. The cost of such procedures are correspondingly high. On a theoretical level, as well, one may question the utility of such refined measures of a drug's reinforcing properties in predicting the actual street abuse of drugs by man. It is clear that pharmacological properties of drugs alone do not determine the incidence of abuse of a compound. A variety of environmental variables can drastically alter the reinforcing properties of any event, including drugs. For instance, using the choice procedure described in the present paper, manipulations of response cost, concurrent punishment, and delay of reinforcement have all been shown to alter preference.[14] Some investigators even contend that the environmental contingencies, particularly the schedule of drug injection, are the major determinants of responding.[32,33] While pharmacological properties of a drug probably do contribute to the incidence of abuse, there is little question that these other factors are overwhelmingly influential. This limits the conclusions and decisions one can make on the basis of even the most refined, quantitative laboratory tests designed to predict the abuse potential of new drugs.

LITERATURE CITED

1. Deneau, G. A., and Seevers, M. H. 1962. Evaluation of morphine-like physical dependence in the rhesus monkey (Macaca mulatta). Bulletin: Drug Addiction and Narcotics (Addendum 2).
2. Villarreal, J. E. 1972. The effects of morphine agonists and antagonists on morphine dependent rhesus monkeys. In: H. W. Kosterlitz, H. O. J. Collier, and J. E. Villarreal (eds.), Agonist and Antagonist Actions of Narcotic Analgesic Drugs. MacMillan, London.
3. Angrist, B. M., and Gershon, S. 1969. Amphetamine Abuse in New York City: 1966–1968. Seminars in Psychiatry 1:195–207.
4. Kiloh, L. G., and Brandon, S. 1962. Habituation and addiction to amphetamines. Br. Med. J. 2:40–43.
5. Kramer, J. C., Fischman, V. S., and Littlefield, D. C. 1967. Amphetamine abuse. J. Am. Med. Assoc. 201:89–93.
6. Tatum, A. J., and Seevers, M. H. 1929. Experimental cocaine addiction. J. Pharm. Exp. Ther. 36:401–410.
7. Schuster, C. R., and Johanson, C. E. 1974. The use of animal models for the study of drug abuse. In: R. J. Gibbins, Y. Israel, H. Kalant, R. E. Popham, W. Schmidt, and R. G. Smart (eds.), Research Advances in Alcohol and Drug Problems, Vol. I, pp. 1–31. John Wiley and Sons, New York.
8. Skinner, B. F. 1938. The Behavior of Organisms. Appleton-Century-Crofts, New York.

9. Schuster, C. R., and Thompson, T. 1969. Self-administration of and behavioral dependence on drugs. Ann. Rev. Pharmacol. 9:483–502.
10. Deneau, G., Yanagita, T., and Seevers, M. H. 1969. Self-administration of psychoactive substances by the monkey: A measure of psychological dependence. Psychopharmacologia 16(1):30–48.
11. Johanson, C. E., Balster, R. L., and Bonese, K. 1976. Self-administration of psychomotor stimulant drugs: The effects of unlimited access. Pharmacol., Biochem. Behav. (In press.)
12. Fischman, M. W., and Schuster, C. R. 1975. Behavioral, biochemical and morphological effects of methamphetamine in the rhesus monkey. In: B. Weiss, and V. G. Laties (eds.), Behavioral Toxicology, pp. 375–399. Plenum Publishing, New York.
13. Ellinwood, E. H., and Duante-Escalante, O. 1972. Chronic methamphetamine intoxication in three species of experimental animals. In: E. H. Ellinwood (ed.), Current Concepts on Amphetamine Abuse pp. 59–68. DHEW Publication No. (HSM) 72-9085. U.S. Government Printing Office, Washington, D.C.
14. Johanson, C. E. 1976. Pharmacological and environmental variables affecting drug preference in rhesus monkeys. Pharmacological Reviews 27:343–355.
15. Johanson, C. E., and Schuster C. R. 1977. A comparison of cocaine and diethylpropion under two different schedules of drug presentation. In: E. Ellinwood and M. M. Kilbey (eds.), Cocaine and Other Stimulants, pp. 545–570; Plenum Press, New York.
16. Wilson, M. C., Hitomi, M., and Schuster, C. R. 1971. Psychomotor stimulant self-administration as a function of dosage per injection in the rhesus monkey. Psychopharmacologia 22:271–281.
17. Balster, R. L., and Schuster, C. R. 1973. A comparison of *d*-amphetamine, *l*-amphetamine, and methamphetamine self-administration in rhesus monkeys. Pharmacol. Biochem. Behav. 1:67–71.
18. Jonsson, C. O. 1969. Behavioral studies of diethylpropion in man. 1969. In: F. Sjoquist and M. Tottie (eds.), Abuse of Central Stimulants, pp. 71–80. Raven Press, New York.
19. Jasinski, D. R., Nutt, J. G., and Griffith, J. D. 1974. Effects of diethylpropion and *d*-amphetamine after subcutaneous and oral administration. Clin. Pharmacol. Ther., 645–652.
20. Findley, J. D. 1962. An experimental outline for building and exploring multi-operant behavior repertoires. J. Exp. Anal. Behav. 5(1):113–166.
21. Johanson, C. E., and Schuster, C. R. 1975. A choice procedure for drug reinforcers: Cocaine and methylphenidate in the rhesus monkey. J. Pharmacol. Exp. Ther. 193(2):676–688.
22. Schuster, C. R., and Balster, R. L. 1972. Self-administration of agonists. In: H. W. Kosterlitz, H. O. J. Collier, and J. E. Villarreal (eds.), Agonist and Antagonist Actions of Narcotic Analgesic Drugs, pp. 243–254. MacMillan, London.
23. Kelleher, R. T., and Morse, W. H. 1968. Determinants of the specificity of behavioral effects of drugs. Ergeb. Physiol. Biol. Chem. Exp. Pharmakol. 60:1–56.

24. Johanson, C. E., Kandel, D., and Bonese, K. F. 1976. The effects of perphenazine on self-administration behavior. Pharmacol. Biochem. Behav. 4:427–433.
25. Schlichting, U. U., Goldberg, S. R., Wuttke, W., and Hoffmeister, F. 1971. *d*-amphetamine self-administration by rhesus monkeys with different self-administration histories. Excerpta Med. Internat. Cong. Ser. 220:62–69.
26. Hoffmeister, F., Goldberg, S. R., Schlichting, U., and Wuttke, W. 1970. Self-administration of *d*-amphetamine, morphine and chlorpromazine by cocaine "dependent" rhesus monkeys. Nauyn-Schmiedelbergsarch Pharmak. 266:359–260.
27. Yanagita, T., Ando, M. A., and Takahashi, S. 1970. A testing method for psychological dependence liability of drugs in monkeys. Committee on Problems of Drug Dependence, NAS-NRC. 6583–6591.
28. Downs, D. A., and Woods, J. H. 1975. Fixed-ratio escape and avoidance-escape from naloxone in morphine-dependent monkeys: Effects of naloxone dose and morphine pretreatment. J. Exp. Anal. Behav. 23:415–427.
29. Goldberg, S. R., Hoffmeister, F., Schlichting, U. U., and Wuttke, W. 1971. Aversive properties of nalorphine and naloxone in morphine-dependent rhesus monkeys. J. Pharmacol. Exper. Ther. 179:268–276.
30. Hoffmeister, F., and Wuttke, W. 1973. Negative reinforcing properties of morphine-antagonists in naive rhesus monkeys. Psychopharmacologia 33:257–258.
31. Hoffmeister, F., and Wuttke, W. 1974. Self-administration: Positive and negative reinforcing properties of morphine antagonists in rhesus monkeys. In: M. C. Braude, L. S. Harris, E. L. May, J. P. Smith and J. E. Villarreal (eds.), Narcotic Antagonists, pp. 361–369. Raven Press, New York.
32. Goldberg, S. R. 1973. Comparable behavior maintained under fixed-ratio and second-order schedules of food presentation, cocaine injection and *d*-amphetamine injection in the squirrel monkey. J. Pharmacol. Exper. Ther. 186:18–30.
33. Goldberg, S. R., and Kelleher, R. T. 1976. Behavior controlled by scheduled injections of cocaine in squirrel and rhesus monkeys. J. Exp. Anal. Behav. 25:93–104.

Brief Review on the Use of Self-Administration Techniques for Predicting Drug Dependence Potential

Tomoji Yanagita

Since the presently used self-administration techniques have been introduced to the field of drug dependence studies, our knowledge of dependence-producing properties of various drugs has increased, and the usefulness and limitation of self-administration experiments in laboratory animals for predicting the drug dependence potentials in man have been well discussed elsewhere.[1-3] Therefore, they are not repeated here, except for the point that the reliability and validity of animal tests for predicting the potentials have been considerably improved since the adoption of the technique. The current test procedures in the self-administration experiments are roughly divided into 3 types: 1) the cross self-administration test of a test drug with active and/or inactive reference agents, 2) the continuous self-administration test, and 3) the test for quantification of the reinforcing property. Therefore, the present status of, and problems in the use of, self-administration techniques for predicting drug dependence potential are discussed with regard to each type.

CROSS SELF-ADMINISTRATION TEST

Many investigators are using this procedure for assessing the reinforcing property of a drug. Animals are first trained to discriminate between a prototype reinforcer and an inactive agent (usually saline) in intravenous self-administration of drugs by pressing a lever at fixed ratios of 1 to 10 or higher. Then, they are tested with cross self-administration of a test drug with the control agents, for a limited time period of a day or a few days, for each agent or each unit dose. Finally, the response rates for the test drug at each unit dose are compared with those for the reference agents in each animal. Any drug that is intravenously injectible can be tested by this procedure, but it is most effective with short-acting drugs, e.g., many of the stimulants and short-acting hypnotics. Some examples of the results in several drugs are illustrated in Figures 1 and 2. The advantage of this test is that it requires a relatively short time period in comparison with the continuous self-administration test. On the other hand, in comparison to the continuous test, this test has such disadvantages as the following: 1) The overt signs of the drug effects at self-maintained dose levels are usually not well observed because of the time limitation of the availability of the drug. 2) Occasionally false negative results may be obtained with such drugs that are weakly reinforcing or long-acting. For example, the reinforcing effect of nicotine, which is clearly

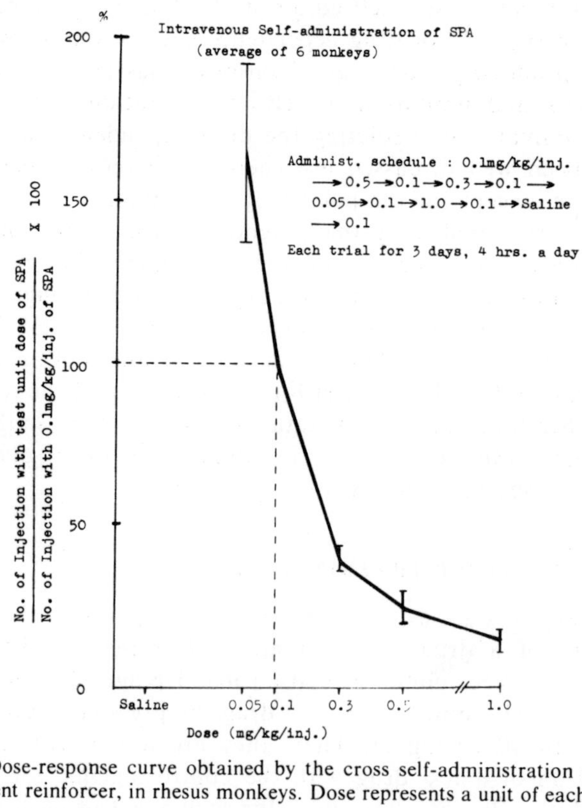

Figure 1. Dose-response curve obtained by the cross self-administration procedure of SPA, a potent reinforcer, in rhesus monkeys. Dose represents a unit of each injection.

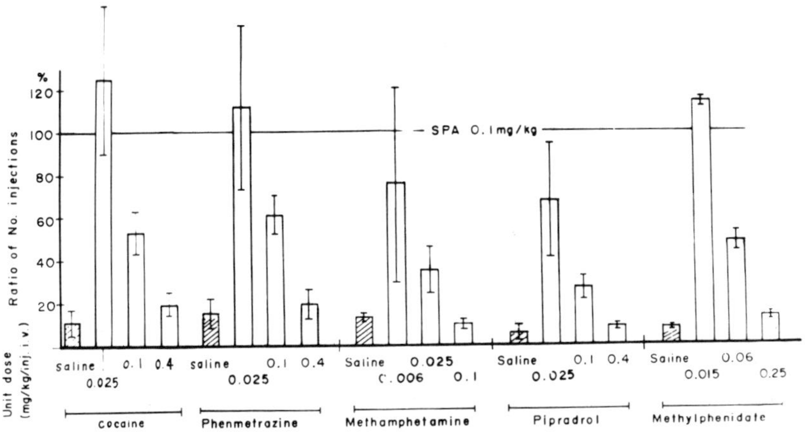

Figure 2. Results of the cross self-administration tests on some stimulants in four rhesus monkeys. Drugs were tested for three days each for each unit dose from high to low doses. Prior to each 3-day trial, the control trials on SPA (at 0.1 mg/kg/inj.) and saline were conducted for three days each. The ratio represents percentage of the number of injections during a test trial to that of SPA.

demonstrable in the continuous test, was not clearly demonstrable by this test when SPA, a potent reinforcer, was used as the active reference drug (Figure 3). 3) Drugs that cannot be prepared in an intravenously injectible form are not applicable because the procedure is not applicable to the intragastric self-administration technique. Concerning point 1 above, one of the most important pieces of information that self-administration experiments can provide is whether or not the drug produces overt behavioral signs at self-maintained dose levels. Occasionally, the overt signs of drug effects will appear in the test, but they may not be sufficient, and the observation should be made on a chronic administration basis.

Concerning point 2, the choice of the active reference drug influences the results greatly, as is illustrated in Figure 4. Therefore, one possible alternative may be to eliminate the use of the active reference drug entirely from this test, and simply compare the response rate for the drug with that of the inactive reference agent. This kind of procedure is being used by several investigators.[4] Concerning point 3, the reason that intragastric self-administration is not suitable for this test is the slow absorption rate and the delayed onset of effects by this administration route, which make it difficult for the animals to follow the quick schedule changes.

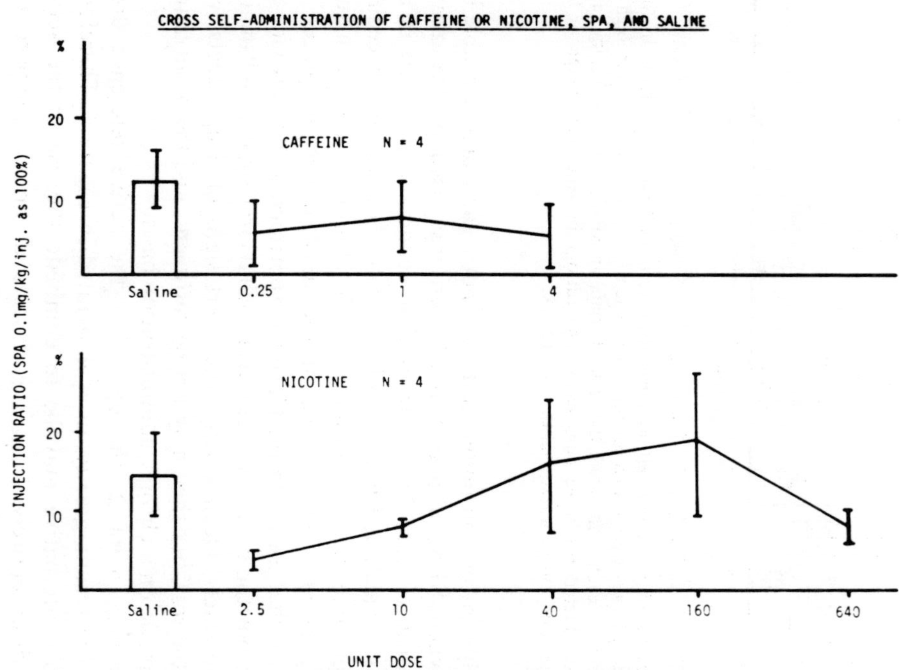

Figure 3. Results of the cross self-administration tests on caffeine and nicotine in rhesus monkeys. The unit dose represents mg/kg for caffeine and μg/kg for nicotine. The injection ratio for nicotine at doses of 40 and 160 μg/kg slightly increased in two monkeys, but the increase was not significant (Yanagita, unpublished).

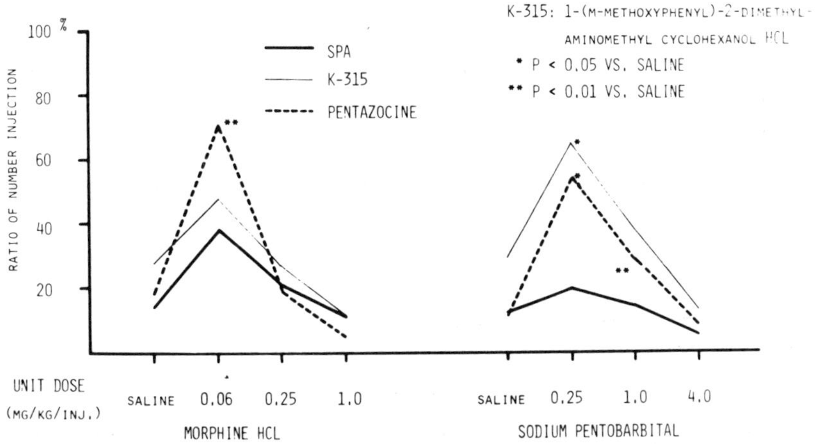

Figure 4. Results of the cross self-administration tests on morphine and pentobarbital-Na in six monkeys. Three drugs were used as reference drugs and six monkeys were tested with the three reference drugs by the latin-square order. The reinforcing effects of morphine and pentobarbital was clearly demonstrated when pentazocine was used as the reference drug (Yanagita, unpublished).

Thus, it was strongly felt that the essential test in self-administration experiments should be the continuous test.

CONTINUOUS SELF-ADMINISTRATION TEST

A standard procedure of the continuous self-administration test is to allow the animal to take the drug for several weeks without time or dose limitation. Both naive and self-administration experienced monkeys are used. At the beginning of the test, the operant levels of the lever pressing behavior of the animals are observed with saline, and when the daily rates become low and stable, saline is replaced with a test drug at an appropriate unit dose. The unit dose used first is determined from the preliminary dose-range finding test, by single manual administration of the drug to normal subjects, and from the results obtained in the cross self-administration test. At fixed intervals, such as every two weeks, the necessity for changing the unit dose and/or imposing forced programmed administration of the drug should be considered. The important information to be obtained from this test concerns the initiation, continuity, and characteristics in self-administration of a test drug by analyzing such parameters as the daily response rate, the daily dose level, and patterns of self-adminis-

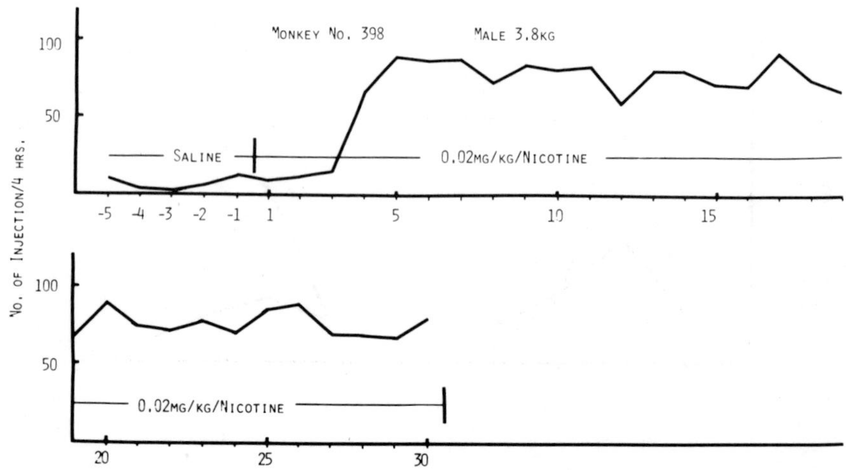

Figure 5. A case of the continuous self-administration test on nicotine in a rhesus monkey. The monkey initiated on the fourth day. Note the stable daily dose levels (Yanagita, unpublished).

tration. A classification of principal drugs by these pattern characteristics is shown in Table 1 and Figures 5 and 6. As mentioned previously, it is also very important to know the behavioral effects at these dose levels. A good example is the case of nicotine. As seen in Figure 5, the monkeys took nicotine at a stable daily dose level. Yet

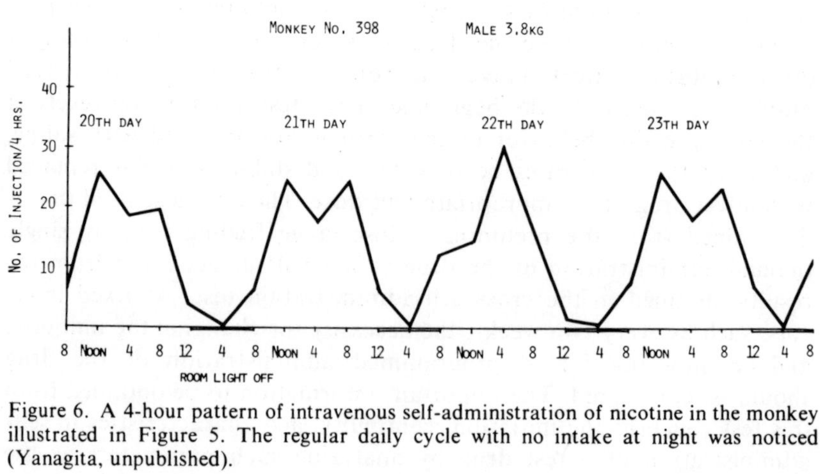

Figure 6. A 4-hour pattern of intravenous self-administration of nicotine in the monkey illustrated in Figure 5. The regular daily cycle with no intake at night was noticed (Yanagita, unpublished).

Table 1. Pattern characteristics of drugs in continuous intravenous self-administration

Reinforcing					
Daily stable			Erratic		
Gradual increase	Transient increase	Flat	Frequent intake	Infrequent	Non-reinforcing
Alcohol[a]	Chlordiazepoxide[a]	Nicotine	Amphetamine	Caffeine	LSD-25
Codeine	Diazepam[a]		Cocaine		Mescaline
Morphine	Nitrazepam[b]		Volatile anesthetics[c]		Nalorphine
Pentobarbital[b]					THC

[a] Both intravenous and intragastric.

[b] Intragastric.

[c] Inhalation.

the monkey never showed the overt behavioral signs. This was a significant difference from those of the principal drugs of nonmedical use, because the overt signs are markedly demonstrable with many stimulants and some sedative-hypnotics.

One disadvantage of this test is the limitation of the unit dose changes within short time periods, since the continuous test procedure requires at least 1 or 2 weeks' observation period before the unit dose is changed. However, the change is very important when an obvious initiation of self-administration is not observed, because if the unit dose is too small, the monkey may not initiate, and if the unit dose is too large, the self-administration rate may become low. Examples of these two cases are illustrated in Figures 7 and 8 respectively.

When a test drug cannot be prepared for intravenous injection, then the intragastric technique must be used. Many of the sedative hypnotics that have been developed recently are water insoluble. Thus the technique has become more important than before. However, the animals are generally less sensitive to the reinforcing effect of the drug by this route. For this reason, the use of experienced monkeys is advantageous for the intragastric self-administration test, because regardless of whether or not the route is intravenous or intragastric, experienced monkeys are more sensitive to drug effects than naive monkeys. One example is shown in Table 2, giving the result of a study with nicotine.

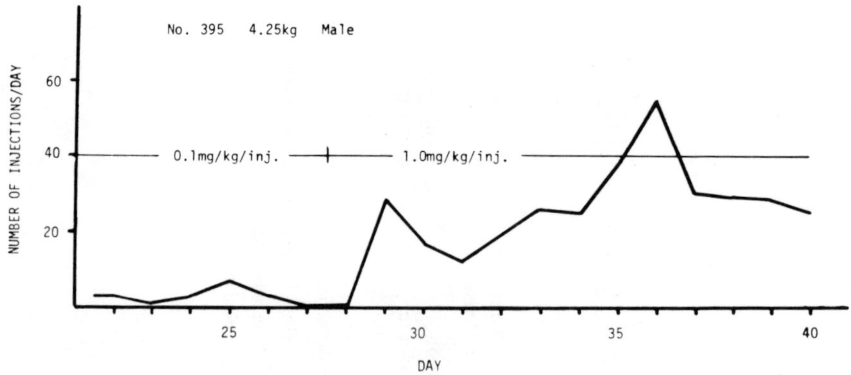

Figure 7. A case of the continuous self-administration test on thebaine in a rhesus monkey. The initiation was observed as the unit dose was increased (Yanagita, unpublished).

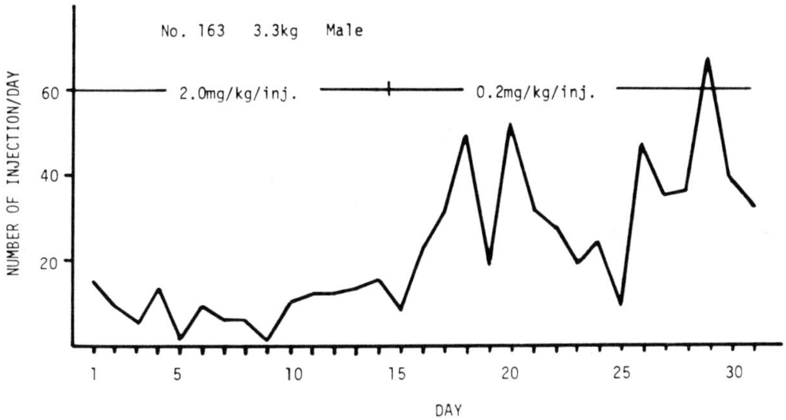

Figure 8. A case of the continuous self-administration test on diazepam by the intragastric technique in a rhesus monkey. The initiation was not clear at the unit dose of 2 mg/kg but became clear as the unit dose was decreased (Yanagita, unpublished).

EXPERIMENTS FOR THE QUANTIFICATION OF THE REINFORCING PROPERTY

Animals may show different interests from man in the subjective effects of the drug; therefore, the mere fact that they self-administer a test drug may not be a strong evidence that the drug has a significant dependence potential for man. But most of the principal drugs of nonmedical use in man seem to possess considerably strong reinforcing effects, as well as gross behavioral effects. Thus, for reliable prediction of the drug dependence potential, the quantification of the reinforcing effect is extremely important. The methods presently under study for this purpose can roughly be categorized according to two techniques. One is the drug choice procedure between two drugs or two different unit doses, which has been intensively studied by Schuster and Johanson.[5] The other is the measurement of the intensity of the animals' drug-seeking efforts, such as the progressive ratio procedure,[3] and the second-order schedule procedure.[6,7] As an example, the results obtained from a progressive ratio test on cocaine and nicotine are illustrated in Table 3. Here, the intensity of the reinforcing effect of nicotine at the unit dose of 200 μg/kg was found to be nearly equal to that of cocaine at 30 μg/kg. One problem of this procedure is the conditioned property of the drug-seeking behavior,

Table 2. Influence of previous experience on intravenous self-administration of nicotine

	Subject	Previous drug	Initiation	Approx. Daily Dose (μg/kg/inj. × No.)	Pattern of intake
Experienced	1[a]	SPA	+	200 × 15	Constant
	2[a]	SPA	+	20 × 100	Constant
	3[a]	SPA	+	20 × 50	Constant
	4[b]	SPA	+	20 × 35	Irregular
	5[a]	Cocaine	+	50 × 40	Constant
	6[a]	Cocaine	+	20 × 100	Constant
Naive	7	None	+	100 × 20	Constant
	8	None	+	200 × 20	Constant
	9	None	+	20 × 80	Constant
	10	None	+	20 × 50	Constant
	11	None	−		
	12	None	−		
	13	None	−		

[a] Time interval longer than 1 month before nicotine study.
[b] Study followed immediately after 9 days' SPA intake.

Table 3. Progressive ratio test on cocaine and nicotine

		Monkey[b]				
Drug	Unit Dose (mg/kg/inj.)	#243 (3.5 kg; female)	#248 (3.8 kg; female)	#281 (4.3 kg; female)	#334 (4.7 kg; male)	Mean of ( )
Saline	0.25[a]	800	400	200	200	*1.0*
Cocaine	0.03	400 (1/2)	800 (2)	800 (4)	1,600 (8)	3.6
	0.12	6,400 (8)	3,200 (8)	6,400 (32)	3,200 (16)	16.0
	0.48	6,400 (8)	6,400 (16)	12,800 (64)	12,800 (64)	38.0
Nicotine	0.05	200 (1/4)	400 (1)	400 (2)	400 (2)	1.3
	0.2	800 (1)	800 (2)	800 (4)	1,600 (8)	3.8

[a] ml/kg.
[b] Numbers in parentheses indicate ratios against the scores for saline.

since animals may come to show high ratios for saline when they are repeatedly used for this test.

For the quantification, some other efforts, such as an attempt to use the conflicting behavior or the resistance in the extinction course, have been made in the past, but these approaches are not yet well developed.

SOME OTHER PROBLEMS

In the present use of self-administration techniques for the prediction of drug dependence potential, monkeys are most often used, but since the supply of monkeys is gradually diminishing, the extent to which other species of animals can be used must be studied. In addition, since the monkey is not necessarily the most similar species to man in pharmacodynamics and pharmacokinetics of individual drugs, some appropriate techniques and procedures for other species must be developed.

Another problem is the limitation of predictability from animal studies, because the dependence potential of some hallucinogens is difficult to demonstrate in animals by using the above procedures.

Although further studies are necessary to establish better methods for predicting dependence potential, at the same time some appropriate measure needs to be established for predicting the extent of social and individual harms that may arise as a result of development of dependence on drugs.

LITERATURE CITED

1. Eddy, N. B. 1973. Bayer-Symposium IV "Psychic Dependence," p. 192. Springer-Verlag, New York.
2. Wikler, A. 1973. Pharmacology and the Future of Man. Proc. 5th Int. Congr. Pharmacology, San Francisco 1972. Vol. 1, p. 18. Karger, Basel.
3. Yanagita, T. 1973. Pharmacology and the Future of Man. Proc. 5th Int. Congr. Pharmacology, San Francisco 1972. Vol. 1, p. 7. Karger, Basel.
4. Winger, G., Stitzer, M. L., and Woods, J. H. 1975. J. Pharmacol. Exp. Ther. 195:505.
5. Johanson, E. E., and Schuster, C. R. 1975. J. Pharmacol. Exp. Ther. 193:676.
6. Goldberg, S. R. 1973. J. Pharmacol. Exp. Ther. 186:18.
7. Goldberg, S. R. et al. 1974. In: Proceedings of the 36th Annual Meeting of the Committee on Problems of Drug Dependence.

Stimulus Self-Administration

Some Implications for the Prediction of Drug Abuse Liability

Nancy K. Mello

One of the issues examined in this volume is the extent to which the relative reinforcing properties of drugs can be predicted from laboratory models. There is little question that there has been dramatic progress in this area over the past twelve years.[1] The sensitivity and sophistication of currently available techniques in behavioral pharmacology have been illustrated by the chapters on self-administration of drugs. Rather than amplify upon the self-evident merit and significance of the presentations by Drs. Brady, Hoffmeister, Johanson, and Yanagita in this text, I would like to discuss some basic behavioral data that have disquieting implications for the way we think about the nature of reinforcement. Since our conceptualization of "reinforcement" is central to strategies evolved for the behavioral assessment of abuse liability with animal models, some continuing examination of basic assumptions is desirable. Self-administration of a psychoactive compound indicates that the compound is "reinforcing" and serves as the primary behavioral index of potential abuse liability.

Although behavioral scientists are usually careful to distinguish between reinforcement and reward, following the conventions established by B. F. Skinner,[2,3] there is a pervasive tendency to equate drug reinforcement with some, usually unspecified, positive or rewarding consequence for the animal or human drug user. "Reinforcing," "rewarding," and "euphorigenic" are often used interchangeably to convey the complex consequences that are believed to follow upon, and in some sense to explain, persistent drug use and abuse. The notion of "reward" in its several variants has a compelling face

---

Preparation of this paper was supported by Grant DA 4RG010 from the National Institute of Drug Abuse, ADAMHA.

validity that does not invite critical examination. Yet there are abundant clinical data that indicate that the reported subjective effects of chronic alcohol abuse and opiate abuse are not "rewarding," in the sense of euphorigenic or relaxing. Chronic alcohol and opiate abuse both appear to be associated with the development of progressive dysphoria, anxiety, irritability, and aggressivity.[4-10,36] Still, drug abuse is maintained despite these seemingly aversive consequences.

The continuation of drug use that produces adverse consequences during intoxication, as well as long-term legal, social, medical, and economic consequences seems antithetical to the idea that drug use is maintained by "rewarding" consequences. It could be argued that the brief and transient positive mood change purportedly associated with the induction of alcohol and heroin intoxication is sufficient to maintain drug self-administration behavior.[cf.8,9,11] These initial changes during intoxication induction have been difficult to characterize in terms of subjective quality or temporal duration.

A second possibility is that drug-induced dissociation results in an inability to recall events that occurred during intoxication and therefore aversive consequences cannot affect the reinitiation and perpetuation of drug use. Alcohol appears to induce such effects clinically,[6,12-15] but the generality of these findings for other drugs of abuse remains to be determined.

A third possibility is that drugs are used to induce some change in subjective state, and the direction of that change—up or down—is far less important than the change itself. This could account for simultaneous and sequential multiple drug use patterns in which drugs with demonstrably different pharmacological effects are used, e.g., methadone + alcohol; amphetamines + barbiturates; marihuana + alcohol, etc. Certainly, anecdotal accounts of voracious polydrug use suggest that the goal is to achieve a rapid change in state, and the direction of the change may be of secondary importance.[16] One limitation of this concept of "state change" is that confirmation or refutation must ultimately rely on accurate descriptions of subjective states by addicted individuals, with all the potential for accidental or deliberate distortion that self-report data inevitably involve. Still, this hypothesis is a more attractive and testable idea than the invocation of masochism or ineffectual hedonism to account for drug abuse.

Comparable ideas about "state change" have been expressed in describing the objectives of a single as well as multiple drug use. In 1953, Wikler and Rasor pointed out that an addict's description of the nature of the "positive" effects of drugs varies considerably in different types of drug addiction.[17] One reason for using drugs advanced by some addicts is to get "off the normal" with the implication that "the normal" is in some way aversive.[17]

Central to the idea that drug-induced "state change" is important in the maintenance of drug self-administration behavior is the notion that the stimulus properties of drugs, rather than the specific qualities of these stimuli, may be important determinants of drug self-administration. State change may be the subjective response to the drug-induced stimulus, whatever that stimulus may be. It is obvious that a drug must have some stimulus properties in order to be self-administered. To the extent that stimulus change effected by drug use may be more important than the inherently positive of negative characteristics of that stimulus, it may be useful to consider drug self-administration within a more general framework of stimulus self-administration. This idea is an extension of, but not identical to, the now familiar idea that drugs have many stimulus properties, i.e., as reinforcing stimuli, discriminative stimuli, and as unconditioned stimuli. This literature has been extensively reviewed and will not be summarized here.[cf.1,18-20] The idea that drug self-administration could be thought of as stimulus self-administration is consistent with contemporary concepts about the nature of reinforcement. These concepts and some data that suggest the reinforcing properties of stimulus presentation are reviewed in the next section.

WHAT IS REINFORCEMENT?

In operant terminology, a reinforcer is an event that maintains behavior, i.e., a reinforcer is a consequence of behavior that increases the probability of the recurrence of that behavior. Food and psychoactive drug self-administration are familiar examples of reinforcers that maintain operant response behavior under certain conditions. Despite the conspicuous absence of "reward" from these definitions, there has been a dominant tendency to think about reinforcers and reinforcement potential in terms of the alleged properties of events, rather than in terms of the functional relations between events and behavior. An alternative framework for differentiating between reinforcement and punishment has been formulated by Morse and Kelleher[21] and is illustrated in Table 1. In this formulation, both reinforcement and punishment are defined in terms of the effect on behavior, rather than in terms of the inherent properties of the reinforcing or punishing stimulus event. The defining characteristics of reinforcers and

Table 1. Reinforcement and punishment differentiated in terms of behavioral effects

Event	Behavioral Effect	
	Increase Behavior	Decrease Behavior
Present Stimulus	Reinforcement	Punishment
Remove Stimulus	Reinforcement	Punishment

Adapted from Morse, W. H., and Kelleher, R. T.: Determinants of reinforcement and punishment. In: W. K. Honig and J. E. R. Staddon (eds.), *Operant Behavior,* 1977.

punishers are how they change behavior. The same stimulus may have either reinforcing or punishing effects, depending upon the conditions under which it is presented. Defining stimulus events in terms of the behavioral effect, rather than in terms of an a priori interpretation of the alleged properties of the stimulus event, represents a radical departure from the insidious dichotomous thinking that has become a convenient convention. The polar extremes of "reward" and "punishment" are as imbedded in our language and our thinking as "good" and "evil" and are often applied with equal fervor and less qualification.

For example, we commonly think of events such as electric shock or the administration of a narcotic antagonist to an opiate-dependent animal as "aversive" events, and there is ample data that animals will work to avoid or escape from the presentation of electric shock or naloxone and nalorphine.[22-26] Moreover, the superimposition of high doses of narcotic antagonists on ongoing response behavior for opiate reinforcement can result in a suppression of that behavior. The superimposition of a response contingent electric shock (2–8 ma) will even suppress cocaine self-administration in monkeys, and the degree of suppression was directly related to increases in shock intensity.[27] There is little question about the effectiveness of these types of events in either suppressing ongoing behavior for another reinforcer or maintaining escape and avoidance behavior. The complex interactions between punished (usually by electric shock) responding and the effects of drugs have been recently reviewed.[26]

RESPONSE-PRODUCED SHOCK

If we think about behavioral control in conventional terms, i.e., in terms of the apparent aversive properties of events such as electric shock, there have been some seemingly anomolous findings that have important implications for our efforts to predict reinforcement potential. *It has been found that the same electric shock event that can maintain escape and avoidance behavior may, under certain conditions, be self-administered by the same monkey.* Identification of this phenomenon, called response-produced shock, developed from the initial observations of Kelleher and co-workers[28] that responding increased during a preshock stimulus and decreased if the terminal shock was removed. Response-produced shock has now been observed in many laboratories, across several species, and has been shown to be a reliable and persistent phenomenon.[29-38] Under certain conditions, monkeys will continue to self-administer electric shock for months and even for years.[35]

An illustration of behavior maintained by response-produced shock is shown in Figure 1.[35] The cumulative response records of the operant performance of a single monkey are shown, and, at the top, behavior on a schedule of shock termination (FI 5 min) is displayed. The first response after 5 minutes has elapsed terminates an electric shock (7 ma), which is presented every 5 minutes. In the lower portion of Figure 1 is shown cumulative responses of the same monkey on a schedule of shock production. Now, instead of terminating a shock presented every 5 minutes, the monkey self-administers a shock of 1 ma every 5 minutes. The diagonal deflections on the cumulative record indicate the 1 ma shock presentations. The rate of responding is higher and the pattern of positively accelerated responding is more marked when responses produce shock than when responses terminate shock. If a response did not produce a shock within 5 seconds after 5 minutes had elapsed, a shock (7 ma) was presented automatically.

Another example of response-produced shock is shown in Figure 2.[35] In the top cumulative record, a monkey with a particular behavioral history receives shocks (5 ma) that are presented every 2 minutes and are independent of response behavior. Each shock is followed by a brief timeout period. In the lower portion of Figure 2, a shock of the same intensity (5 ma) is scheduled to occur upon the first response after a fixed interval of 2 minutes (FI 2 min) and is followed by a brief timeout. Response behavior is obviously maintained by shock presentation and the rate of responding increases, and the pattern of responding is more positively accelerated on a shock presentation schedule than on a shock termination schedule.

The specifics of the schedules of reinforcement that are required to develop response-produced shock behavior are of less concern here than the fact that this phenomenon must be preceded by some

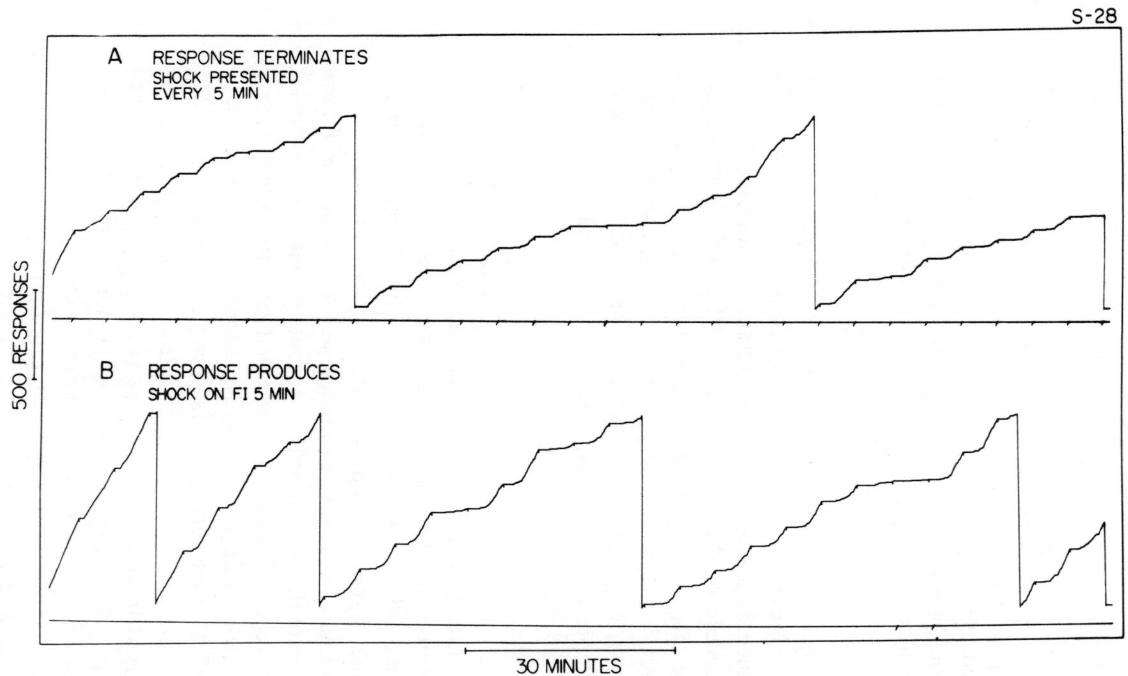

Figure 1. Performance under an FI 5 min schedule of termination of electric shock and an FI 5 min schedule of presentation of electric shock (Monkey S-28). *A*: Short diagonal strokes in the event record (bottom) indicate successive electric shock presentations (7 ma); diagonal strokes on the cumulative record (top) indicate the termination of shock. *B*: Strokes on the cumulative record indicate 1 ma electric shock presentations. If a response did not produce shock within 5 seconds after 5 minutes had elapsed, a 7-ma shock was presented automatically. When responses produced shock, rates of responding became higher and patterns of positively accelerated responding became more marked. From Morse, W. H., and Kelleher, R. T. 1970. Schedules as fundamental determinants of behavior. In: W. N. Schoenfeld (ed.), The Theory of Reinforcement Schedules, pp. 139–185. Appleton-Century-Crofts, New York. Reprinted by permission of Prentice-Hall, Inc., Englewood Cliffs, New Jersey.

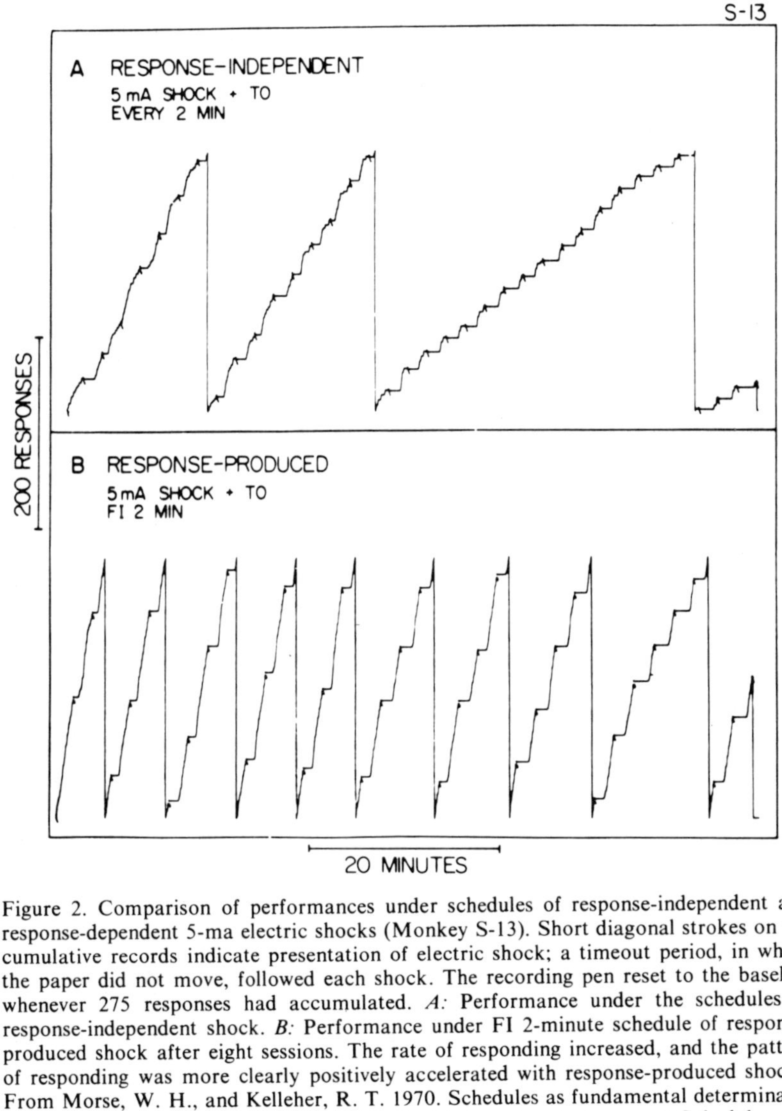

Figure 2. Comparison of performances under schedules of response-independent and response-dependent 5-ma electric shocks (Monkey S-13). Short diagonal strokes on the cumulative records indicate presentation of electric shock; a timeout period, in which the paper did not move, followed each shock. The recording pen reset to the baseline whenever 275 responses had accumulated. *A:* Performance under the schedules of response-independent shock. *B:* Performance under FI 2-minute schedule of response-produced shock after eight sessions. The rate of responding increased, and the pattern of responding was more clearly positively accelerated with response-produced shocks. From Morse, W. H., and Kelleher, R. T. 1970. Schedules as fundamental determinants of behavior. In: W. N. Schoenfeld (ed.), The Theory of Reinforcement Schedules, pp. 139–185. Appleton-Century-Crofts, New York. Reprinted by permission of Prentice-Hall, Inc., Englewood Cliffs, New Jersey.

specified behavioral history. There has been a continuing debate about the optimal schedule to facilitate response-produced shock, and the technicalities involved preclude a full discussion here.[30,39] However, one effective procedure is to maintain an animal on an avoidance schedule (a schedule in which each response postpones the occurrence of a shock for some period of time), then to superimpose a schedule of response-contingent shock presentation concurrently with the avoidance schedule (e.g., a fixed interval of ten seconds), then to eliminate the avoidance schedule. This procedure has been used effectively by a number of investigators.[29,31-35,37] However, it is important to emphasize that a history of avoidance-responding is not essential for response-produced shock. Kelleher and Morse[31] introduced a concurrent fixed-interval 10-minute shock production schedule after animals had learned to obtain food on a variable interval of 2-minute schedule (VI 2 min). Subsequently, response-produced shock maintained schedule performance after the food schedule had been eliminated. These data are two illustrations from an extensive series of experiments that testify to the fact that electric shock, the favorite "aversive" event of generations of psychologists, can under certain conditions be a reinforcing stimulus.

There have been several studies of the effects of various drugs on response-produced shock that further illustrate that this is a reliable and reproducible phenomenon. These data have been recently reviewed by McKearney.[39] One dramatic illustration of the effects of methamphetamine on response-produced shock is shown in Figure 3, which displays cumulative response records from a single monkey. The top row shows response-produced shock performance by the monkey and the second row shows the effects of 0.17 mg/kg methamphetamine on response-produced shock behavior. The rate of response acceleration is very impressive.[40] Morphine (0.03–1.0 mg/kg) and *d*-amphetamine (0.01–1.0 mg/kg) also increase rates of response in a shock self-administration paradigm, and only chlorpromazine has so far been shown to decrease response rates for electric shock.[41] More recently it has been shown that some doses of morphine, methadone, nalorphine, and naloxone increase responding on schedules of shock termination as well as schedules of shock presentation.[42]

Between 1967 and 1970, several investigators confirmed and extended the original observations of response-produced shock.[29,31-33,35-38] Then, perhaps because the basic phenomenon is quite difficult to think about and to integrate with our familiar ideas about what maintains behavior and what does not, these data did not have the

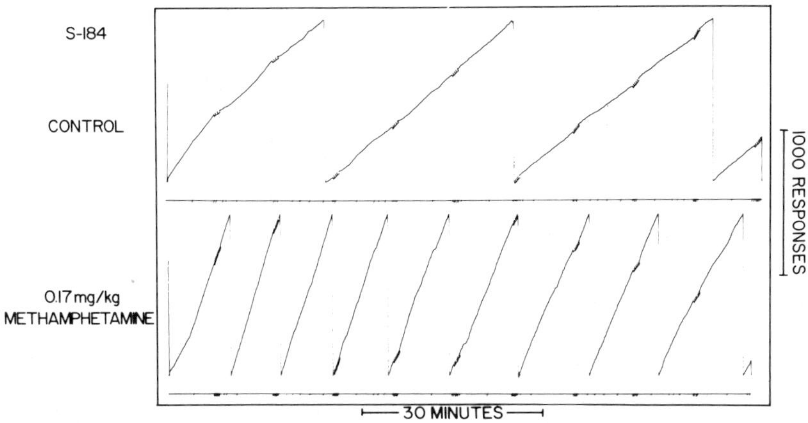

Figure 3. Effects of methamphetamine (0.17 mg/kg) on responding under a multiple 3-minute variable-interval 10-response fixed-ratio schedule of shock presentation (Monkey S-184). *Ordinate:* cumulated responses. *Abscissa:* time. The recording pen was displaced downward during fixed-ratio (FR) components. All shocks were recorded as downward deflections of the event marker, and shocks during FR periods are indicated by an upward deflection of the recording pen as well. Note that methamphetamine increased responding under both schedule components. From McKearney, J. W. 1973. Methamphetamine effects on responding under a multiple schedule of shock presentation. Pharmacol. Biochem. Behav. 1: 547–550. Reprinted with permission of the publisher and author.

impact on behavioral science that might have been anticipated from such significant findings. The implications of these data for the questions addressed in this volume are obvious. If an animal will work to self-administer a seemingly noxious electric shock, indeed, the same shock that he previously worked to avoid or to escape from, how do we think about drug self-administration behavior and the assessment of abuse liability?

NARCOTIC ANTAGONIST SELF-ADMINISTRATION

These fascinating findings on response-produced shock have recently been extended to response-produced narcotic antagonist administration in opiate-dependent monkeys. The parallels between these two paradigms are striking. Although opiate-dependent monkeys will work to escape from and to avoid the infusion of antagonists,[22,24,25] under certain conditions the same animals will work to produce narcotic antagonist administration. The first studies in this area were by Goldberg and co-workers,[23,43] and these findings have recently been confirmed and extended by Woods and colleagues.[44] In 1972, Goldberg, Hoffmeister, and Schlichting reviewed the data on modification of behavioral effects by morphine dependence following administration of morphine antagonists.[43] During studies in which either saline or nalorphine was substituted for morphine over a 7½-hour session, it was found that responding that was followed by nalorphine injections decreased less rapidly than responding followed by saline injections. The rate of response distribution decline within successive 2½-hour segments of the 7½-hour saline and nalorphine substitution sessions is shown in Figure 4. It is clear that nalorphine-maintained responding occurred at a rate not only higher than saline-maintained responding, but also higher than morphine-maintained responding. The authors interpreted these results with caution, suggesting that under certain conditions, response-produced nalorphine injections can maintain responding of animals physiologically dependent upon morphine. The authors concluded that these findings illustrate that the experimental history of the organism and the behavioral schedule under which a stimulus event is presented, rather than the type of events, may determine the effect that an event will have on behavior.[43]

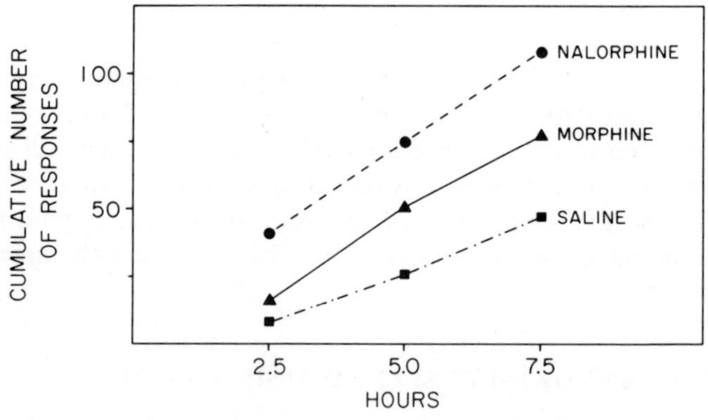

Figure 4. Distribution of responses within the last three saline substitution sessions and nalorphine-substitution sessions (100 mcg/kg injection), compared to the distribution of morphine-maintained responses at comparable times on control days. *Abscissa:* successive 2.5-hour segments of 7.5-hour saline or nalorphine substitution sessions. *Ordinate:* cumulative number of responses during successive 2.5-hour segments. Each point represents the mean of results of three sessions with two monkeys. From Goldberg, S. R., Hoffmeister, F., and Schlichting, U. U. 1972. Morphine antagonists: Modification of behavioral effects by morphine dependence. In: J. M. Singh, L. Miller, and H. Lal (eds.), Drug Addiction, I. Experimental Pharmacology pp. 31–48. Futura Publishing Co., Mount Kisco, New York. Reprinted with permission of the publisher.

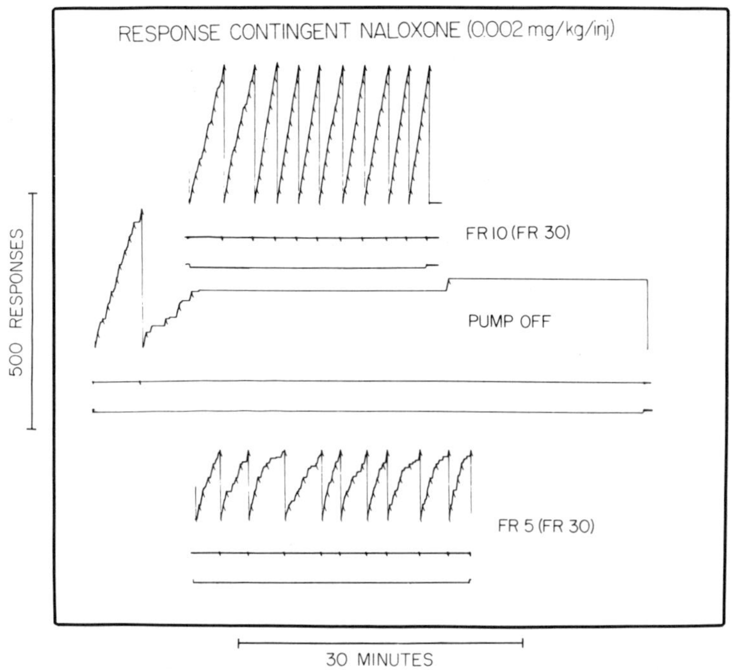

Figure 5. Cumulative records of responding maintained by naloxone in a morphine-dependent monkey. The upper record shows the eighth session of responding when every completed FR 30 unit produced a 1.5-sec flash of the house light and every tenth completed FR 30 unit produced an injection of naloxone (0.002 mg/kg per injection) plus a 1-min time-out accompanied by house light illumination. The center record shows performance in the third session with the naloxone infusion pump disconnected. All other aspects of the procedure were as described above. The lower record shows reinstatement of naloxone-maintained responding in the first session with the naloxone pump reconnected. In this and subsequent sessions, the schedule value was reduced to FR 5 (FR 30). Injections of naloxone or saline are indicated by downward deflections of the center event pen. Each session was terminated after 10 injections or about 1 hour. From Woods, J. H., Downs, D. A., and Carney, J. 1975. Behavioral functions of narcotic antagonists: Response drug contingencies. Fed. Proc. 34(9):1777–1784. Reprinted with permission of the publisher.

In 1975, the parallel between response-produced shock and response-produced antagonist administration was further extended by the investigations of Woods, Downs and Carney.[44] In the top row of Figure 5 are shown the cumulative records of performance by a monkey when every 30 responses produced a secondary reinforcing stimulus (i.e., a 1.5 second flash of light), and every 300 responses produced an injection of naloxone (0.002 mg/kg) followed by a 1-minute timeout and a light signal. The downwards deflections on the event marker indicate the delivery of each successive naloxone injection. The center of Figure 5 shows the effect of disconnecting the naloxone infusion pump when the secondary reinforcing stimuli, i.e., the light signal, the timeout, etc., remain unchanged. The monkey responded briefly and then stopped. At the bottom of Figure 5 we see the reinstatement of naloxone-maintained responding during the first session after the naloxone pump was reconnected. Notice that the schedule was reduced from 300 responses to 150 responses required for naloxone reinforcement. Under these conditions, morphine-dependent monkeys could earn about ten naloxone injections over the course of an hour.[44]

CONCLUSIONS

These data on response-produced shock and response-produced antagonist administration in opiate-dependent monkeys challenge all of our comfortable assumptions about what constitutes a "positive" and an "aversive" event, and what classes of events will be reinforcing. These data argue strongly that it is not the inherent properties of the event per se, but the way in which the event is scheduled that determines the subsequent effect on behavior. The schematic formulation presented in Table 1, which defines reinforcement and punishment in terms of behavioral effects, can account for these data on response-produced shock and antagonist self-administration as well as comparable phenomena. For example, recent reports that amphetamine can be reinforcing and also serve as an aversive stimulus in the same animals[45] can be accommodated within this framework.

If behavioral histories and schedules of stimulus presentation can be arranged so that animals will self-administer electric shock and narcotic antagonists, then clearly we must be very careful about the type of reinforcement schedules we use to assess a new compound for addiction liability. It is well known that ongoing behavior is a powerful determinant of the behavioral effects of drugs. This fundamental principle deriving from the early works of Dews,[46] and extended in the work of Morse and Kelleher[21,47] and many others, has become generally recognized and appreciated.[19] These data indicate the power of schedules of reinforcement as analytic tools.

A schematic summary of these ideas is shown in Table 2. Perhaps the most important implication of these data on response-produced shock and response-produced antagonist self-administration is to provide a different way of thinking about reinforcement. Stimuli are

Table 2. Schematic representation of the functional relationship between antecedent events and behavioral consequences

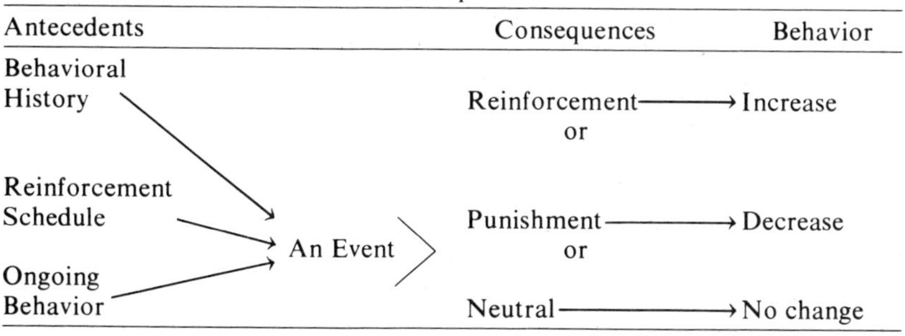

not inherently positive or aversive, but the reinforcing or punishing properties of stimulus events are dependent upon the behavioral history of the organism, the schedule of presentation of that event, and the ongoing behavior at the time. It is clearly impossible to assume an invariant effect of any particular stimulus event.

These data from basic behavioral science and from behavioral pharmacology may be very relevant to the human condition. The initial consequences of drug use for the naive user, as summarized in Table 3, are not consistent with any effects that most of us would consider a priori to be reinforcing. Opiates, barbiturates, and alcohol each produce a variety of somatic and emotional effects that appear

Table 3. Some reported acute effects of drugs in naive users

	Drugs		
Effects	Opiates	Barbiturates	Alcohol
Nausea	X		X
Vomiting	X		X
Dysphoria	X	X	X
Emotional Liability		X	X
Aggressivity			X
Impairments in:			
Concentration	X	X	X
Thinking	X	X	X
Comprehension		X	X
Memory		X	X
Judgment		X	X
Drowsiness	X	X	X
Lethargy	X	X	X

Adapted from Jaffe, J. H.[50] and Mello, N. K., and Mendelson, J. H.[48]

disadvantageous to the user. Yet, despite these consequences of initial acute drug use, many individuals persist in using these agents to the point of abuse and addiction. This behavior is somewhat analogous to response-produced shock. In the case of alcoholism, it has been observed that alcohol addicts tend to have a clear recollection of their "first drink."[48] However, numerous clinical impressions indicate that the first drink was not necessarily memorable because of its relaxing, euphorigenic, tension-reducing, and self-actualizing effects on the user.[49,50] It is more likely that the future alcoholic drank to the point of intoxication and became nauseated and vomited.

Traditional explanations of both the episodic reinitiation and the perpetuation of drug abuse have often been structured in terms of various hypothetical constructs such as "craving" and "drug hunger." The circularity inherent in these constructs, which are defined by the behavior that they are invoked to explain, and the lack of empirical support for alcohol "craving" has been discussed elsewhere.[57] This is not the appropriate forum in which to reexamine the utility of those constructs that have tended to constrain our thinking about the determinants of human drug abuse.

Another way of thinking about drug abuse is to consider drug administration as a form of stimulus self-administration. Perhaps, under some conditions, in individuals with a certain behavioral history, drug self-administration has less to do with the pharmacological properties of the compound or with its anticipated effect than with its properties as a definite stimulus event that has as a consequence some change in subjective state. The hypothesis is that probably any drug that has definite stimulus properties, i.e., behavioral effects for the user, is a drug that has abuse potential. If change, rather than any particular direction of change, is the goal this certainly complicates the prediction of drug abuse liability. At present, the evidence relating to this hypothesis is primarily anecdotal, although it is known that both alcohol and opiates produce progressive dysphoria, anxiety, and irritability as a function of chronic use by addicts.[4,5,6,8,9,10]

The parallels between human drug use, response-produced shock, and comparable phenomena are provocative. Under certain conditions of behavioral history and schedule control, substances that were so noxious that animals would work to avoid them undergo a transition from punishing to reinforcing stimuli as a function of the schedule of presentation. There are numerous nonpharmacological factors that affect drug use and response to drugs in man and experimental animals. Examination of schedule-controlled behavior is perhaps one way of studying these issues and of increasing the predictive power of the assessment of abuse liability with animal models.

ACKNOWLEDGMENT

I am grateful to Drs. Goldberg, Kelleher, Morse, McKearney, and Woods for permission to reprint their data and for supplying photographs.

LITERATURE CITED

1. Schuster, C. R., and Johanson, C. E. 1974. The use of animal models for the study of drug abuse. In: R. J. Gibbins et al. (eds.), Research Advances in Alcohol and Drug Problems, Vol. 1, pp. 1–31. Wiley & Sons, New York.
2. Skinner, B. F. 1938. The Behavior of Organisms, An Experimental Analysis. Appleton-Century-Crofts, Inc., New York.
3. Skinner, B. F. 1953. Science and human behavior. Macmillan Company, New York.
4. Haertzen, C. A., and Hooks, N. T. 1969. Changes in personality and subjective experience associated with the chronic administration and withdrawal of opiates. J. Nerv. Ment. Dis. 148:606–614.
5. McNamee, H. B., Mello, N. K., and Mendelson, J. H. 1968. Experimental analysis of drinking patterns of alcoholics: Concurrent psychiatric observations. Am. J. Psychiatr. 124:1063–1069.
6. Mello, N. K. 1972. Behavioral studies of alcoholism. In: B. Kissin and H. Begleiter (eds.), The Biology of Alcoholism: Vol. II. Physiology and Behavior, pp. 219–291. Plenum Publishing Corp., New York.
7. Mendelson, J. H. (ed.). 1964. Experimentally induced chronic intoxication with withdrawal in alcoholics. Quart. J. Stud. Alc. Suppl. #2.
8. Mirin, S. M., Meyer, R. E., and McNamee, H. B., 1976. Psychopathology, craving and mood during heroin acquisition: An experimental study. Int. J. Addict., 11:525–543.
9. Mirin, S. M., Meyer, R. E., and McNamee, H. B. 1975. Psychopathology and mood during heroin use: Acute vs. chronic effects. In: Proceedings of the 37th Annual Scientific Meeting, Committee on Problems of Drug Dependence, pp. 300–319. NAS-NRC, Washington, D.C.
10. Nathan, P. E., O'Brien, J. S., and Norton, D. 1971. Comparative studies of the inter-personal and affective behavior of alcoholics and non-alcoholics during prolonged experimental drinking. In: N. K. Mello and J. H. Mendelson (eds.), Recent Advances in Studies of Alcoholism, pp. 619–646. U.S. Government Printing Office, Washington, D.C.
11. Davis, D. 1971. Mood changes in alcoholic subjects with programmed and free-choice experimental drinking. In: N. K. Mello and J. H. Mendelson (eds.), Recent Advances in Studies of Alcoholism. Publ.

No. (HSM)71-9045, pp. 596–618. U.S. Government Printing Office, Washington, D.C.

12. Goodwin, D. W. 1971. Blackouts and alcohol induced memory dysfunction. In: N. K. Mello and J. H. Mendelson (eds.), Recent Advances in Studies of Alcoholism, pp. 508–536. Publ. No. (HSM)71-9045. U.S. Government Printing Office, Washington, D.C.
13. McGuire, M. T., Mendelson, J. H., and Stein, S. 1966. Comparative psychosocial studies of alcoholic and non-alcoholic subjects undergoing experimentally induced ethanol intoxication. Psychosom. Med. 28:13–25.
14. Mello, N. K. 1973. Short-term memory function in alcohol addicts during intoxication. In: M. M. Gross (ed.), Alcohol Intoxication and Withdrawal: Experimental Studies, pp. 333–344. Proc. 30th Internat. Congress on Alcoholism and Drug Dependence. Plenum Publishing Corp., New York.
15. Tamerin, J. S., Weiner, S., and Mendelson, J. H. 1970. Alcoholics' expectancies and recall of experiences during intoxication. Amer. J. Psychiatr. 126:1697–1704.
16. Goldman, A. 1974. Ladies and Gentlemen—Lenny Bruce. Random House, New York.
17. Wikler, A., and Rasor, R. W. 1953. Psychiatric aspects of drug addiction. Am. J. Med. 14:566–570.
18. Goldberg, S. R. 1976. The behavioral analysis of drug addiction. In: S. D. Glick and J. Goldfarb (eds.), Behavioral Pharmacology, pp. 283–316. C. V. Mosby Co., St. Louis.
19. Kelleher, R. T., Goldberg, S. R., and Krasnegor, N. (eds.). 1975–76. Control of Drug Taking Behavior by Schedules of Reinforcement. Pharmacological Reviews 27(3 + 4):291–548.
20. Thompson, T., and Pickens, R. 1971. Stimulus Properties of Drugs. Appleton-Century-Crofts, New York.
21. Morse, W. H., and Kelleher, R. T. 1977. Determinants of reinforcement and punishment. In: W. K. Honig and J. E. R. Staddon (eds.), Operant Behavior. Prentice-Hall, Englewood Cliffs, New Jersey.
22. Downs, D. A., and Woods, J. H. 1975. Fixed-ratio escape and avoidance-escape from naloxone in morphine-dependent monkeys: Effects of naloxone dose and morphine pretreatment. J. Exp. Anal. Behav. 23(3):415–427.
23. Goldberg, S. R., Hoffmeister, F., Schlichting, U. U., and Wuttke, W. 1971. Aversive properties of nalorphine and naloxone in morphine-dependent rhesus monkeys. J. Pharmacol. Exp. Therap. 179(2):268–276.
24. Hoffmeister, F., and Wuttke, W. 1973. Self administration: Positive and negative reinforcing properties of morphine antagonists in rhesus monkeys. In: M. C. Braude, L. S. Harris, E. L. May, J. P. Smith and J. E. Villarreal (eds.), Narcotic Antagonists. Advances in Biochemical Psychopharmacology, Vol. 8, pp. 361–369. Raven Press, New York.
25. Hoffmeister, F., and Wuttke, W. 1973. Negative reinforcing properties of morphine antagonists in naive rhesus monkeys. Psychopharmacologia 33:247–258.

26. McMillan, D. E. 1975. Determinants of drug effects on punished responding. Fed. Proc. 34(9):1870–1879.
27. Grove, R. N., and Schuster, C. R. 1974. Suppression of cocaine self-administration by extinction and punishment. Pharmacol. Biochem. Behav. 2:199–208.
28. Kelleher, R. T., Riddle, W. C., and Cook, L. 1963. Persistent behavior maintained by unavoidable shocks. J. Exp. Anal. Behav. 6:507–517.
29. Byrd, L. D. 1969. Responding in the cat maintained under response-independent electric shock and response-produced electric shock. J. Exp. Anal. Behav. 12:1–10.
30. Eubanks, J. L., Killeen, P., Hamilton, B., and Wald, B. A. 1975. The effect of timeout on performance on a variable-interval schedule of electric-shock presentation. J. Exper. Anal. Behav. 23(3):457–463.
31. Kelleher, R. T., and Morse, W. H. 1968. Schedules using noxious stimuli. III. Responding maintained with response-produced electric shocks. J. Exp. Anal. Behav. 11:819–838.
32. McKearney, J. W. 1968. Maintenance of responding under a fixed-interval schedule of electric shock presentation. Science 160:1249–1251.
33. McKearney, J. W. 1969. Fixed-interval schedules of electric shock presentation: Extinction and recovery of performance under different shock intensities and fixed interval durations. J. Exp. Anal. Behav. 12:301–313.
34. McKearney, J. W. 1972. Maintenance and suppression of responding under schedules of electric shock presentation. J. Exp. Anal. Behav. 17:425–432.
35. Morse, W. H., and Kelleher, R. T. 1970. Schedules as fundamental determinants of behavior. In: W. N. Schoenfeld (ed.), The Theory of Reinforcement Schedules, pp. 139–185. Appleton-Century-Crofts, New York.
36. Morse, W. H., Mead, R. N., and Kelleher, R. T. 1967. Modulation of elicited behavior by a fixed-interval schedule of electric shock presentation. Science 157:215–217.
37. Stretch, R., Orloff, E. R., and Dalrymple, S. D. 1968. Maintenance of responding by fixed-interval schedule of electric shock presentation in squirrel monkeys. Science 162:583–586.
38. Stretch, R., Orloff, E. R., and Gerber, G. J. 1970. Multiple interruption of responding maintained by a fixed-interval schedule of electric-shock presentation in squirrel monkeys. Can. J. of Psychol. 24:117–125.
39. McKearney, J. 1972. Schedule-dependent effects: Effects of drugs, and maintenance of responding with response-produced electric shocks. In: R. M. Gilbert and J. D. Keehn (eds.), Schedule-Effects: Drugs, Drinking, and Aggression, pp. 3–25. University of Toronto Press, Toronto.
40. McKearney, J. W. 1973. Methamphetamine effects on responding under a multiple schedule of shock presentation. Pharmacol. Biochem. Behav. 1:547–550.
41. McKearney, J. W. 1974. Effects of *d*-amphetamine, morphine and chlorpromazine on responding under fixed-interval schedules of food presentation or electric shock presentation. J. Pharm. Exp. Ther. 190(1):141–153.

42. McKearney, J. W. 1975. Effects of morphine, methadone, nalorphine and naloxone on responding under fixed interval (FI) schedules in the squirrel monkey. Fed. Proc. 34(3) (abstr.).
43. Goldberg, S. R., Hoffmeister, F., and Schlichting, U. U. 1972. Morphine antagonists: Modification of behavioral effects by morphine dependence. In: J. M. Singh, L. Miller and H. Lal (eds.), Drug Addiction I. Experimental Pharmacology, pp. 31–48. Futura Publishing Co., Mount Risco, New York.
44. Woods, J. H., Downs, D. A. and Carney, J. 1975. Behavioral functions of narcotic antagonists: Response-drug contingencies. Fed. Proc. 34(9):1777–1784.
45. Wise, R. A., Yokel, R. A., and DeWitt, H. 1976. Both positive reinforcement and conditioned aversion from amphetamine and from apomorphine in rats. Science 191:1273–1275.
46. Dews, P. B. 1975. Studies on behavior. I. Differential sensitivity to pentobarbital of pecking performance in pigeons depending on the schedule of reward. J. Pharm. Exp. Ther. 113:343–401.
47. Kelleher, R. T., and Morse, W. H. 1968. Determinants of the specificity of behavioral effects of drugs. Reviews of Physiol., Biochem. Exper. Pharmacol. 60:1–56.
48. Kuehnle, J. C., Anderson, W. H., and Chandler, E. 1974. Report on first drinking experience in addictive and nonaddictive drinkers. Arch. Gen. Psychiatr. 31:521–523.
49. Catanzaro, R. J. 1968. The disease: Alcoholism. In: R. S. Catanzaro (ed.), Alcoholism, The Total Treatment Approach, pp. 5–25. Charles C Thomas, Springfield, Ill.
50. Mello, N. K., and Mendelson, J. H. 1976. The development of alcohol dependence: A clinical study. McLean Hospital Journal 1(2):64–88.
51. Mello, N. K. 1975. A semantic aspect of alcoholism. In: H. D. Cappell and A. E. Lablanc (eds.), Biological and Behavioral Approaches to Drug Dependence, pp. 73–87. Addiction Research Foundation of Ontario, Ontario, Canada.

Evaluating The Abuse Potential of Psychotropic Drugs in Man

Marian W. Fischman

A traditional approach to the assessment of a drug's abuse potential is the utilization of a variety of pharmacological and behavioral procedures to characterize its spectrum of action. This pattern is compared to the known actions of drugs of abuse and an estimate of the abuse potential of the unknown compound is made. In 1972 the Committee on Problems of Drug Dependence[1] published an account of currently acceptable procedures for estimating the abuse liability of drugs. A major theme of that paper was the comparison of the actions of lesser known or unknown drugs with the established actions of morphine (for narcotics) or sodium barbital (for barbiturates). Thus, according to their guideline, once a profile of the physiological and behavioral effects of a standard known drug of abuse is established, that profile can be used as a template against which the abuse liability of other drugs in the same class is assessed. There is no attempt to state that any drug will or will not be abused. It is only possible to say that the drug being tested is like, or unlike, the prototype. Since we do not know which of the many actions of drugs are those responsible for its abuse, it is necessary to test a wide spectrum of its actions. Clearly, many environmental and physiological variables are relevant in determining potential abuse. In order to accurately evaluate the spectrum of a drug's action, data must be collected using a broad range of measures. There are, unfortunately, no single tests that can be done in the laboratory that will provide sufficient information. Results must be combined from many different procedures to yield a broad profile of empirical information with which to make the comparison.

There appear to be relatively clear-cut procedures for assessing the physical dependence capacity of a drug.[2,3,4] Evaluation of the

This research was supported by FDA 223-72-3042 (E. H. Uhlenhuth, Principal Investigator); ADM-45-165, (C. R. Schuster, Principal Investigator); and DA-00250, (D. X. Freedman, Principal Investigator).

abuse potential of drugs that do not produce physical dependence is less straightforward. Most of the procedures currently in use, such as the self-administration procedure,[5,6] are well suited to the animal laboratory, but have a limited utility when the experimental organisms are human, for ethical as well as practical reasons. The difficulties of extrapolating from data collected on infra-human organisms to predict effects in man are obvious, but the self-administration procedures have thus far been shown to have reasonably good predictive value, as long as their underlying assumptions and techniques are precisely defined and kept in mind.

What are needed to complement the animal laboratory methodology are a series of reliable procedures with which data can be obtained to describe the profile of a drug's action in man. Some of these procedures are available and in use, some are in the process of development and, of course, many have yet to be developed. For many years now, drug testing with humans at the Addiction Research Center in Lexington, Kentucky has included some physiological measures, gross behavioral observations, subjective effects, questionnaires, and, where applicable, measures of physical dependence. This battery has produced a substantial amount of data on narcotic drugs.[7,8] In addition, data on other classes of drug, such as the stimulants, have been collected,[9,10] although the methods for characterizing these other classes have not yet been as extensively used and systematically validated.

At The University of Chicago, my colleagues Eberhard Uhlenhuth and Charles R. Schuster and I have begun to develop human laboratory operant procedures for studying drug-behavior interactions. By measuring fine-grained behavioral effects with a methodology that has been shown to be highly reliable in the animal laboratory, we hope to develop a battery of behavioral tests that show selective sensitivity to specific classes of drugs. These results, when added to the physiological and subjective effects of a specific drug should provide a multi-dimensional pattern of drug action. When prototypical drugs from several different classes of abused drugs are thus evaluated, we should be able to take other drugs from those same classes, assess their effects utilizing the same battery of physiological, subjective, and behavioral effects, and rank them on their similarity to the standard drug. Employing known drugs of abuse in our test procedures as the standards would enable us to correlate the data engendered by our methods with human abuse of those drugs. Thus, we would expect that a compound with a profile of action that correlated highly with our standard heavily abused drugs would be a potential drug of abuse. On the other hand, a drug of the same class with many dissimilar actions might well promise to have less abuse potential. It is also relevant to make comparisons with drugs of abuse from other classes for the same reasons. In addition, comparing our test compounds to drugs with little or no known abuse potential will assure us of the specificity of our procedures.

This paper is a report of ongoing research in the development of a battery of physiological and behavioral tests for the assessment of the effects of stimulant and depressant drugs. Table 1 indicates the scope of the test battery currently being developed. We are attempting to develop procedures for humans that are selectively sensitive to the spectrum of action of different classes of drugs. This review is a report of early data obtained utilizing some of the physiological and behavioral measures included in our test series. Much of the data are

Table 1. Drug evaluation in man

A. Measures of Physiological Effects
   1. electrocardiograph
   2. heart rate
   3. diastolic and systolic blood pressure
   4. skin temperature
   5. core body temperature
   6. respiration rate
   7. galvanic skin response

B. Measures of Behavioral Effects
   1. Questionnaires
      a. addiction research center inventory
      b. profile of mood states
      c. drug effects questionnaire
      d. experimenter conducted interview
      e. observation of subject
   2. Psychomotor Performance
      a. reaction time
      b. tapping time
   3. Schedule Controlled Performance
      a. free operant avoidance
      b. punishment
      c. differential reinforcement of low rate
   4. Discrimination and Memory
      a. signal detection
      b. vigilance

preliminary, and are included here only as examples to show the potential of this approach to the assessment of a drug's profile of action in man.

PHYSIOLOGICAL MEASURES

Male volunteer subjects ranging in age from 21–35 were subjects in an experiment comparing the physiological effects of 10 mg of intravenously administered *d*-amphetamine with doses of intravenous cocaine ranging from 4 to 32 mg (see Reference 11 for a complete description of this study). Each subject had a long history of illicit intravenous cocaine use, as well as other stimulant use, and was judged to be psychologically and physiologically fit prior to beginning the study. Subjects were hospitalized for the duration of the two-week experiment, and were evaluated daily on a series of physiological and behavioral measures before, during, and after intravenous injections of cocaine, *d*-amphetamine, and saline. A full description of the procedures used and measures taken is available in Fischman et al.[11] Although heart rate, electrocardiograph, respiration rate, blood pressure, and skin and core body temperature were all measured, consistent drug effects were obtained on only blood pressure and heart rate. In addition, no dose of cocaine or *d*-amphetamine caused any clinical abnormalities in subjects' EEG recordings.

Data showing the cardiovascular effects of cocaine and *d*-amphetamine in 12 subjects are presented in Figures 1–4. Intravenous cocaine produced a dose-related increase in heart rate in all subjects tested. Thirty minutes of predrug baseline data were collected each day prior to the injection of any test solution. Median percent change in heart rate from this thirty-minute baseline is shown in Figure 1. Four milligrams of cocaine did not differ in effect from saline, 8 mg had an intermediate effect, with a median peak increase in heart rate of 21%, while 16 and 32 mg had very similar effects, with median peak increases of 30–37.5%.

In general, increases in heart rate began within 2–5 minutes after the drug injection and peaked at 8–10 minutes regardless of the dose administered. Heart rate had returned to predrug baseline by 60 minutes following 4 and 8 mg of cocaine, but not always at 16 or 32 mg. Figure 2 shows that median peak percent change in heart rate increased in a generally linear fashion with dose, leveling off between 16 and 32 mg. These two measures (dose and peak heart rate) are significantly correlated (F-test, $p < 0.05$).

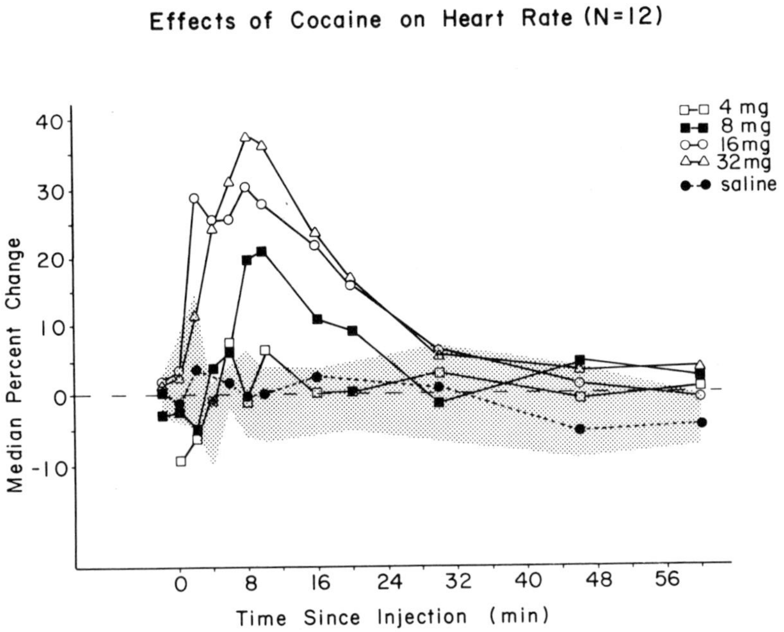

Figure 1. Median percent change in heart rate for one hour after saline or 4–32 mg cocaine. Percent change was calculated for each dose of cocaine with reference to its own thirty minute predrug baseline. The sale function represents data collected on day 8 of the experimental series; the shaded area around it indicates the semi-interquartile range of those data.

A dose-related increase in blood pressure after intravenously administered cocaine was also observed. The changes in diastolic and systolic blood pressure were highly correlated; only systolic blood pressure changes are shown in Figures 2 and 4. The median percent change in systolic blood pressure was no different from placebo after 4 and 8 mg of cocaine (Figure 3). Both 16 and 32 mg caused a peak of approximately 15% (140 mm Hg) which generally occurred 4–10 minutes after drug administration. There was a monotonic linear relationship (F-test, $p < 0.01$) between dose and peak systolic blood pressure. This is shown in Figure 2.

The effects of intravenous cocaine and *d*-amphetamine on blood pressure and heart rate are compared in Figure 4. There was a median increase in both heart rate and systolic blood pressure of 10–15% after *d*-amphetamine. This effect on blood pressure was closest to that seen after 24 or 32 mg of cocaine, both in terms of peak and duration of

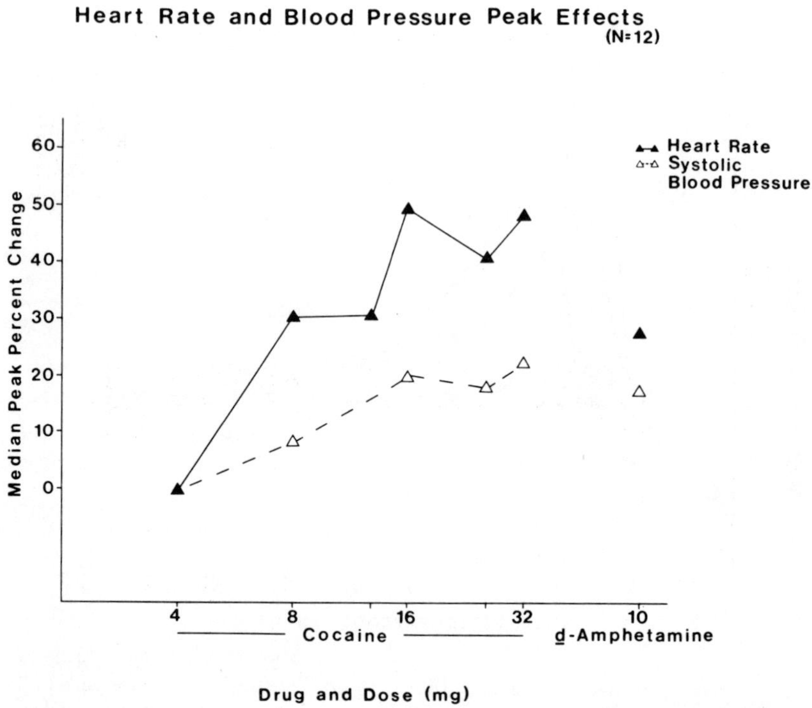

Figure 2. Median peak percent change in heart rate and systolic blood pressure after intravenous injections of saline, 4–32 mg cocaine and 10 mg *d*-amphetamine. Percent change was calculated for each dose and drug with reference to baseline data collected for thirty minutes before injection of that dose of drug.

effect. There was no dose of cocaine that closely resembled the *d*-amphetamine effect on heart rate. The effects of 8 mg of cocaine were similar, but it caused a greater median peak percent change and had a shorter duration of action. Neither heart rate nor systolic blood pressure returned to baseline levels at sixty minutes after injection of 10 mg *d*-amphetamine.

SUBJECTIVE MEASURES

The twelve male volunteer subjects evaluated the effects of intravenous cocaine, *d*-amphetamine, and saline. Questionnaires were administered twice during every drug or placebo (saline) session. One of these was a short form of the 550-item Addiction Research Center Inventory (ARCI).[12] This was made up of forty-nine questions compiled by Martin et al.[9] in their study of some effects of a variety of psychomotor stimulant drugs in man. They were taken from the Morphine-Amphetamine (MBG), Pentobarbital, Chlorpromizine, Alcohol (PCAG), LSD, and Benzedrine (BG) scales. These are described[9] as including measures of sedation and euphoria, an estimate of dysphoric and psychotomimetic changes and an empiric amphetamine scale. A difference score (post-drug minus predrug) was computed for each scale at each drug or saline condition. These scores are shown in Figure 5. Scores on these scales were very stable when saline was administered; virtually no change was measured after injection. However, scores on the five separate scales were consistently related to drug dose. Amphetamine (A), Morphine-Benzedrine (MBG), Benzedrine (BG), and LSD scale scores all increased after cocaine injection in a dose-related fashion. PCAG scores decreased at all doses of cocaine except 4 mg. Ten mg of *d*-amphetamine caused similar,

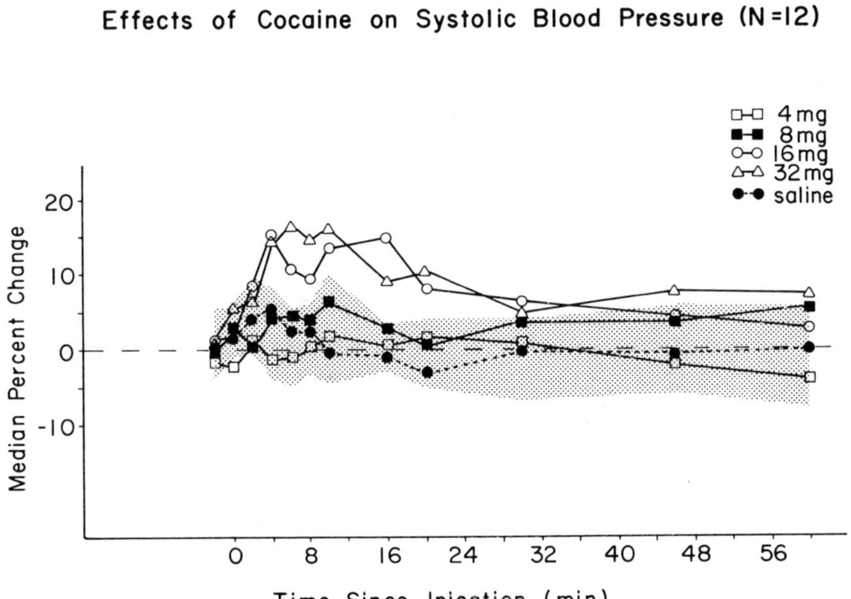

Figure 3. Median percent change in systolic blood pressure for one hour after intravenous injection of saline or 4–32 mg cocaine. Percent change was calculated for each dose of cocaine from the predrug baseline measured during the thirty minutes prior to injection of that dose. The saline function represents data collected on day 8 of the experimental series; the shaded area indicates the semi-interquartile range for those data.

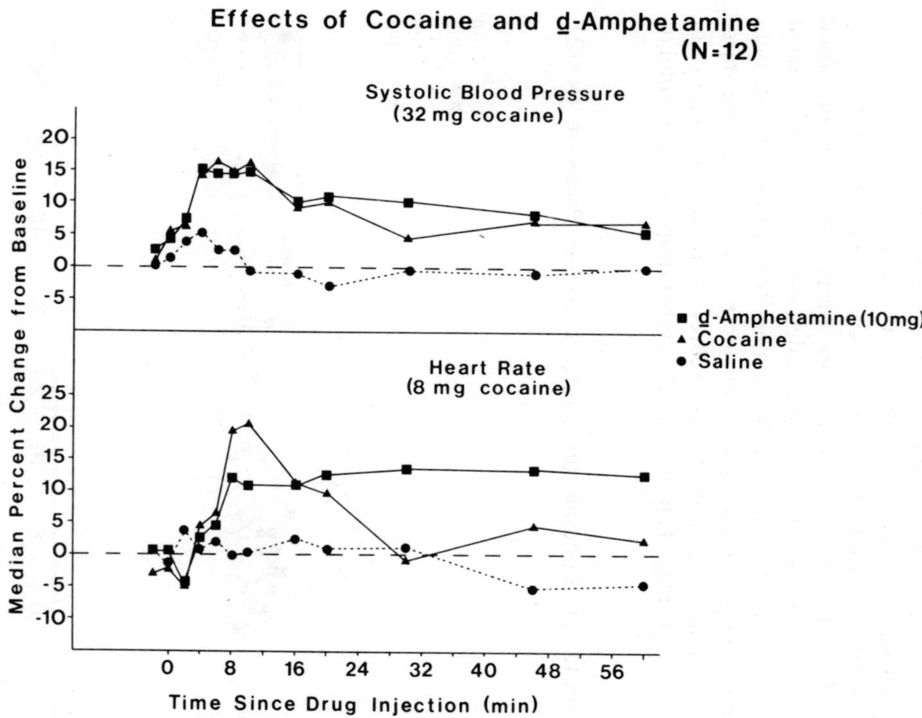

Figure 4. A comparison of the effects of intravenous cocaine and *d*-amphetamine on heart rate and systolic blood pressure. Median percent change is shown after 10 mg *d*-amphetamine compared with 8 mg cocaine for heart rate effects and 32 mg cocaine for blood pressure effects.

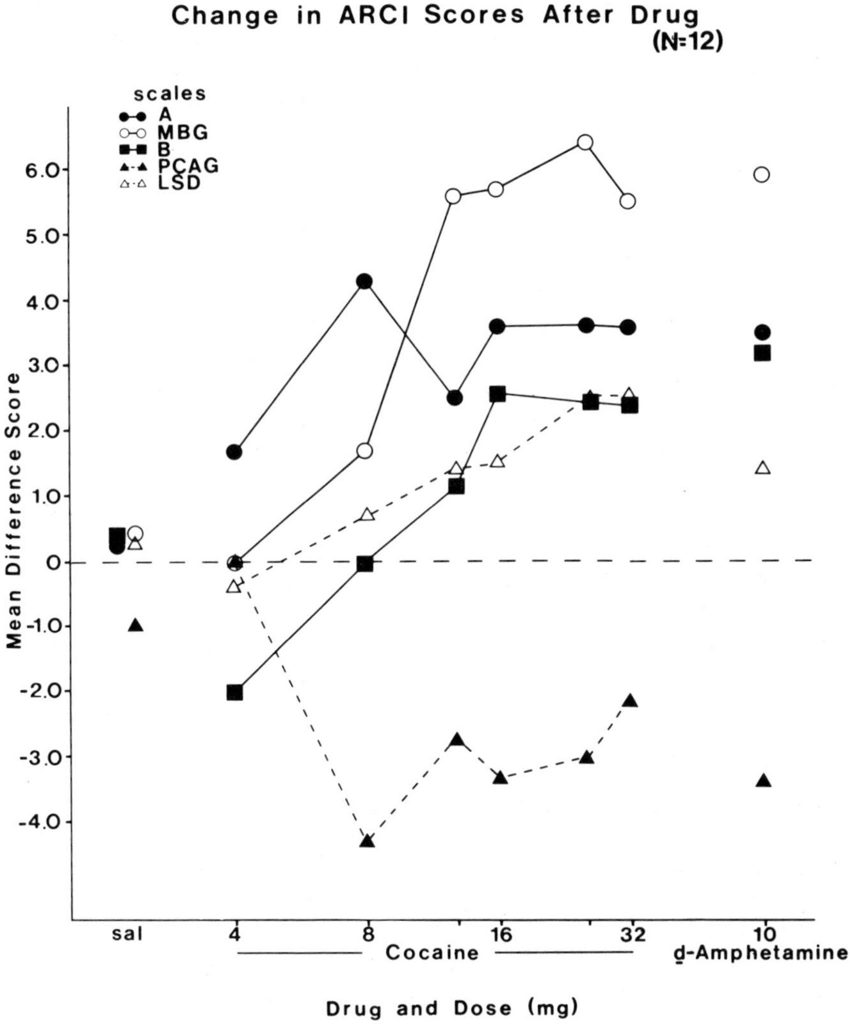

Figure 5. Mean change in scores on five separate scales of the Addiction Research Council Inventory. A short form of the Inventory was answered prior to drug or saline injection and again fifteen minutes after injection. The scales were: Amphetamine (A), Morphine-Benzedrine (MBG), Benzedrine (B), Lysergic Acid (LSD) and Pentobarbital-Chlorpromizine-Alcohol (PCAG).

although not identical effects on these scores. The pattern of increase of the scores for each of the scales was the same as that seen after cocaine. Thus, the greatest increase after both drugs was in the MBG scale, followed by A, BG, and LSD. The effect of 10 mg of amphetamine most closely mimics the scores obtained after 16 mg cocaine.

In addition to this questionnaire, subjects were required to fill out a drug effects questionnaire (see Fischman et al. for a description[11]). Among other questions, they were asked to identify the drug they had been given that day and to compare it on a scale from 0–10 (0 = no drug, 5 = same as average on the street, 10 = the highest ever taken) with the illegally acquired stimulants that they usually self-administered for recreational purposes. Those data are shown in Figure 6. A dose of 16 mg cocaine was generally rated as similar to the average dose that subjects were self-injecting on the street. Doses of 24 and 32 mg of cocaine were rated as among the highest these subjects had ever taken. There was a generally dose-related increase in subjective rating, with *d*-amphetamine rated as having a subjective effect comparable to 16 mg of cocaine. With few exceptions, subjects were able to correctly discriminate all doses of cocaine above 4 mg, as well as 10 mg of *d*-amphetamine, from placebo. They were less able to discriminate between cocaine and *d*-amphetamine. Cocaine was administered a total of 60 times and was correctly identified on 47 occasions, identified as amphetamine on six occasions (four times at 16 mg, twice at 32 mg) and saline on seven occasions (four times at 4 mg and once each at 8, 12, and 16 mg). *d*-Amphetamine was administered 14 times, correctly identified on four occasions, identified as cocaine on nine occasions and as saline once. The subjects' judgment of what drug was administered was confounded by the fact that cocaine was given more frequently than either *d*-amphetamine or saline. However, it has been suggested[13] on the basis of anecdotal evidence, that although the immediate effects of intravenous amphetamine and cocaine may be indistinguishable, a distinction can be made by experienced users because the effects of cocaine are dissipated more rapidly. The cues that people use in discriminating these drugs are not known, but perhaps if subjects were allowed to wait longer than sixty minutes after drug administration, giving time for the effects of cocaine but not *d*-amphetamine to dissipate, their drug discriminations would have been better. On the other hand, it was not always true in our studies that the effects of cocaine dissipated more rapidly than those of *d*-amphetamine.

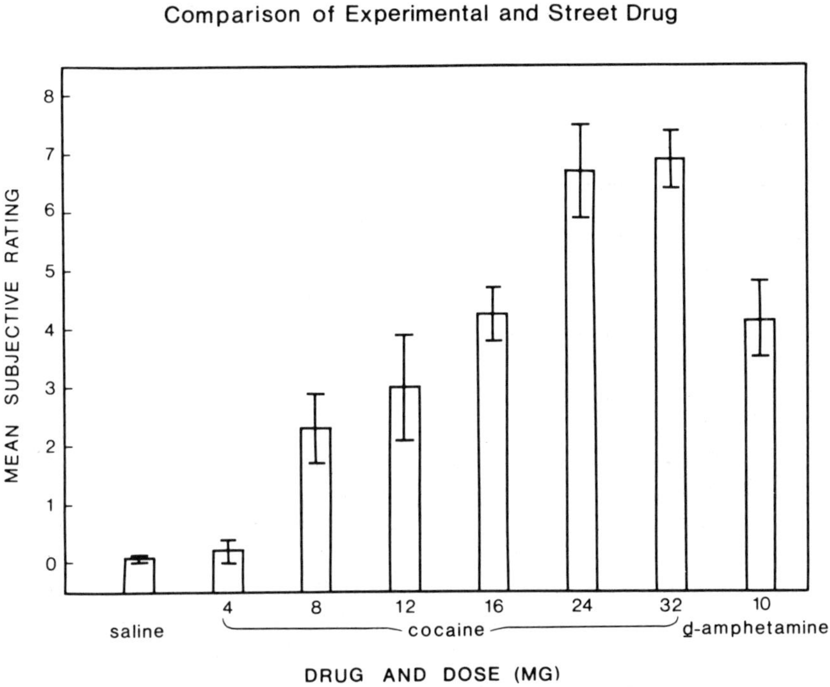

Figure 6. Subjective ratings for intravenous injections of saline, cocaine and *d*-amphetamine. Subjects were asked to rate each intravenous injection on a 0–10 point scale (0 = no drug, 5 = average dose, 10 = the highest ever taken), comparing it to the dose of stimulant drug they were accustomed to self-administer when the drug was illicitly acquired. Means were calculated for each subject; the *bars* represent the mean rating for all 12 subjects. *Brackets* indicate the standard errors of those means.

The profile of cocaine action derived from these data indicates that its stimulant actions clearly mimic those reported for other stimulant drugs such as the amphetamines, diethylpropion and methylphenidate.[9,10,14,15,16] This similarity in behavioral effect has also been reported when these two drugs were tested in the animal laboratory.[17,18] Ten milligrams of *d*-amphetamine appeared to have a potency comparable to 8–16 mg cocaine. Heart rate peak effect was similar to that produced by 8 mg of cocaine, while measures of blood pressure peak effect, the ARCI stimulant scale scores, and subjective ratings were similar to those produced by 16 mg of cocaine. In addition, the time course of the pressor effect appeared most similar to that seen after 32 mg cocaine. If one had to equate the abuse potential of a dose of cocaine with 10 mg of *d*-amphetamine, 16 mg would be the most likely choice.

BEHAVIORAL MEASURES

Free Operant Avoidance

Conditioned avoidance behavior has been investigated in a variety of studies concerned with drug-behavior inter-actions.[19,20] Despite considerable differences in experimental design, it has been found that the phenothiazine compounds and narcotic analgesics decrease responding which postpones the delivery of shock at doses that do not suppress escape responding.[21-23] Because the avoidance-escape paradigm has provided a means of differentiating classes of drugs in infrahuman organisms, it seemed logical to determine if similar selectivity could be demonstrated using man as the experimental organism.

Thirteen volunteer subjects, ranging in age from 21 to 30, were the subjects in this experiment. They were seated in a small cubicle in front of a stimulus response console containing lights, two levers, and a point counter. At the beginning of each four-hour experimental session, the counter registered 3600 points that could, at the end of the session, be converted to money at the rate of 0.05 cents/point. Subjects could press the right hand lever in front of them to avoid or escape point loss which was programmed on a modified free operant avoidance schedule.[24] A diagram of this schedule is presented in Figure 7. If the subject did not respond at all, every 30 seconds, 10 points were subtracted at the rate of 1 point per second. If the subject made an avoidance response by pressing the lever during the 30-second interval, point loss was delayed for 30 sec. Any response that occurred during the 10-second period when points were being subtracted terminated that period of point loss and delayed its reoccurrence for 30 seconds.

Each experimental session began with one hour of baseline data collection before the administration of drug or placebo. Subjects then drank 30 ml of a flavored quinine-based solution in which drug was sometimes mixed. This was followed by three more hours of testing. The following drugs were evaluated in this procedure: *d*-amphetamine (5, 10, 15, and 20 mg), diazepam (5, 10, 15, and 20 mg), pentobarbital (50, 100, 150, and 200 mg), chlorpromazine (50, 75, and 100 mg), and imipramine (75 and 150 mg). Not all doses were tested in all subjects.

Subjects were not given any information concerning the temporal

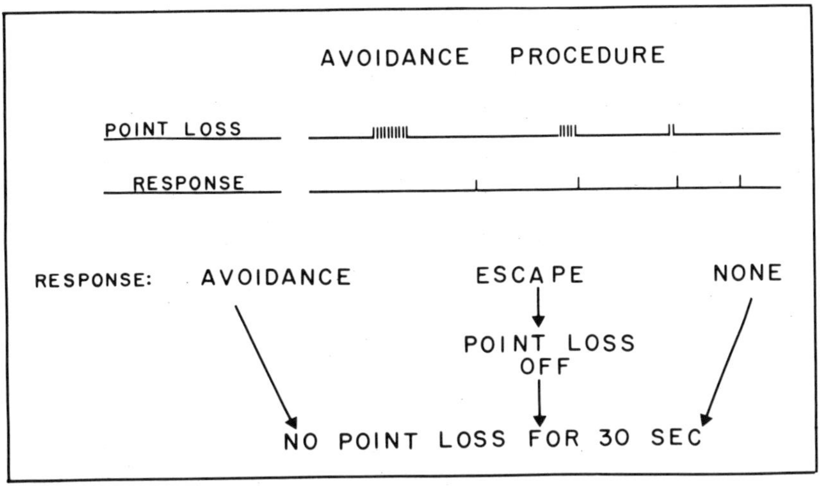

Figure 7. Diagram of the modified free operant point loss avoidance paradigm.

parameters of this study. They were told only that point loss could be postponed with a lever press and/or temporarily terminated with a lever press. Although spacing of lever press responses varied between subjects, there was a pattern of responding for each subject that remained relatively constant across sessions. Interresponse time (IRT) distributions were calculated for each hour of every four-hour experimental session. An IRT is the time (in seconds) between avoidance responses or between the last point subtracted and the next avoidance response. These were calculated in intervals of two seconds, and are graphed as the percent of the total number of avoidance responses per hour in Figures 8–10. The data collected after one dose each of *d*-amphetamine, diazepam, chlorpromazine, pentobarbital, and imipramine, as well as placebo, are shown for one subject.

Figure 8A presents data when placebo was administered. This subject had a moderately high rate of responding. The obtained IRT distributions peaked at 5–6 seconds and were quite steep. There were rarely any points lost in placebo sessions and a point loss sequence was always terminated after the first point was subtracted. When 15 mg of *d*-amphetamine was administered (Figure 8B) there was a sharp increase in the number of avoidance responses emitted and an abrupt shift of the IRT distributions to the shorter latencies. During the second hour after drug (hour 3), this subject was responding on the average of once per second as opposed to once every 4–5 seconds dur-

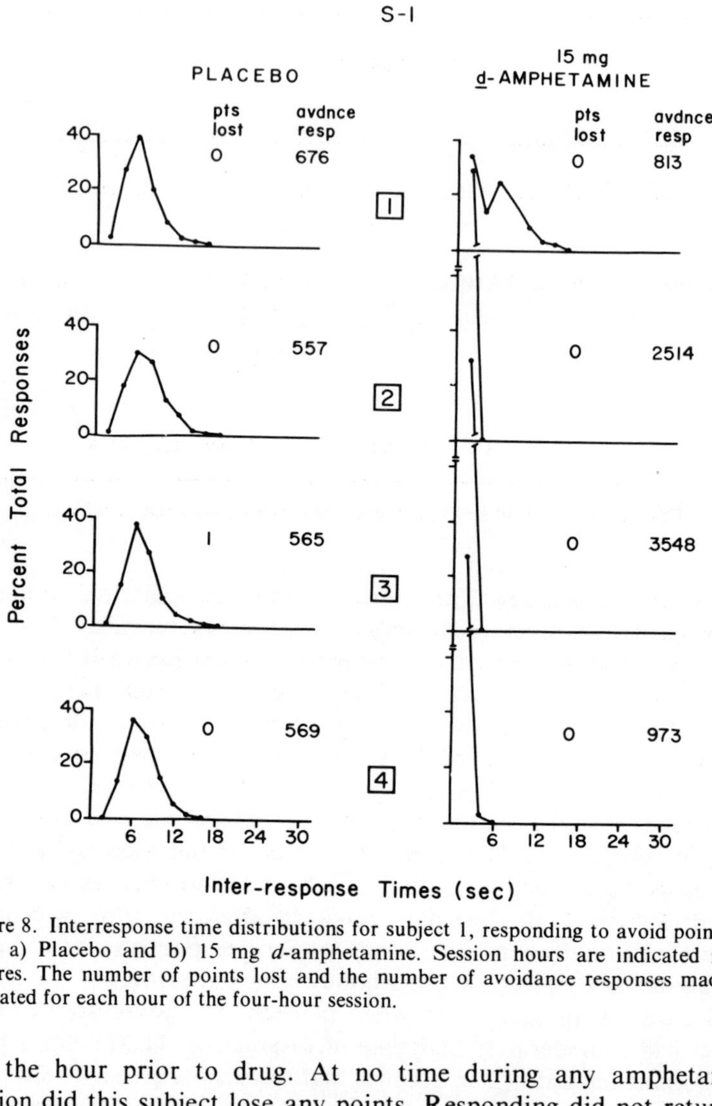

Figure 8. Interresponse time distributions for subject 1, responding to avoid point loss, after a) Placebo and b) 15 mg *d*-amphetamine. Session hours are indicated in the squares. The number of points lost and the number of avoidance responses made are indicated for each hour of the four-hour session.

ing the hour prior to drug. At no time during any amphetamine session did this subject lose any points. Responding did not return to baseline rates by the end of the four-hour session.

In Figure 9A data are presented showing the effects of 100 mg of chlorpromazine on avoidance responding. The patterning of this responding was severely disrupted; the interresponse time distributions in the third and fourth hours are flattened over the usual model IRT of 5–6 seconds. During the third hour, 46% of the avoidance responses were separated by two seconds or less but fewer responses were made. Because of the decreased avoidance response rates, 95 points were lost during this hour; however, there was no period of point loss that was not escaped. This trend was even more marked during the fourth hour. The short IRTs disappeared, but there was a greater decrease in the number of avoidance responses made (less than half the number made in the first hour). Ninety-eight points were lost, but again, no periods occurred in which point loss was not escaped. These data are a clear example of the selective suppressant effect of chlorpromazine on avoidance but not escape behavior. The effects of 150 mg of

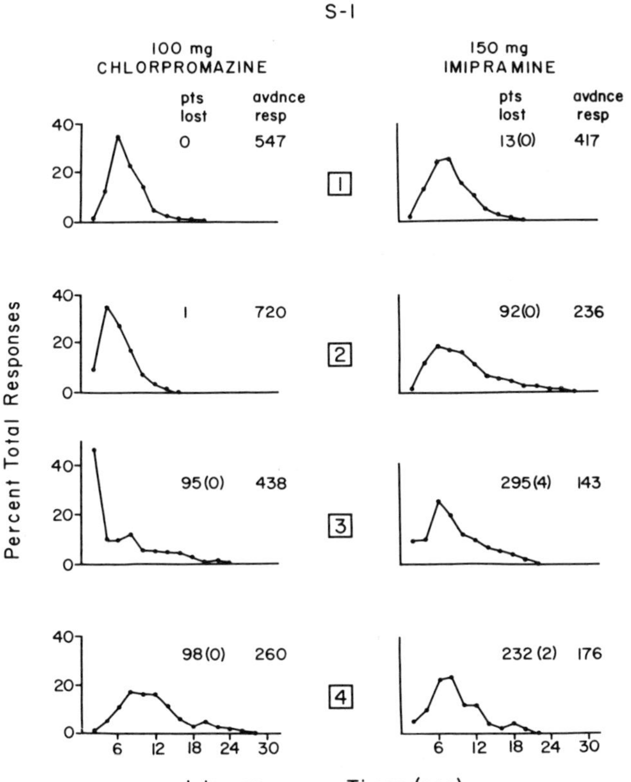

Figure 9. Interresponse time distributions for subject 1, responding to avoid point loss, after a) 100 mg chlorpromizine, b) 150 mg imipramine. Session hours are indicated in the squares. The number of points lost and the number of avoidance responses made are indicated for each hour of the four-hour session. Numbers in parenthesis are the number of 10 second periods in which no escape response was made.

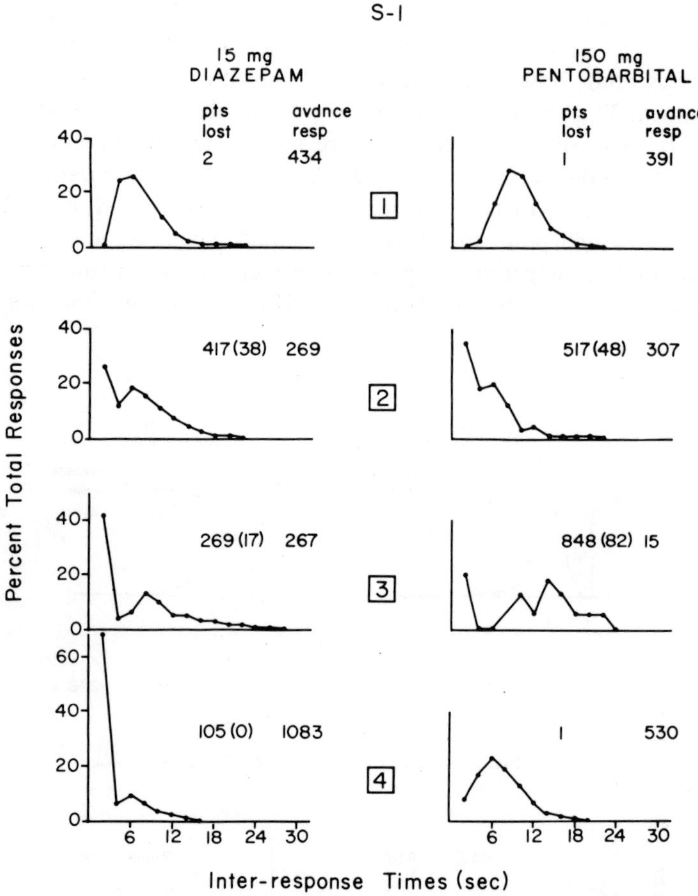

Figure 10. Interresponse time distributions for subject 1, responding to avoid point loss, after a) 15 mg diazepam, b) 150 mg pentobarbital. Session hours are indicated in the squares. The number of points lost and the number of avoidance responses made are indicated for each hour of the four-hour session. Numbers in parentheses are the number of 10 second periods in which no escape response was made.

imipramine (Figure 9B) were somewhat similar to those seen after 100 mg chlorpromazine, except responding was more severely suppressed. During the second hour, avoidance responding decreased to almost half that seen in the first hour, and 92 points were lost. There were no periods of no escape. During the third and fourth hour, avoidance responding decreased still more and point loss increased. At the same time there were very few periods of no escape—four in the third hour and two in the four hour.

Diazepam and pentobarbital had suppressant effects on both avoidance and escape responding. In the first hour after 15 mg of diazepam (Figure 10A), avoidance responding decreased to almost half that seen during the predrug hour and 417 points were lost; 380 of these points were lost during the 38 ten-second periods when no escape responses were made. This effect, although lessened, was still present during the second hour after drug. During the last hour, this subject showed an abrupt increase in avoidance responding to almost three times its initial value. The increase was unlike that seen after *d*-amphetamine because concomittant with the increase in avoidance responding was the continued high level of point loss (105 in the last hour).

The disruptive effects of 150 mg of pentobarbital were also evident in the first hour after drug (Figure 10B). Although avoidance responding was not initially suppressed, there was a shift to shorter IRTs and an increase (to 517) in the number of points lost and the number of periods of no escape (48). In the second hour after drug, this subject made only 15 responses and sat through 82 periods of point loss (out of possible 90) without making any escape responses. By the last hour, response rate was increased and the IRT distribution was similar to that seen prior to drug, approaching baseline levels.

The data collected in the free operant point loss avoidance paradigm clearly show differences depending on the drug being administered. It is impressive that not only are the stimulant and depressant drugs differentiable on the basis of their behavioral effects, but other drugs with more mixed effects can also be differentiated on the basis of their selective effects. Chlorpromazine and imipramine, drugs with little or no abuse liability, were readily differentiated from the other drugs tested. These data replicate the selective suppressant effects found by others testing the phenothiazines,[21,23] and clearly show the rate increasing effects of the amphetamines[25,26] and the more general suppressant effects of pentobarbital and diazepam.[26-28] It is now important to test other drugs from these classes to extend the generality of these findings in humans and establish broader profiles of behavioral action for these drugs.

Differential Reinforcement of Low Rate (DRL)

It has been well established that the behavioral effects of a specific dose of a compound are dependent on the environmental contingencies prevailing at a given time (see Ref. 20 for a discussion of this). Thus, for example, when the contingencies generate different baseline rates, it has been shown that there is an inverse relationship between operant response output and dose of amphetamine.[29-31] It is therefore important when describing a spectrum of action of a specific compound to include behavioral measures with differing contingencies. In the avoidance paradigm present in this paper, no consequences are attached to response rate as long as that rate is at least 2 responses per minute. In the differential reinforcement of low rate schedule of reinforcement, responses must be spaced by a minimum interval programmed by the experimenter. Responses made during the interval reset the timing contingencies and the full-time interval must again pass before a response is reinforced. The clock runs continuously, and is reset with every response. In order to make the task reported here more interesting to the subjects, the DRL schedule of reinforcement was utilized within the framework of a vigilance paradigm.[32] Subjects were seated in front of a blank television screen and given two push buttons to depress. They were told to monitor the screen so that a "1" always appeared on the screen. Whenever a zero was on the screen they were instructed that they could earn a point by depressing the right-hand button within 2 seconds, thereby changing the "0" to a "1." Points were convertible to money at the rate of 8¢ per point. Initially the screen was blank. The subject could monitor it (turn on the "0" or "1") for 0.5 seconds by pressing the left-hand button. Zeros were programmed to occur with 75% probability on a DRL 20 sec with a 20-second limited hold. That is, observing responses occurring with a latency of less than 20 sec or more than 40 sec always illuminated a "1" on the television screen. When 20–40 sec had elapsed since the last response, there was a 75% probability that a "0" would be illuminated. If a "0" appeared on the screen, it could be changed to a "1" and a point could be earned if the subject pressed the right hand push button within 2 sec. If a "1" appeared on the screen, it was not possible to earn a point. The subject had to wait at least 20 seconds more before checking the screen in order to possibly (75% probability) see a "0."

Subjects were tested on this procedure for one hour and were then administered an oral dose of diazepam (5, 10, 15 mg) or *d*-amphetamine (5, 10, 15 mg) dissolved in 30 ml of a flavored quinine-based solution, or the flavored solution alone (placebo). When amphetamine was administered, 90 minutes elapsed between drinking the drug and beginning the second experimental session. When the drug was diazepam, only 45 minutes elapsed. Placebo sessions interspersed in the amphetamine series occurred after 90 minutes; those in the diazepam series occurred after 45 minutes.

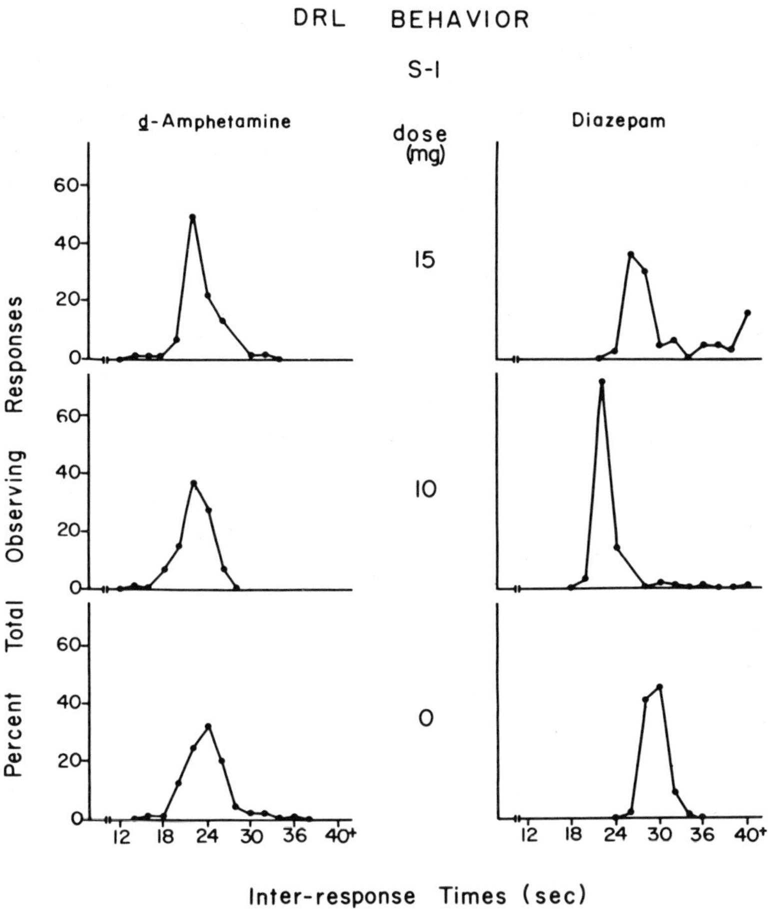

Figure 11. Interresponse time distribution for subject 1, making an observing response maintained on a DRL schedule of point presentation after a) two doses of *d*-amphetamine and b) two doses of diazepam as well as placebo.

Data are presented in Figure 11 showing the IRT distributions obtained during the DRL schedule for the same subject used to illustrate results with the avoidance paradigm. Each IRT distribution represents data collected during a one-hour session after drug or placebo was administered and an appropriate length of time had elapsed. The amphetamine series was conducted first. No information was given to this subject concerning the temporal requirements of the schedule. If, however, IRT distributions are compared under placebo conditions for this paradigm and the avoidance paradigm, a clear example of the schedule control of behavior can be seen. When no consequences were attached to response rate (within the limits of two per minute) this subject pressed the lever an average of nine times per minute (range 6–13) during baseline conditions with IRT distributions peaking at 6–8 sec. This pattern of responding was quite steady over the eleven months that she was tested. When the behavioral task was changed and the DRL schedule of reinforcement was in effect, IRT distributions shifted rapidly, to peak between 20 and 40 sec. After placebo on the third day that this schedule was in effect (6th session) her IRT distribution peaked at 25–26 sec. When the task required a specific rate of response, it did not take very long for behavior to shift.

Amphetamine was administered in the order 10, 5, 15 mg; the placebo data shown in Figure 11A were taken from the session that was run between the 10 and 5 mg sessions. Fifteen mg of *d*-amphetamine caused a small 2 second peak shift to the left. In addition, the distribution was considerably narrowed after 15 mg *d*-amphetamine. The shift to more rapid responding was minimal compared to that seen after the same dose of *d*-amphetamine when the avoidance paradigm was in effect. Then, (Figure 9) all IRT's occurred within 0–4 sec. Dews and Morse[33] also found that human subjects, working on a DRL schedule of reinforcement, showed a small shift to slightly shorter interresponse times after ingesting amphetamine. Like the subject illustrated here, their subjects did not obtain a significantly different number of reinforcements when placebo and amphetamine sessions were compared.

The IRT distribution shown in Figure 11B for a placebo session during the diazepam series reflects a general shift to longer interresponse times seen during all the baseline sessions in the diazepam series. After diazepam, the modal IRT was shortened, but still longer than the required 20 seconds. In addition, response patterning was disrupted after 15 mg diazepam, as reflected in the increased number of longer IRTs and particularly IRTs longer than 40 seconds. This same disruption in patterning was seen when 15 mg diazepam was administered during the avoidance paradigm (Figure 10). Then, an increase in short IRTs was seen, but many points were lost and periods of no escape responding occurred. In both the DRL and avoidance paradigms, although there was an increase in the percent of shorter interresponse times, there were also many missed opportunities for response. These were manifested as points lost or responses separated by more than 40 seconds.

The behavioral data presented here clearly illustrate the interaction of drug effects with ongoing behavior. Human subjects usually volunteer because they need the money, and generally will work hard to overcome any drug effects that might interfere with their earning that money. Therefore, frequently only small changes in behavior are apparent. In addition, the subjects we have been testing are generally graduate students with long past histories of reinforcement for earning maximal number of points or performing at close to perfect levels despite fatigue, boredom, etc. Despite the fact that this group is unlikely to show any large amount of behavioral toxicity, except at very debilitating drug doses, we have been able to show selective drug effects that, with further research, we hope will be generalizable to other drugs within the same classes. The data from these procedures should be useful additions to the overall profile of a drug's actions in comparing it to other known drugs of abuse.

GENERAL DISCUSSION

The battery of measures described in this chapter show great promise for use in the evaluation of the actions of psychotropic drugs in man. The prediction of a new drug's abuse potential may be possible by comparing its profile of effects to those shown by known drugs of abuse. It should be clear that no single set of measurements is sufficient to differentiate among many classes of drugs. For example, the effects of opiates and phenothiazines on avoidance responding of rats are indistinguishable,[21,23] and it is likely that this would also be true for man. Therefore, it is important to make additional measurements to provide those data necessary to distinguish between these two classes of drugs. They appear to have, for example, very different subjective effects, as measured by a variety of questionnaires, such as the ARCI. The necessity for multiple measures to distinguish between classes of drugs is also shown by the fact that chlorpromazine and imipramine produced similar effects on escape-avoidance responding of normal human volunteers in this study. Data have recently been collected, however, indicating that these two drugs can be differentiated on the basis of their subjective effects in normal subjects.

Comparison of the effects of cocaine and *d*-amphetamine is an example of the way in which multi-dimensional profiles of drug action can be used to predict abuse potential. If cocaine were an unknown drug, it could be concluded from the physiological and behavioral data reported here that cocaine would be comparable to the amphetamines in terms of its abuse liability. This is, of course, true. Thus, by comparing standard drugs in this manner, it is possible to validate the battery of measures presented in this paper as potential predictors of a new drug's abuse potential. Further research along these lines that combines many of the suggested procedures is clearly necessary before the long-range goal of predicting abuse potential can be met. Nevertheless, the research to date is promising.

LITERATURE CITED

1. Committee on Problems of Drug Dependence. 1972. Testing for Dependence Liability in Animals and Man. Bulletin on Narcotics. 25:25–39.
2. Deneau, G. A., and Seevers, M. H. 1962. Evaluation of morphine-like physical dependence in the rhesus monkey (macaca mulatta). Bulletin, Drug Addiction and Narcotics (Addendum 2).
3. Fraser, H. F. 1968. Methods for assessing the addiction liability of opioids and opioid antagonists in man. In: A. Wikler (ed.), The Addictive States, pp. 176–187. Williams and Wilkins, Baltimore.
4. Villarreal, J. E. 1973. The effects of morphine agonists and antagonists on morphine-dependent rhesus monkeys. In: H. W. Kosterlitz, H. O. J. Collier, and J. E. Villarreal (eds.), Agonist and Antagonist Actions of Narcotic Analgesic Drugs, pp. 73–93. University Park Press, Baltimore.
5. Schuster, C. R., and Thompson, T. 1969. Self-administration of and behavioral dependence on drugs. Ann. Rev. Pharmacol. 9:483–502.
6. Schuster, C. R., and Johanson, C. E. 1974. The use of animal models for the study of drug abuse. In: R. J. Gibbins, I. Yedy, H. Kalant, R. E. Popham, W. Schmidt, and R. G. Smart (eds.), Research Advances in Alcohol and Drug Problems, Vol. I. J. Wiley and Sons, Inc, New York.
7. Martin, W. R., and Fraser, H. F. 1961. A comparative study of physiological and subjective effects of heroin and morphine administration intravenously in post-addicts. J. Pharmacol. Exp. Ther., 133:388–398.
8. Jasinski, D. R. 1973. Assessment of the Dependence Liability of Opiates and Sedative-Hypnotics. In: L. Goldberg and F. Hoffmeister (eds.), Psychic Dependence, pp. 160–170. Springer-Verlag, Berlin.
9. Martin, W. R., Sloan, J. W., Sapira, J. D., and Jasinski, D. R. 1971. Physiological, subjective and behavioral effects of amphetamine, methamphetamine, ephedrine, phenmetraxine and methylphenidate in man. Clin. Pharmacol. Ther. 12:245–58.
10. Jasinski, D. R., Nutt, J. G., and Griffith, J. D. 1974. Effects of diethylpropion and *d*-amphetamine after subcutaneous and oral administration. Clin. Pharmacol. Ther. 645–652.
11. Fischman, M. W., Schuster, C. R., Resnekov, L., Fennel, W., Shick, J. F. E., and Krasnegor, N. A. 1976. Cardiovascular and subjective effects of intravenous cocaine in man. Arch. Gen. Psych. 33:983–989.
12. Haertzen, C. A. 1966. Development of scales based on pattern of drug

effects, using the Addiction Research Center Inventory (ARCI). Psychological Reports, 18:163–194.
13. Kramer, J. C., Fischman, V. S., and Littlefield, D. C. 1967. Amphetamine abuse. JAMA 201:305–309.
14. Jonsson, L. E., and Gunne, L. M. 1970. Clinical studies of amphetamine psychosis. In: E. Costa and S. Garattini (eds.), International Symposium on Amphetamines, and Related Compounds. Raven Press, New York.
15. Griffith, J. D., Cavenaugh, J., Held, J., and Oates, J. A. 1972. Dextroamphetamine: Evaluation of psychomimetic properties in man. Arch. Gen. Psych. 26:97–100.
16. Martin, W. R. 1973. Assessment of the abuse potentiality of amphetamines and LSD-like hallucinogens in man and its relationship to basic animal assessment programs. In: L. Goldberg and F. Hoffmeister (eds.), Psychic Dependence, pp. 146–155. Springer-Verlag, Berlin.
17. Smith, C. B. 1964. Effects of *d*-amphetamine upon operant behavior of pigeons. Enhancement by resperine. J. Pharmacol. Exp. Ther. 146:167–174.
18. McMillan, D. E., Dearstyne, M. R., and Engstrom, T. G. 1975. Some effects of local anesthetic on schedule-controlled behavior. Pharmacol. Ther. Dent. 2:57–64.
19. Cook, L., and Catania, A. C. 1964. Effects of drugs on avoidance and escape behavior. Federation Proceedings, 23:818–835.
20. Kelleher, R. T., and Morse, W. H. 1968. Determinants of the specificity of behavioral effects of drugs. Ergebnesse der Physiologia. 60:1–56.
21. Cook, L., and Weidley, E. 1957. Behavioral effects of some psychopharmacological agents. Annals of the New York Academy of Science 66:740–752.
22. Verhave, T., Owen, J. E., and Slater, O. H. 1958. Effects of various drugs on escape and avoidance behavior. Prog. Neurobiol. 3:267–301.
23. Heise, G. A., and Boff, E. 1962. Continuous avoidance as a baseline for measuring behavioral effects of drugs. Psychopharmacologia 3:264–282.
24. Sidman, M. 1956. Time discrimination and behavioral interaction in a free operant situation. J. Comp. Physiol. Psychol. 49:469–473.
25. Dalrymple, S. D., and Stretch, R. 1971. Effects of amphetamine and chlorpromazine on second-order escape behavior in squirrel monkeys. Psychopharmacologia 21:268–282.
26. Longoni, A., Mandelli, J., and Pessotti, I. 1973. Study of anti-anxiety effects of drugs in the rat, with a multiple punishment and reward schedule. In: S. Garattini, E. Mussini and L. O. Randall (eds.), The Benzodiazepines, pp. 347–354. Raven Press, New York.
27. Bignami, G., deAcetis, L., and Gatti, G. L. 1971. Facilitation and impairment of avoidance responding by phenobarbital sodium, chlordiazepoxide and diazepam—The role of performance baselines. J. Pharmacol. Exper. Ther. 176:725–732.
28. Cook, L., and Sepinwall, J. 1975. Reinforcement schedules and extrapolations to humans from animals in behavioral pharmacology. Fed. Proc. 34:1889–1897.

29. Dews, P. B. 1958. Analysis of effects of psychopharmacological agents in behavioral terms. Fed. Proc. 17:1024.
30. Clark, F. C., and Steele, B. J. 1966. Effects of *d*-amphetamine on performance under a multiple schedule in the rat. Psychopharmacologia 9:157–169.
31. McMillan, D. E. 1968. The effects of sympathomimetic amines on schedule-controlled behavior in the pigeon. J. Pharmacol. Exp. Ther. 159:315–325.
32. Holland, J. G. 1958. Human vigilance. Science. 128:61.
33. Dews, P. B., and Morse, W. H. 1958. Some observations on an operant in human subjects and its modification by dextro-amphetamine. J. Exper. Anal. Behav. 1:359–364.

Clinical Evaluation of Sedative-Hypnotics for Abuse Potential

Donald R. Jasinski

One valid means of evaluating agents for morphine-like abuse potential is to demonstrate that single doses of the agents produce a characteristic profile of subjective effects and euphoria in nontolerant, nondependent narcotics addicts.[1-3] A similar approach has been utilized in evaluating agents for amphetamine-like abuse potential.[4,5]

In a series of studies, Martin and his colleagues[6,7] demonstrated that nontolerant narcotic addicts: 1) distinguish pentobarbital from placebo and morphine, and 2) report euphoria with pentobarbital. These investigators further observed that pentobarbital produced a dose-related facilitation of post-rotatory nystagmus. They subsequently utilized the electro-oculogram and bioassay techniques to compare the increased frequency and duration of post-rotatory nystagmus produced by pentobarbital and meprobamate.

These studies by Martin and his colleagues[6,7] suggested that sedative-hypnotics might be evaluated for barbiturate-like abuse potential by assessing their ability to produce pentobarbital-like subjective effects, euphoria, and facilitation of post-rotatory nystagmus in nontolerant, nondependent subjects. On this basis, two studies have been conducted 1) to compare intramuscularly administered pentobarbital, secobarbital, phenobarbital, and placebo, and 2) to compare orally administered pentobarbital, secobarbital, and placebo (Table 1).

The measures of drug effect were, with slight modification, those developed by Martin and his colleagues[6,7] to measure the effects of pentobarbital. These were 1) electro-oculographs of post-rotational nystagmus,[7] 2) the "subjects' and observers' single dose opiate questionnaires,"[1] and 3) a subjective drug effect questionnaire[8] containing 40 items from the Morphine-Benzedrine Group Scale (MBG), the

Table 1. Characteristics of the two studies in which single doses of the drugs were administered to nondependent, nontolerant narcotic addicts at minimum 7-day intervals utilizing the double-blind crossover technique

	Study Number	
	I	II
Number of Subjects	10	9
Design	Latin Square	Randomized Block
Route of Drug Administration	Intramuscular	Oral
Drugs and Doses	(A) Placebo	(A) Placebo
	(B) Pentobarbital	(B) Pentobarbital
	50 mg	60 mg
	120 mg	120 mg
	288 mg	240 mg
	(C) Secobarbital	(C) Secobarbital
	75 mg	60 mg
	180 mg	120 mg
	432 mg	240 mg
	(D) Phenobarbital	
	150 mg	
	360 mg	
	557.1 mg	

Pentobarbital-Chlorpromazine-Alcohol Group Scale (PCAG), and the LSD Specific Scale. Each item in the MBG and PCAG Scales that showed dose-related responses was placed in a subset of a Euphoria Scale for the MBG items and a Sedation Scale for the PCAG items to obtain scale scores that were dose responsive.

Pentobarbital administered orally or intramuscularly produced effects similar to those described by Martin and his colleagues. In both studies pentobarbital was 1) identified as a barbiturate, 2) produced dose-related scores on the symptom, sign, "liking," euphoria and sedation scales, and 3) increased the frequency and duration of post-rotatory nystagmus in a dose-related manner (Figures 1 and 2).

Secobarbital produced a profile of effects similar to those of pentobarbital (Figures 1 and 2) with a similar onset and duration of action. Relative potencies were calculated from the dose effect curves for pentobarbital and secobarbital utilizing the standard statistical methods for parallel line bioassay (Figures 1 and 2). These relative potencies were in concordance across the various measures and indicated that secobarbital is equipotent to pentobarbital when administered intramuscularly or orally.

Phenobarbital also produced a profile of effects similar to those of pentobarbital (Figure 1). The onset and duration of effects for phenobarbital were indistinguishable from pentobarbital and secobarbital. In contrast to secobarbital, phenobarbital was clearly less potent than pentobarbital (Figure 1), and again there was concordance of potency estimates across the various measures of subjective effects. Phe-

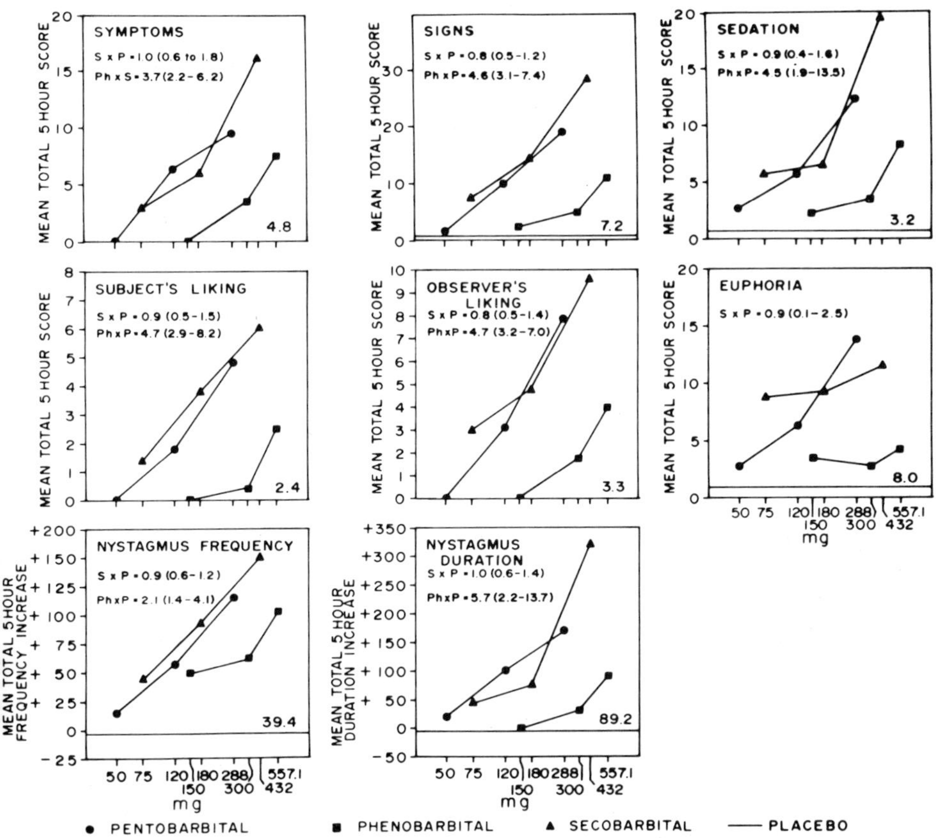

Figure 1. Dose-response curves for the comparison of intramuscularly administered pentobarbital, secobarbital, phenobarbital, and placebo for 1) symptoms and subjects' liking scale scores from the subjects' single dose opiate questionnaires, 2) sign and observers' liking scale scores from the observers' single dose opiate questionnaires, 3) the sedation and euphoria scale scores from the subjective drug effect questionnaires, and 4) the change in frequency and duration of post-rotatory nystagmus. Numbers in upper left-hand corner of each graph represent the relative potency and 95% confidence limits expressed as mg of secobarbital (S $\times$ P) or mg of phenobarbital (Ph $\times$ P) equivalent to 1 mg of pentobarbital. The number in the lower right hand corner of each graph represents the standard deviation (square root of the error mean square in the analysis of variance).

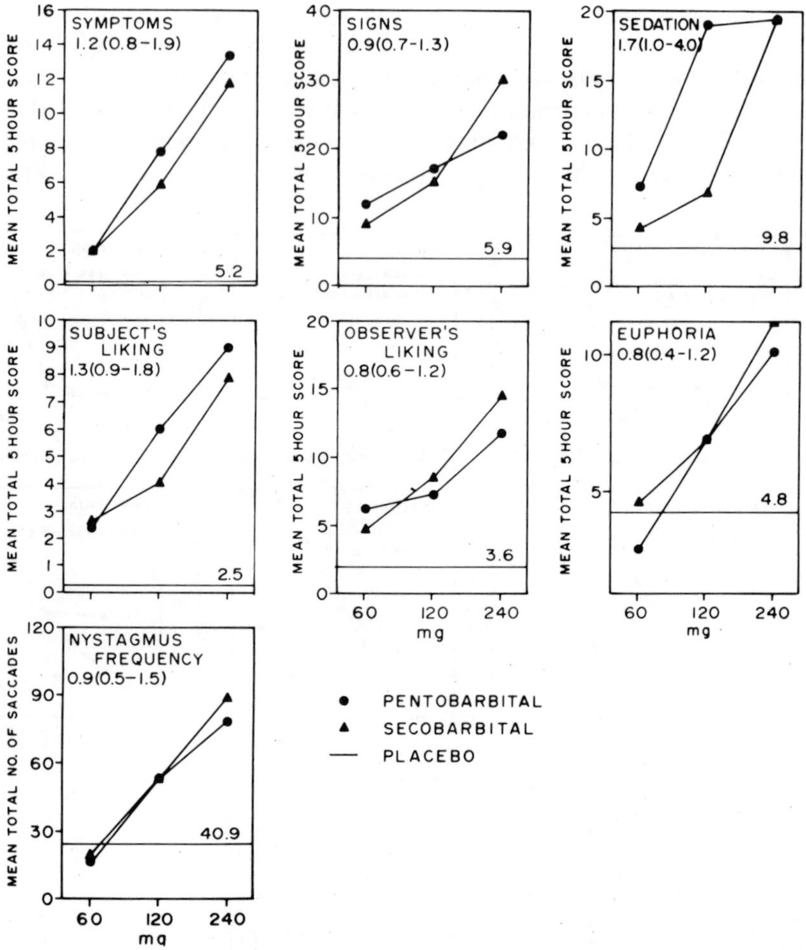

Figure 2. Dose response curves for the comparison of orally administered pentobarbital, secobarbital, and placebo for 1) symptom and subjects' liking scale scores from the subjects' single dose opiate questionnaires, 2) sign and observers' liking scale scores from the observers' single dose opiate questionnaires, 3) euphoria and sedation scale scores from the subjective drug effect questionnaires, and 4) the changes in frequency of post-rotatory nystagmus. Numbers in upper left-hand corner of each graph represent the relative potency and 95% confidence limits expressed as mg of secobarbital equivalent to 1 mg of pentobarbital. The number in the lower right-hand corner of each graph represents the standard deviation (square root of the error mean square in the analysis of variance).

nobarbital appeared to be more potent in increasing the frequency of post-rotatory nystagmus than in producing subjective effects or increasing the duration of nystagmus.

The studies conducted to date suggest that the abuse potential of sedative hypnotics could be evaluated by assessing their ability to produce pentobarbital-like subjective effects, euphoria, and post-rotatory nystagmus; the studies have indicated 1) that pentobarbital reproducibly produces a characteristic profile of effects, 2) that valid measures of these effects exist, and 3) that secobarbital and phenobarbital can be bioassayed for these effects.

LITERATURE CITED

1. Fraser, H. F., Van Horn, G. D., Martin, W. R., Wolbach, A. B., and Isbell, H. 1961. Methods for evaluating addiction liability. (A) "Attitude" of opiate addicts toward opiate-like drugs, (B) A short term "direct" addiction test. J. Pharmacol. Exp. Ther. 133:371–387.
2. Martin, W. R., and Fraser, H. F. 1961. A comparative study of physiological and subjective effects of heroin and morphine administered intravenously in post-addicts. J. Pharmacol Exp. Ther. 133:388–399.
3. Martin, W. R. 1966. Assessment of the dependence-producing potentiality of narcotic analgesics. In: L. Lasagna and C. Radouco-Thomas (eds.), International Encyclopedia of Pharmacology and Therapeutics. Pergamon Press, New York.
4. Martin, W. R., Sloan, J. W., Sapira, J. D., and Jasinski, D. R. 1971. Physiologic, subjective and behavioral effects of amphetamine, methamphetamine, ephedrine, phenmetrazine, and methylphenidate in man. Clin. Pharmacol. Ther. 12:245–258.
5. Jasinski, D. R., Nutt, J. G., and Griffith, J. D. 1974. Effects of diethylpropion and *d*-amphetamine after subcutaneous and oral administration. Clin. Pharmacol. Ther. 16:645–652.
6. Martin, W. R., Thompson, W. O., and Fraser, H. F. 1974. Comparison of graded single intramuscular doses of morphine and pentobarbital in man. Clin. Pharmacol. Ther. 15:623–630.
7. McClane, T. K., and Martin, W. R. 1976. Subjective and physiologic effects of morphine, pentobarbital, and meprobamate. Clin. Pharmacol. Ther. 20: 192–198.
8. Jasinski, D. R., Martin, W. R., and Sapira, J. D. 1968. Antagonism of the subjective, behavioral, pupillary, and respiratory depressant effects of cyclazocine by naloxone. Clin. Pharmacol. Ther. 9:215–222.

Co-Variance of Neuroendocrine Function and Behavior

A Potential Technique for Assessing Drug Abuse Liability

Jack H. Mendelson

and

Nancy K. Mello

An examination of reported patterns of polydrug abuse suggests that the actual choice of drugs among polydrug abusers does not always correspond to the reported rationale for their drug of choice. Statements of preference for a specific drug (e.g., marihuana in preference to alcohol or to narcotics) are often inconsistent with observed behaviors. Moreover, multiple substance use often produces effects that are the opposite of the effect associated with the preferred drug. There is little doubt that polydrug abuse is related to the local availability of specific substances. However, substance availability cannot account for the paradoxical abuse of readily available agents, such as alcohol and marihuana, which appear to have different subjective and pharmacological effects. Heroin addicts may perpetuate the abuse of opiates to achieve feeling states associated with the reduction of sexuality and aggression. Yet, these same individuals may become addicted to alcohol while on methadone maintenance, even though alcohol is usually associated with increases in aggressive behavior and libidinal drives.

Perhaps one way of resolving the apparent paradox that opposite

---

This study was supported in part by Grant DA 4RG010 from the National Institute on Drug Abuse, ADAMHA, Dept. of Health, Education, and Welfare, Washington, D.C.

behavioral states are induced by sequential or concurrent use of different types of drugs is that the drugs do not necessarily make the user feel better but do make him feel "different." The notion that drug abusers employ substances to induce quantitative rather than qualitative change in feeling state is not an original one. Dostoevski pointed out in *Notes from the Underground* that one of man's most "advantageous advantages" is the ability to induce changes even when such changes are neither necessary nor rewarding in a socially conventional sense.

A perusal of case records and biographies of polydrug abusers suggests that alterations in self-induced changes in feeling states may be a very important goal for those who use drugs. Use of "uppers" followed by "downers" or the converse is not uncommon. Some of this behavior may be accounted for by an attempt to titrate certain qualitative, subjective drug effects. However, it is also possible that eclectic alterations in feeling states may be preferred to more predictable changes in moods and feelings that might be produced by use of a single drug.

Although the range of changes induced by a large number of stimulant and depressant drugs used by humans is probably enormous, there are two central or core areas of behavior that appear to be very important. These are the facilitation or attenuation of sexual and aggressive feeling states and behavior. Drug-induced changes in these behaviors may be overt, such as the phenomena of alcohol-induced belligerence and bravado or narcotic-induced suppression of libidinal drive. In a more subtle way, alcohol may enhance feelings of masculinity and power and narcotics may decrease an individual's ability to respond to provocation with anger. It is perhaps not important whether a drug accentuates or diminishes sexuality or aggression if "turning on" or "turning off" enhances an individual's ability to fulfill a wish or desire toward "self-actualization." But if drugs are used to modulate feeling states and behavior associated with sex and aggression, such drugs achieve their mechanism of action in part through perturbations of the central nervous system, pituitary-gonadal-hormonal axis.

There is probably little doubt that pituitary-gonadal hormones play a crucial role in the regulation of sexual behavior as well as the processes of sexual differentiation in a large number of species, ranging from rodents to subhuman primates.[1] Because the repertoire of behaviors associated with procreative function and aggression are so closely linked in a number of animal species, it has been postulated that the biological mechanisms that regulate sexual function must also be associated with the processes of aggression. Evidence derived from human studies is less definitive regarding the regulatory actions of sex hormones on sexual and aggressive behavior, in part because of the methodological problems for carrying out well-controlled studies. However, there is some evidence that aggressive behavior in human adult males may bear a relationship to plasma testosterone levels.[2-4] Most recently it was found that increments in circulating luteinizing hormone levels and follicle-stimulating hormone levels occurred in normal males during periods of sexual arousal.[5] This study is important since it is the first time that serial hormone levels were determined over short intervals of time and correlated with standardized presentation of erotic stimuli. Even more important was the finding that the elevation in LH levels was directly related to the duration of sexual arousal. It therefore appears that there is a significant relationship between plasma luteinizing hormone levels in human males and libidinal drive. If there is concordance between hormonal regulation of drive states related to aggression and sexuality in humans, it would also be postulated that LH levels would co-vary with aggressive behaviors.

Figure 1 is a schematic depiction of the stimulatory and feedback relationships between the hypothalamus, pituitary, and target organs regulated by pituitary gonadotrophins. The regions of the brain that appear crucial for secretion of gonadotrophin-releasing hormone are the most rostral medial preoptic areas of the hypothalamus, the anterior hypothalamus, and the more caudal arcuate median eminence region. All of these areas exhibit some sensitivity for the "short loop" negative feedback effects of luteinizing hormone. There is also a "long loop" negative feedback produced by testosterone. It is generally believed that the dopaminergic as well as norepinephrine-regulated synapases in the arcuate median eminence region are important in negative feedback effects of testosterone on gonadotrophin-releasing hormone. The negative feedback influence of testosterone on gonadotrophin-releasing hormone probably involves inhibition of synaptic activity as a consequence of decrements in plasma levels of testosterone. It is also of interest that gonadotrophin-releasing hormone release can be stimulated by both dopamine and by pituitary peptides when administered intraventricularly. It is now also known that receptor sites for sex steroids exist in various regions of the

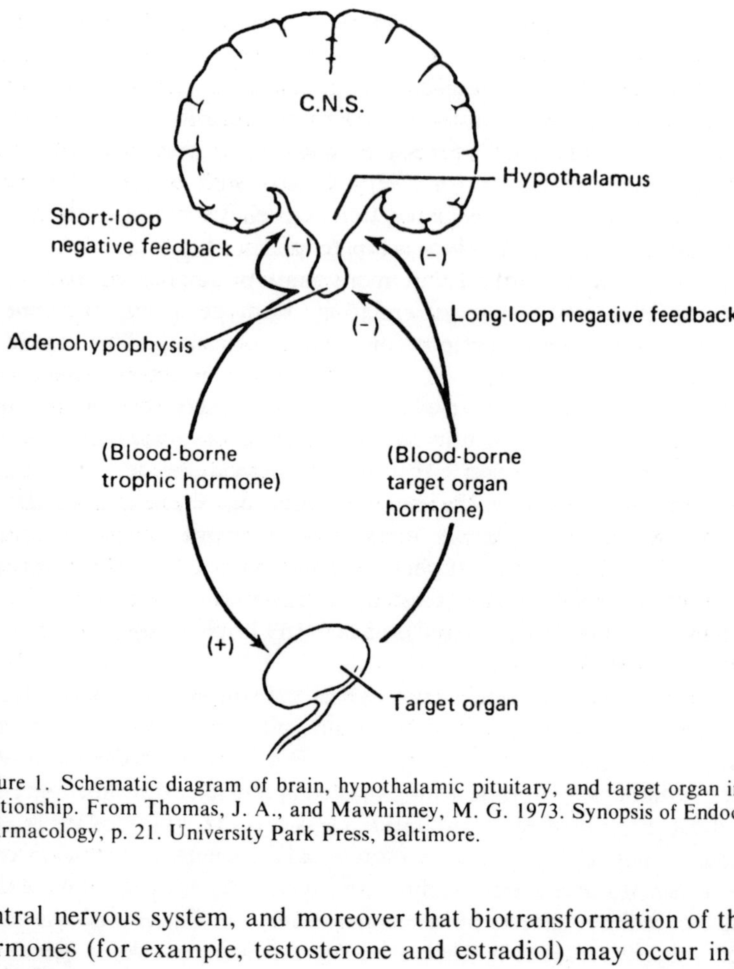

Figure 1. Schematic diagram of brain, hypothalamic pituitary, and target organ interrelationship. From Thomas, J. A., and Mawhinney, M. G. 1973. Synopsis of Endocrine Pharmacology, p. 21. University Park Press, Baltimore.

central nervous system, and moreover that biotransformation of these hormones (for example, testosterone and estradiol) may occur in the brain.[21]

In a series of careful and comprehensive experimental animal studies, Cicero and his associates found that chronic morphine or methadone administration to male rats produced a significant decrement in serum testosterone levels.[7,8] They also found that both morphological structure and physiological activity of the secondary sex organs (the seminal vesicles and prostate glands) are altered and deranged following chronic administration of narcotics. Similar findings in studies with mice have been reported by Thomas and Dombrowski.[9] The most recent reports from Cicero's laboratory[10] demonstrate that both dose and potency of narcotics are significant determinants of suppression of plasma testosterone levels and luteinizing hormone levels in rats.

Cicero and co-workers[10] showed that a dose-response relationship can be established for a number of narcotic drugs as a function of drug-induced suppression of plasma testosterone levels in rat. These dose-response relationships are highly correlated with the potency of the same drugs for suppressing activity of the isolated electrically stimulated guinea pig ileum and mouse vas deferens.

Cicero has also shown that suppression of plasma testosterone by narcotics is stereospecific. It was found that the − isomer of methadone was significantly more potent than the + isomer in suppressing plasma testosterone levels. In chronic studies of narcotic-induced suppression of plasma testosterone levels, Cicero and colleagues[10] found that tolerance developed to narcotic-induced hormone suppression. Finally, it was reported that narcotic antagonists (naloxone) inhibited the effects of narcotics on suppression of plasma testosterone levels.[10]

If narcotic-induced suppression of plasma testosterone levels is to be employed as a means of assessing drug abuse liability in humans, it is important to determine if chronic narcotic use is associated with the development of tolerance, or perhaps irreversible impairment of the pituitary-gonadal system. In a study of heroin-dependent males in Hong Kong, we examined the relationship between plasma testosterone levels and the time course of chronic heroin use and protracted abstinence.[13] All subjects except one had normal testosterone levels 1 to 12 months following cessation of drug use. The single subject who showed abnormally low testosterone levels at 2 to 3 months following cessation of heroin use, was a 15-year-old boy who initiated heavy heroin use at age 12, prior to the onset of puberty. Animal studies have shown that morphine administration at a critical developmental stage can result in long-lasting effects on neuroendocrine function.[11] Consequently, we conducted a more detailed study of plasma testosterone levels in young adult males who began heroin use before or at the onset of puberty, in order to determine the generality of our previous observation.

Data obtained in this follow-up study were concordant with our previous findings that chronic heroin use is associated with a decrease in plasma testosterone levels.[12] However, there did not appear to be a permanent impairment in gonadotrophins or testosterone secretion in abstinent males who became addicts prior to puberty. Testosterone and luteinizing hormone levels returned to normal after cessation of heroin use in all males studied. Consequently, although heroin acutely suppresses testosterone and pituitary-gonadotrophin levels, this suppression is transient, and following cessation of heroin use these hormone levels return to normal.[12,13] In recent clinical studies,[16] we have found a dose-response relationship between narcotic dose and degree of suppression of plasma testosterone levels in man. This finding is in agreement with the animal studies of Cicero and co-workers.[10]

We believe that still another criterion should be added to those advanced by Cicero and co-workers[10] for evaluating the effects of narcotics on the pituitary-gonadal system. The *duration of effect* of a narcotic on a biological system should have a time-course that parallels the duration of action of the drug. For example, methadone should produce a more protracted suppression of plasma testosterone levels than an equally potent dose of morphine. Moreover, it would be predicted that L-alpha-acetylmethadol, which has an even longer duration of action, would produce a more protracted suppression of plasma testosterone levels. This hypothesis was substantiated in collaborative studies of effects of L-alpha-acetylmethadol (LAAM) on plasma testosterone levels in adult males.[14]

Data obtained by Cicero in studies with rodents[7,8,10] and our findings in studies with humans,[12-16] converge to suggest that the pituitary-gonadal-hormonal axis is very sensitive to the effects of narcotic drugs.

Figure 2 depicts the effects of heroin on the hypothalamus and possibly the pituitary in blocking the secretion of blood-borne trophic hormones from the anterior pituitary. Under these conditions both "short" and "long loop" negative feedback systems are affected. Since suppression of LH occurs following heroin administration, plasma testosterone levels also fall. The decrement in plasma testosterone levels without morphine blockade would ordinarily result in increased GnRH and LH output. However, a decrement in testosterone levels following initial suppression of luteinizing hormone may have other significant neural consequences.

On the basis of our observations of heroin-induced suppression of the episodic secretory rate of luteinizing hormone and testosterone,[6] we have formulated the following hypotheses.

1. Narcotic-induced suppression of plasma luteinizing hormone levels co-varies with the magnitude and time course of opiate-induced suppression of libidinal drive and aggressive behaviors.
2. Altered pituitary-gonadal function and changes in sexual and aggressive behavior produced by heroin are related to the action of the

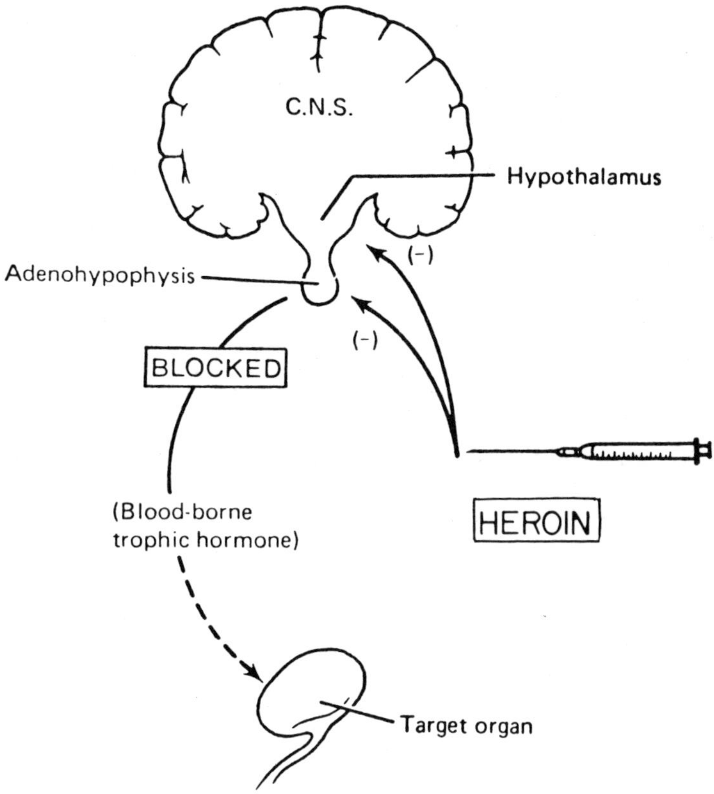

Figure 2. Schematic diagram of heroin blockade of hypothalamic-pituitary trophic hormones. Adapted from Thomas, J. A., and Mawhinney, M. G. 1973. Synopsis of Endocrine Pharmacology, p. 23. University Park Press, Baltimore.

drug at hypothalamic sites that regulate secretion of gonadotrophin-releasing hormone.

3. The rapid decrement in LH secretory pulses following narcotic use is probably due to a prior decrement in GnRH release.

4. A decrement in GnRH release with a concomitant decrease in luteinizing hormone release would not only produce a significant decrement in testosterone secretion, but also affect "short loop" and "long loop" feedback mechanisms.

5. The immediate effects of narcotics in dramatically suppressing LH release co-vary with the immediate effects of narcotics to induce the "rush" or "high" or orgasmic-like experience.

6. Longer term narcotic effects on suppressing LH, testosterone, and plasma cortisol levels co-vary with states of quiescence, lack of libidinal and aggressive drive, and satiation commonly reported following the more immediate and dramatic heroin-induced "rush."

Recent research also indicates that alcohol may affect both central and peripheral mechanisms of testosterone secretion and biotransformation in male experimental animals and humans.[17,18] We have carried out determinations of plasma LH and testosterone in healthy adult males during the time course of ascending, peak, and descending limbs of the blood alcohol curve. Because of the large circhoral variations in both LH and testosterone secretion,[19] consecutive 20-minute serial determinations of hormonal levels prior to and following ethanol intake were made.

Data obtained in these studies are shown in Table 1. A significant fall in plasma levels ($p < 0.05$) occurred during the ascending limb of the blood alcohol curve as contrasted to pre-alcohol (0 time) levels. At peak blood levels, plasma testosterone levels were even more significantly depressed ($p < 0.01$). Luteinizing hormone levels were not significantly different during the ascending phase of the blood alcohol curve when compared with 0 time values. However, LH values were significantly elevated at peak alcohol levels ($p < 0.01$). During the descending phase of the blood alcohol curve, plasma testosterone levels remained significantly depressed ($p < 0.01$) and LH levels decreased. Changes in plasma luteinizing hormone levels and testos-

Table 1. Plasma testosterone and LH during ascending, peak, and descending blood alcohol levels

	0	Ascending	Peak	Descending
Testosterone				
(ng/100 ml) $\bar{X}$	857.73	756.17	689.38	704.11
±S.E.	63.61	47.04	51.81	42.23
LH				
(ng/ml) $\bar{X}$	48.22	51.21	62.49	54.92
±S.E.	4.28	4.97	5.25	5.44
Time of Alcohol Intake				
(minutes) $\bar{X}$	−15	+36	+84	+216
±S.E.	0	3.3	4.4	2.4
Blood Alcohol				
(mg/100 ml) $\bar{X}$	0	81	109	59
±S.E.	0	7.2	4.6	2.3

terone levels observed in this study occurred when blood alcohol levels were not inordinately high. Blood alcohol levels observed in this study (109 mg/100 ml) are those usually associated with mild to moderate inebriation in social drinkers.

Findings obtained in this study are consistent with data previously obtained in our laboratory[20] that alcohol intake lowers plasma testosterone levels in human males. The findings of this study also support reports of others that alcohol-induced alterations in androgens may occur as a consequence of the effects of ethanol on the gonads directly[18] or on biotransformation mechanisms in the liver.[17] If central supression of gonadotrophin secretion by ethanol caused reduction of plasma testosterone levels, an initial decrement of plasma luteinizing hormone levels should have been observed prior to the fall in plasma testosterone levels at peak blood alcohol levels.

These data are consistent with predicted effects of the "long loop" feedback mechanisms that have been described for the reciprocal relationship between plasma testosterone and luteinizing hormone levels.[21] Rapid feedback stimulation of LH output would be expected to occur if peripheral levels of testosterone fell and central hypothalamic-pituitary mechanisms were not inhibited.

Our data and data obtained by others suggest the following hypotheses:

1. Ethanol-induced changes in plasma testosterone may reflect or perhaps modulate alterations in sexual and aggressive behavior associated with acute and chronic alcohol intake.
2. Decreased testosterone levels at peak blood ethanol concentrations may produce decrements in male sexual behavior and performance.
3. Increments in plasma luteinizing hormone levels during peak blood ethanol levels may be important for neural processes that regulate expression of aggression and sexual desire.
4. Heightened aggressivity and sexual desire during peak alcohol levels may in turn be dependent upon the peripheral actions of ethanol on the gonads and/or the liver, which determine plasma testosterone levels and concomitant "long loop" feedback effects on hypothalamic and pituitary function.

Figures 3 and 4 compare opiate- and alcohol-induced changes in androgen function in males with respect to possible mechanisms of action of the drugs (Figure 3) and reported behavioral correlates of drug effects (Figure 4). Both alcohol and opiates produced a suppression in testosterone levels but via different mechanisms. Opiate

DRUG INDUCED CHANGES IN ANDROGEN FUNCTION IN MALES

DRUG	TESTOSTERONE	LH	POSSIBLE MECHANISMS
OPIATES	↓	↓	CENTRAL INHIBITION
ALCOHOL	↓	↑	PERIPHERAL - DECREASED SYNTHESIS

Figure 3. Effects of opiates and alcohol on testosterone and LH levels and plasma and possible mechanisms for these effects.

suppression of plasma testosterone levels is a consequence of initial suppression of luteinizing hormone. However, alcohol suppression of testosterone level is the result of peripheral actions, the drug and plasma LH levels are increased via feedback "long loop" effects. Behavioral correlates of decreased libido, aggression, and sexual performance are consistent with a decrement in both testosterone and LH produced by opiates, whereas libido and aggression are increased following alcohol intake. Alcohol-induced aggression and sexual desire would co-vary with an increment in LH levels, whereas a decrease in sexual performance during alcohol intoxication would co-vary with a decrement in plasma testosterone levels.

Although a number of useful techniques and methods are cur-

DRUG INDUCED CHANGES IN ANDROGEN FUNCTION IN MALES

DRUG	TESTOSTERONE	LH	REPORTED BEHAVIORAL CORRELATES: LIBIDO	AGGRESSION	SEXUAL PERFORMANCE
OPIATES	↓	↓	↓	↓	↓
ALCOHOL	↓	↑	↑	↑	↓

Figure 4. Effects of opiates and alcohol on testosterone and LH levels in plasma and reported behavioral correlates with such changes.

rently available for determination of drug abuse liability for opiate compounds there are no comparable methods for a wide range of stimulants and depressants.[22-26] Martin and Jasinski have pointed out that:

> No single technique used in a single species will allow a valid assessment of the abuse potentiality of psychoactive drugs. With the enormous growth of the chemical and pharmaceutical industries and their impact upon health, it is to society's self-interest to identify the abuse potentiality of new drugs and chemicals prior to their introduction into the open market or medical practice. Broad-based studies of new and useful drugs and chemicals in several species using a variety of techniques are not only justified but indicated.[24]

The challenge for both behavioral and biological science research is to identify and accurately measure variables that may be especially relevant for understanding drug abuse liability in humans.

We have aruged that a crucial aspect of the behavioral mechanism of action of drugs that are abused by humans is the ability of such drugs to attenuate or facilitate sexual and aggressive behaviors. We have further argued that drug effects on sexual and aggressive behaviors co-vary with drug-induced changes in pituitary-gonadal hormones. With respect to drugs such as opiates, a good correlation exists between hormonal (testosterone and LH) changes, addictive potency, dose-time factors, and development of tolerance. Early studies with ethyl alcohol indicate that predictable alterations occur on the pituitary-gonadal axis following ingestion of this agent by humans. It would appear reasonable to carefully explore the covariance between behavior changes and alterations in hormonal levels with a variety of psychoactive compounds. If concordance between drug-induced changes in behavior and biological function (hormonal levels) is found in both experimental animals and humans, a new and powerful behavioral and bioassay procedure will be available for assessing drug abuse liability.

LITERATURE CITED

1. Floody, O. R., and Pfaff, D. W. 1974. Res. Publ. A.R.N.M.D. 52:149.
2. Ehrenkrantz, J., Bliss, E., and Sheard, M. H. 1974. Psychosom. Med. 36:469.
3. Persky, H., Smith, K. D., and Basu, G. K. 1971. Psychosom. Med. 33:265.
4. Rose, R. M. In: J. R. Tinklenberg (ed.), Marihuana and Health Hazards, p. 63. Academic Press, New York.

5. Laferla, J. J., Anderson, D. L., and Schalach, D. S. 1976. Psychosom. Med. 38:62.
6. Mirin, S. M., Mendelson, J. H., Ellingboe, J., and Meyer, R. E. 1976. Psychoneuroendocrinology 1:359–369.
7. Cicero, T. J., Meyer, E. R., Bell, R. D., and Wiest, W. G. 1974. Res. Com. Chem. Path. Pharmacol. 7:17.
8. Cicero, T. J., Meyer, E. R., Wiest, W. G., Olney, J. W., and Bell, R. D. 1975. J. Pharmacol. Exp. Ther. 192:542.
9. Thomas, J. A., and Dombrowski, J. T. 1975. Arch. Int. Pharmacodyn. Ther. 215:215.
10. Cicero, T. J., Wilcox, C. E., Bell, R. D., and Meyer, E. R. 1976. J. Pharmacol. Exp. Ther. 198:340–346.
11. Zimmermann, E., Branch, B., Newman Taylor, A., Young, J., and Pang, C. N. 1974. In: E. Zimmermann and C. N. Pang (eds.), Narcotics and the Hypothalamus, p. 183. Raven Press, New York.
12. Mendelson, J. H., and Mello, N. K. (1976). (In preparation.)
13. Mendelson, J. H., and Mello, N. K. 1975. Clin. Pharmacol. Therap. 17:529.
14. Mendelson, J. H., Inturrisi, C. E., Renault, P., and Senay, E. C. 1976. Clin. Pharmacol. Therap. 19:371.
15. Mendelson, J. H., Mendelson, J. E., and Patch, V. D. 1975. J. Pharmacol. Exp. Ther. 192:211.
16. Mendelson, J. H., Meyer, R. E., Ellingboe, J., Mirin, S. M., and McDougle, M. 1975. J. Pharmacol. Exp. Ther. 195:296.
17. Rubin, E., Lieber, C. S., Altman, K., Gordon, G. G., and Southren, A. L. 1976. Science 191:563.
18. Van Theil, D. H., Gavaler, J. S., and Lester, R. 1974. Gastroenterology 67:1188.
19. De Lacerda, L., Kowarski, A., Johanson, A. J., Athanasiou, R., and Migeon, C. J. 1973. J. Clin. Endocrinol. Metab. 37:366.
20. Mendelson, J. H., and Mello, N. K. 1974. Res. Publ. A.R.N.M.D. 52:225.
21. Greep, R. O., Astwood, E. B., Knobil, E., Sawyer, W. H., and Geiger, S. R. (eds.). 1974. Handbook of Physiology: The Pituitary Gland and Its Neuroendocrine Control, Vol. IV, Section 7, Parts 1 and 2. The Williams & Wilkins Co., Baltimore.
22. Cochin, J. 1968. In: Selected Pharmacological Testing Methods. Medical Research Series, No. 3, p. 121. Marcel Dekker Publ., New York.
23. Fraser, H. F. 1968. Res. Publ. A.R.N.M.D. 46:176.
24. Martin, W. R., and Jasinski, D. R. In: W. R. Martin (ed.), Handbook of Experimental Pharmacology. Springer-Verlag, Heidelberg (In press.)
25. Schuster, C. R., and Johanson, C. E. 1974. In: R. J. Gibbins, Y. Israel, H. Kalant, R. E. Popham, W. Schmidt and R. G. Smart (eds.), Research Advances in Alcohol and Drug Problems, p. 1. John Wiley and Sons, New York.
26. Seevers, M. H., and Deneau, G. A. 1963. In: W. S. Root and F. G. Hofmann (eds.), Physiological Pharmacology, p. 565. Academic Press, New York.

Testing For Dependence Liability of Stimulants and Depressants in Animals and Man

Committee on

Problems of Drug Dependence

Assembly of Life Sciences

National Research Council

In 1966, the Committee on Problems of Drug Dependence of the National Academy of Sciences-National Research Council prepared a document entitled, "Testing for Dependence Liability in Animals and Man."* That document was updated in 1972.** Since then, not only have the Committee's interests in abuse potential of drugs continued to broaden, but abuse of a wide variety of substances that act on the central nervous system has increased. Before the 1966 report, nearly all published research was concerned with testing morphine-like drugs in physically dependent monkeys and human addicts. However, very significant advances have occurred in developing new techniques for predicting the abuse liability of a broader range of drugs, including stimulants and depressants.

In all probability no single method will have such substantial predictive validity that drug abuse liability can accurately be assessed

Prepared with support from the Drug Enforcement Administration, the Food and Drug Administration, and the National Institute on Drug Abuse, under contract 271-76-3322.

* Committee on Problems of Drug Dependence, Addendum I: Testing for dependence liability in animals and man. 1966. pp I–X. Bulletin, Problems of Drug Dependence. National Academy of Sciences-National Research Council, Washington, D.C.

** Committee on Problems of Drug Dependence, Testing for Dependence Liability in Animals and Man (Revised 1972), Bulletin on Narcotics XXV, pp. 25–39, 1973.

using one measure. Moreover, the relative weighting attached to various predictors may vary considerably from one drug class to another. Thus, in considering the various predictive tools, one must be constantly wary of single approaches (e.g., using solely self-administration or physical-dependence methods). Finally, in drug development, abuse potential must always be considered in the context of therapeutic efficacy. That is, a unique and critically needed compound should not be discarded solely because early laboratory testing predicts some dependence liability; but a newly developed drug that is shown by several laboratory predictors to have a very high abuse potential would be difficult to justify if it were not absolutely essential to medical practice.

The purpose of this document is to present a brief resume of the current state of knowledge concerning prediction of abuse liability of central nervous system stimulants and sedative-hypnotics. Predictive procedures in four categories will be considered: 1) testing for physical dependence in animals, 2) self-administration in animals, 3) psychological and behavioral evaluation in man, and 4) behavioral toxicity and other predictive procedures in animals.

PHYSICAL DEPENDENCE IN ANIMALS

Central nervous system stimulants are not known to cause physical dependence in animals. However, central nervous system depressants that have been abused by man generally produce physical dependence in some animal models. These compounds include the barbiturates, ethanol, the nonbarbiturate sedative-hypnotics, and the minor tranquilizers. Testing for physical dependence in animals is important in order to identify the pharmacological profile of the test drug in comparison with the profiles of prototypic drugs that are abused by man, to predict the individual and social harm that might result from the abuse of the test drugs, and to predict the extent to which withdrawal need may be associated with drug-seeking behavior. As with centrally acting narcotic analgesics and their antagonists, there are three principal ways of determining physiological dependence capacity, the likelihood that a depressant will produce physical dependence: 1) direct development of dependence on chronic administration, by the animal or by an operator; 2) the effect of a substitute drug on withdrawal symptoms in a dependent animal; and 3) the effect of a single dose of the drug on withdrawal symptoms.

Several measures of withdrawal-symptom severity are available, so reproducibility has been generally satisfactory. The methods now used were developed with dogs, monkeys, cats, and mice, and have been validated with standard drugs such as sodium barbital (dogs and monkeys), pentobarbital (cats), and ethanol (mice). Although most, but not all, depressants that are abused by man produce physical dependence in these animal models, physical dependence may not be as useful an other pharmacological properties in predicting abuse potential. Nevertheless, determination of physical dependence recommends itself as a relatively rapid, economical, and fairly reliable preliminary screen.

Depressants with abuse potential are widely divergent in chemical structure. It therefore seems appropriate to examine different prototypic drug standards, whose abuse potential in man is known, to enhance predictability. These might include secobarbital, pentobarbital, amobarbital, chloral hydrate, glutethimide, methaqualone, diazepam, meprobamate, and ethanol.

Because the type of physical dependence and the severity of withdrawal symptoms depend in large measure on the pharmacodynamic and pharmacokinetic properties (biologic half-life, metabolism, etc.) of a drug, it is desirable to use standards whose pharmacokinetics are well established or can be readily determined, such as hexobarbital, phenobarbital, chlorodiazepoxide, oxazepam, and bromide ion.

SELF-ADMINISTRATION IN ANIMALS

A primary pharmacological property of drugs germane to predicting abuse liability is their ability to reward or reinforce self-administration behavior. There is substantial face validity to the use of drug-taking behavior in laboratory animals as a method of studying important aspects of drug-seeking and drug-taking behavior in man.

It must be recognized that the reinforcing action of a drug is only one of the pharmacological properties that eventually dictate the public health consequences of its use. Other properties of the drug—such as physical dependence liability, toxicity, and range of therapeutic uses—are also important determinants of abuse liability, as are social factors.

Over the last 15 years, laboratory methods have been developed and perfected for studying the reinforcing properties of drugs in laboratory animals. Basically, these procedures arrange conditions so that a discrete behavioral response is followed by the administration of the drug. For example, intravenous drug self-administration studies have typically used animals with chronic venous catheters attached to a remotely operable infusion pump. The pump can be made to operate in response to an action, such as a lever press, and infuse a fixed quantity of drug solution. Systematic changes in the performance required to produce an infusion yield detailed quantitative data on the drug's reinforcing properties. Such techniques have become increasingly refined and have been applied in a variety of species of laboratory animals, including rats, cats, dogs, and nonhuman primates.

Most compounds that serve as reinforcers in laboratory animals and that are used by man are abused by man. This isomorphism is clearest in the case of opioid analgesics: analgesic agonists with demonstrated abuse liability in man are readily self-administered by both naive and physically dependent animals. Furthermore, narcotic antagonists, such as nalorphine and cyclazocine, are devoid of abuse liability in man and are not positive reinforcers under most conditions in which they have been studied in laboratory animals. The narcotic agonists, morphine, codeine, meperidine, heroin, and propoxyphene, have been shown to serve as positive reinforcers in rhesus monkeys. In the initial studies, the subjects were made physically dependent before any opportunity for self-administration; later studies have demonstrated conclusively that a state of physical dependence is not necessary for narcotic agonists to serve as positive reinforcers, although the reinforcing efficacy of a centrally acting analgesic is generally increased if the subjects are physically dependent.

The agonist-antagonists pentazocine and propiram fumarate serve as positive reinforcers in nondependent monkeys, but not, under most conditions, in monkeys physically dependent on morphine. In contrast, neither the partial agonists nalorphine and cyclazocine nor the antagonist naloxone serves as positive reinforcers in nondependent monkeys. These findings correlate well with the available data on human abuse, suggesting that self-administration procedures are useful in predicting the abuse liability of the narcotic analgesics and their antagonists in man.

Self-administration procedures have been widely used to study psychomotor stimulant drugs. The data on psychomotor stimulants are consistent in that cocaine, the amphetamines, methylphenidate, phenmetrazine, and diethylpropion serve as reinforcers in a number of species. These compounds have all been reported to be abused by man. Fenfluramine and chlorphentrazine, however, are not reliably self-administered by animals; this corresponds with clinical reports that their abuse potential differs from that of the more typical psychomotor stimulants. In short, present evidence suggests that self-administration procedures are useful in evaluating abuse liability of psychomotor stimulant drugs.

A number of barbiturates and minor tranquilizers serve as reinforcers in animal self-administration procedures; however, they have not been studied extensively and systematic comparisons among drugs have not been carried out. In spite of the limited validation of self-administration procedures for studying the abuse liability of depressants, it seems that all drugs shown to be reinforcers in infrahuman self-administration are also abused by man.

A common approach to the sequential evaluation of the abuse liability of a stimulant or depressant involves the procedures described below.

Substitution

Animals are trained to self-administer a prototypic drug at a dose previously determined to be effective in producing repeated lever-pressing. Typically, daily experimental sessions last for several hours, during which the drug is delivered once for every *n* (e.g., 10) responses. After establishment of a stable rate and pattern of drug-reinforced responding, test drugs may be substituted for the standard drug. The rate and pattern of response generated by the test drug are compared with those observed with the prototypic drug and with saline (vehicle) substitution. A test drug is considered to be a positive reinforcer if it maintains a higher rate of responding than that observed when saline is substituted. Is is essential that a broad range of doses be tested, because a dose that is higher or lower than optimal may not maintain a response rate above that observed with saline or vehicle.

The substitution procedure permits evaluation of a range of test doses in a relatively short period. If a drug maintains a response rate significantly above that with saline, initial evidence of abuse potential is thereby established. In interpreting such initial evidence, the environmental and pharmacological history of the test subject, the schedule of drug delivery, the duration of access to the drug, the species, and the route of administration must be considered; all have been shown to influence the degree to which drugs may serve as reinforcers.

Continuous Self-Administration

Animals are allowed to self-administer drugs without dose or time limitation every day for several weeks. The initial test dose is based on the results obtained in the substitution procedure, which allows a determination of the amount of drug taken and the pattern of daily intake. The procedure is especially useful for assessing toxicity, tolerance, and physical dependence development at self-regulated doses. Food intake and water intake are measured concurrently. Measures of conditioned and unlearned behaviors can be obtained concurrently.

The use of experimentally naive animals in this procedure has the added advantage of demonstrating that prior drug history is not needed for the test drug to serve as a reinforcer. The use of naive animals, however, is complicated by the fact that learning the drug-reinforced response is influenced by a number of variables. For example, failure to obtain self-administration may reflect inadequate experimental procedures, rather than a lack of reinforcing effect of the drug. The continuous access procedure yields primarily qualitative information and does not readily lend itself to refined quantitative comparison of the reinforcing strength of different drugs.

Procedures Designed to Compare the Effectiveness of Different Drugs as Reinforcers

In general, attempting to quantify the relative reinforcing strengths of drugs within a class is more useful than comparison among drug classes. Two approaches appear to have merit in the prediction of the relative abuse liability of stimulant and depressant drugs: the progressive ratio procedure, and the choice procedure. A third approach, involving second-order schedules of reinforcement, shows great promise, but has not been studied sufficiently to allow statements concerning predictive validity.

Progressive Ratio Procedure This is perhaps the most widely used self-administration assessment procedure. A baseline performance is obtained with a standard drug, the test drug is substituted, and the response requirement systematically increased. For example, the number of responses required for drug reinforcement could be progressively doubled. The response requirement that the animal fails to meet (e.g., 100 responses) is called the breaking point. It has been shown, with this procedure, that the breaking point can be used to rank-order some psychomotor stimulant drugs according to reinforcing strength. The rank order of these drugs correlates highly with their reported dependence liability in man. Dose and duration of action appear to be important variables in the effective use of this procedure.

Choice Procedures This procedure permits the experimental animal to choose between two drug solutions. Two measures can be derived: percent choice of one solution compared with the other, and rate of response maintained by the two solutions. Animals are trained to choose between a prototypic drug and saline. After initial training, the test drug may be substituted at various doses. To ensure exposure to each of the drug solutions, a period of self-administration of each drug alone may be provided. Animals choose various psychomotor stimulant drugs over saline, higher doses of a given drug over a lower dose, and, finally, one drug over another, regardless of doses. This procedure appears to have considerable promise in the rank ordering of drugs.

Second-Order Schedule Procedure Animals are trained to respond on a simple schedule of reinforcement producing a brief stimulus presentation (e.g., a light or tone). Periodically, the brief stimulus is presented concurrently with a drug. The brief stimulus is able to maintain impressively large amounts of behavior, even when only intermittently coupled with drug delivery. This procedure has not been applied to the prediction of relative abuse liability of drugs. Because such second-order schedules maintain high rates of responding, it may be possible to use this procedure in a manner analogous to the progressive ratio procedure. This could be done by determining how infrequently drug reinforcement could be given while still maintaining response. A primary advantage of this procedure is that extended samples of behavior leading to drug reinforcement can be maintained with little or no confounding effect of previous drug administration (e.g., earlier the same day).

BEHAVIORAL TOXICITY IN ANIMALS

Behavioral toxicology usually is considered within the context of environmental and occupational exposure although no logic limits it to those bonds. Indeed, nontherapeutic actions of drugs helped to spur the development of behavioral toxicology, a historical alliance that meshes it with the issues discussed here. Even if therapeutic effects are accompanied by conjoint adverse responses, the latter are tolerated, in view of some subjective equation of risks and benefits. The same effects, if produced by administration outside a therapeutic context, can be conceived of as toxic—they would not be acceptable if they arose from an environmental agent.

Conventional Screening

Chronic or long-term, as well as acute, behavioral observations seem a compelling necessity, given our current appreciation of long-term consequences of drug exposure. Prolonged amphetamine abuse, for example, is believed by clinicians to lead to presistent behavioral or psychological changes. Experiments on drug administration in animals indicate that it is possible to produce a long-term residual supersensitivity that predisposes to behavioral and motor disorders as responses to later pharmacological or environmental manipulations.

Such tests require that the behavior under observation at least be sensitive to acute levels of the doses that will be studied chronically and others should be sensitive to toxic side effects unrelated to the desired clinical effects. Techniques range from tests of simple locomotor activity to tests using reinforcement schedules, complex behavioral surveys, and examinations of specific sensory and motor systems and learning. For example, punishment procedures, such as those sensitive specifically to barbiturates and minor tranquilizers, would be useful in assessing compounds of that class.

Circumstances of Use

Patterns of abuse are not always easily included in the toxicological categories of "acute," "subacute," and "chronic." For many circumstances, a more accurate descriptive term is "episodic," which is more congruent with the abuse patterns often associated with amphetamines, cocaine, sedative-hypnotic agents, and solvents. Even opiate use many be more accurately characterized by such a term.

Acute Phase While a person is experiencing the peak effects of drug administration, the prime toxicologic focus is on functions that are maximally disabled, that is, functions so impaired that the subject's capacity to deal adequately with the environment is compromised. We are most interested in relatively specific functions for such an assessment: learning, sensory intactness, motor coordination, and complex behavioral sequences.

Postepisodic Phase The course of recovery of the functions impaired during an episode must be specified. Rates of recovery vary from function to function, and generalizing from one to another is likely to be unprofitable.

A second question concerns the extent to which additional

impaired functions intrude into the postepisodic phase that may have played negligible roles in the acute phase. For example, rebound phenomena might well produce a pattern of effects distinctly different from those seen during the acute phase (cf. repeated administration of amphetamine at short intervals). In addition, nonspecific blunting of functional integrity may occur—a slightly out of focus behavioral capacity, rather than sharply defined impairments. Such changes are difficult to assess; techniques for gauging behavioral function in everyday environments are badly needed.

Chronic Phenomena If episodic abuse is considered a common pattern with centrally acting drugs, the term "chronic" takes on further connotations. Instead of referring only to a relatively stable exposure situation, it describes one overlaid with the fluctuating pattern of administration and recovery, and it turns our attention toward the way in which successive episodes and their immediate recovery phases are modified through an extensive history of such episodes. An alternative approach may be chronic exposure to just sublethal doses.

These issues are complicated by two apparently opposing processes. One is the development of tolerance, which is characteristic of many substances of abuse. The other is the progressive modification of central nervous system mechanisms to sensitize the organism to further administration of the same or different drugs. These two manifestations of prolonged use may be reflections of the same process. Also demanding attention are the possible irreversible neurochemical and neurophysiological manifestations associated with behavioral abnormalities in chronic stimulant intoxication.

Consequences of Exposure Schedules

The consequences of long-term chemotherapy in psychiatry exemplify some of the problems relevant to a consideration of stimulants and depressants. A major side effect of neuroleptic therapy is the production of movement disorders. Early in treatment, these closely mimic the symptoms of Parkinson's disease: retardation of movement (akinesia), a peculiar motor restlessness (akathisia), and sometimes a resting tremor. Prolonged use sometimes induces a movement disorder known as tardive or persistent dyskinesia, a syndrome now evoking increasing concern. There is emerging evidence that a variety of chronically administered compounds may induce a residual excessive sensitivity to stimulants.

The development of motor disorders and psychosis, the persistence of delusional ideation, and the residual sensitivity to reactivation of psychosis by moderately high doses may also constitute a series of abuse liabilities in the chronic use of stimulants. Existing evidence from experimental animals indicates that there are evolving chronic behavioral disorders and dyskinesia, including residual effects, and warrants continued investigation with behavioral methods. Although current behavioral surveys are not completely satisfactory, methods for assessing behavior of experimental animals offer sensitive indexes of the development of behavioral and motor disorders, as well as of the sensitization to drug effects and residual effects.

Behavioral Toxicology and Abuse Liability

Behavioral observations focusing on impaired function represent a major avenue of assessing dependence liability. Because conventional assays, even in their chronic form, are not congruent with patterns of drug abuse, and because abuse is such a socially important feature of the use of centrally active drugs, behavioral toxicology in this sense may represent an even more important facet than in its more conventional toxicological framework.

Two pertinent parameters of abuse patterns cannot be predicted from usual preclinical test results: dosages that maintain self-administration, and the associated temporal parameters of self-administration behavior.

Doses and administration patterns for behavioral toxicology should ideally be chosen on the basis of the parameters found in self-administration studies. These are probably the best preclinical guides available. Although tolerance and dependence studies are also relevant, they possesses a less immediate relationship to the core problem.

An additional reason for using self-administration patterns as a guide is the impossibility, as indicated earlier, of separating, in one situation, the reinforcing properties of a substance from its general behavioral effects, such as blunting of stimulus control.

Appropriate Behavioral Techniques

Anticipated advances in behavioral technologies argue against the desirability of making any recommendations that would tend to institutionalize current practices. Any behavioral function can be assessed by a broad variety of procedures and, for maximal validity, must be evaluated in the most appropriate species. Although it is becoming more and more a standard practice, behavioral teratology should not and must not be neglected. Lifetime studies are indispensable for determining many of the most vital features of toxicity and also serve to amplify toxic effects that in another context would remain covert.

Depending on the nature of initial surveys, a variety of sensitive behavioral assessments are available, including sensory capability, motor coordination, and activity levels. Acquisition and retrieval of learned responses and maintenance of schedule-controlled behavior are also important indicators of toxicity. Observation techniques occupy an important role in the assessment of behavioral and motor disorders.

BEHAVIORAL EVALUATION IN MAN

Important factors in the choice of agents for evaluation in man will be the results of animal testing and the proposed therapeutic use. In this regard, there are differences among species in reactivity to psychoactive drugs and in the metabolism and kinetics of the drugs. It is necessary to evaluate the abuse potential of psychoactive agents in man before they are used therapeutically. In general, an agent should be evaluated for dependence potential if it is found during clinical trials to have hypnotic or sedative effects, to modify mood, to intoxicate, to disturb cognitive processess, or to alter the subject's control over his own functioning.

Subject Selection

The risk to a human subject from an evaluation of an amphetamine-like or sedative-hypnotic drug during a well-designed study of dependence liability is quite small. Idiosyncratic toxicity can be minimized by choosing subjects who have already used these drugs—whether in benign or substantial patterns of abuse. Their reaction tends to resemble that of a hypothetical population that may be described as "susceptible." A valid test of dependence liability can be obtained with fewer such subjects, because they interpret the effects of a drug in terms of their past experience and are less likely to give "placebo" responses.

Sedative and psychostimulant drugs can become incorporated into patterns of dependence among those in various walks of life, so such drugs should be evaluated in populations that are "normal" in terms of behavior alterations or impairments that may arise in ordinary life circumstances.

Any such experiments should be subject to peer review, and the customary constraints and safeguards, based both on common sense and ethical considerations, must be observed. Initiation and continuation of a subject's participation in a study should be voluntary; all subjects should be informed of the purpose of the study and the associated risks and must have the opportunity to withdraw consent without jeopardy.

Kinetics

Study of the kinetics of depressant drugs is essential in predicting their dependence potential and the type of withdrawal reaction that they will evoke.

The drugs most likely to produce dependence are those whose effects are swift, sure, and short. The more rapid the onset of a clearly discernible effect, the more likely that the drug will be used for intoxicating purposes. Rapid absorption and short duration of action meet these needs.

The development of physical dependence requires a sustained pharmacological effect over a finite period. Drugs with a high degree of lipid solubility, a large apparent volume of distribution, and a long half-life (either of the parent drug or an active metabolite), generally meet these requirements. The severity of the withdrawal reaction is inversely related to the rate of decline. Conceivably, a drug with a sufficiently large cumulative effect and a slow disappearance rate would produce no withdrawal symptoms, despite the fact that it might induce physical dependence.

The most frequently abused drugs are those that are rapidly absorbed and that have a moderately long half-life (12–24 hours), e.g., secobarbital, meprobamate, and ethanol. Drugs that are slowly absorbed and long-acting are less frequently abused. Thus, analysis of the kinetics of a new sedative drug during phase 1 or 2 clinical studies might predict potential abuse.

Profiles of Abused Drugs

The traditional approach in assessing human drug-dependence potential is to compare the subjective, behavioral, and physiological effects of an unknown compound with those of known compounds with well-established dependence potential. Profiles of pharmacological action of prototypical stimulant and depressant drugs appear to be useful models. If a new compound displays a pharmacological profile similar to that of a drug with established dependence liability, considerable dependence liability of the new compound would be expected.

A number of measures of drug effects are currently used for such purposes. Subjective effects of drugs are assessed with questionnaires, such as the Addiction Research Center Inventory. From scale scores, drugs can be categorized according to their euphoric or sedative effects. Subjective effects are also assessed through unstructured observations by the subject. Behavioral tasks used in establishing profiles for predicting dependence liability include performance tests (reaction time, tapping time) and measures of perceptual-motor functioning. Operant tasks, which are highly sensitive in assessing drug effects in animals, are being investigated, as are such other phenomena as changes in risk-taking behavior, social interaction, sexual functioning, appetite, vigiliance, and arousal. Physiological measures—including electrocardiography, electroencephalography, heart rate, blood pressure, temperature, respiration, evoked potentials, pupillary changes, and postrotational nystagmus—are also being employed to establish profiles of drug effects.

Self-Administration

Another general approach for predicting drug-dependence liability may involve the use of human self-administration for assessing the reinforcing effects of drugs. As with animal models, human self-administration studies appear likely to be useful in predicting dependence liability and with appropriate proper ethical considerations, this approach may prove successful as a predictive technique in its own right or as a useful adjunct with other techniques.

Toxicity Assessment

Evaluation for dependence liability includes an assessment of the toxicity of a psychoactive drug, the dose at which toxic effects occur (compared with therapeutic and reinforcing doses), and the degree to which behavioral toxicity may be affected by other psychoactive substances. Among the toxic effects that must be considered are the following:

1. The degree to which the substance produces ordinarily nonreinforcing side effects (e.g., dysphoria) that will tend to limit self-administration. In general, dependence potential will be greater if such untoward side effects occur only at doses well above those that are

substantially reinforcing. It must be recognized that some events are unpleasant for most persons, yet positively reinforcing for other persons.

2. The capacity of the drug to produce aberrations in behavior associated with stimulation or depression; changes in perception, mood, consciousness, cognitive processes, or judgment; and decrements in motor coordination. In general, abuse potential will be greater if a drug's capacity to produce such changes is greater.

3. The degree to which symptoms occur, when drug use is discontinued, that tend to reinforce further drug taking (e.g., changes in mood or feeling states, psychic distress, and physical discomfort), whether or not such symptoms are associated with physical dependence itself or with other drug-related phenomena.

4. The degree to which behavioral toxicity or reduction in motor coordination results from one or two therapeutic doses of a drug alone or in combination with a blood alcohol content of 30 mg percent or higher.

Validation

The validation of methods involving human subjects to predict dependence liability of a drug will initially involve demonstrating the ability to measure both the reinforcing properties of prototypical drugs, and the equivalence of the test drug to prototypical drugs. Ultimately, predictions made on the basis of experimental studies can be validated only by the actual occurrence of drug-related problems when the test drug is generally available. Because drugs are introduced under various circumstances of availability and in various social and cultural settings, it is imperative that monitoring programs be established in order to produce data for validation of predictive methods and to reveal unanticipated drug-related problems related to changes or differences in mores.

RECOMMENDATIONS FOR FURTHER RESEARCH

1. Drug interactions and cross-substitutions should be studied as factors in multiple drug use and as contributors to the development of withdrawal manifestations.

2. Differences and similarities between animals and man, with regard to tolerance, physical dependence, and withdrawal, should be investigated.

3. Objective measures of withdrawal symptoms should be developed.
4. The relationship of withdrawal characteristics to dependence liability should be studied.
5. Specific antagonists to the depressant drugs should be developed.
6. Because there is some diversity of opinion as to the role of physical dependence in determining the abuse potential of depressants (sedative-hypnotics and minor tranquilizers), more experience must be gained regarding the extent of abuse of widely used, prototypical drugs.
7. There is considerable need for further research in drug self-administration by nonintravenous routes; in particular, methods for chronic intragastric and oral self-administration of drugs that are not water-soluble require exploration.
8. With the increasing cost of rhesus and squirrel monkeys, it becomes more important to develop improved methods for chronic parenteral self-administration of drugs in rodents and less expensive primates. A large body of information on rhesus monkeys has already been gathered; therefore, consideration should be given to developing mechanisms for maintaining continuing colonies of these species.
9. Far greater emphasis should be placed on concurrent or interpolated measures of other behavioral actions of self-administered drugs; this is particularly important in chronic studies in which drugs are continuously available for self-administration.
10. Despite the considerable advances in our knowledge of the variables that influence drug self-administration, a great many issues remain to be resolved, such as the role of pharmacological and environmental histories and the significance of the duration of access to drugs and of schedules of drug self-administration.
11. Care must be taken to distinguish drug-taking from drug-reinforced behavior—i.e., drug self-administration in animals and humans may be induced, not by the drug, but by another inducing condition (e.g., a sweet-flavored solution for liquid-deprived rats); it is essential that drug self-administration be demonstrated in the absence of other inducing conditions.
12. Greater emphasis should be placed on validating data on infrahuman self-administration in controlled situations, so that they may be properly compared with data on humans in the same situations.
13. Research with human subjects should not be limited to long-term

hard-core abusers of multiple drugs, but should include subjects with various patterns of drug abuse.

14. The relations between subjective ratings of drug effects (e.g., the Addiction Research Center Inventory) and objective behavioral measures of drug actions (e.g., operant tasks) should be investigated in human subjects.

15. Acute, postepisodic, and long-term effects of abused drugs on objectively measurable aspects of natural and conditional responses of animals should be investigated.

16. Methods of assessing subtle behavioral effects of abused drugs (e.g., on complex discrimination, problem-solving, and learning of complex tasks) should be improved.

17. Behavioral teratological effects of administration of high doses of abused drugs to pregnant female animals and their offspring should be investigated.

Index